Expert
Consultations
in Breast
Cancer

BASIC AND CLINICAL ONCOLOGY

Editor

Bruce D. Cheson, M.D.

National Cancer Institute
National Institutes of Health
Bethesda, Maryland

ADDITIONAL VOLUMES IN PREPARATION

Cancer Screening: Theory and Practice, *edited by Barnett S. Kramer, John K. Gohagan, and Philip C. Prorok*

Supportive Care in Cancer: A Handbook for Oncologists: Second Edition, Revised and Expanded, *edited by Jean Klastersky, Stephen C. Schimpff, and Hans-Jorg Senn*

Integrated Cancer Management: Surgery, Medical Oncology, and Radiation Therapy, *edited by Michael H. Torosian*

The Graft Versus Leukemia Effect in Allogeneic Stem Cell Transplantation, *edited by John Barrett and Yin-Zheng Jiang*

AIDS-Related Cancers and Their Treatment, *edited by Ellen Feigal, Alexandra Levine, and Robert Biggar*

Expert Consultations in Breast Cancer

Critical Pathways and Clinical Decision Making

edited by

William N. Hait
David A. August

UMDNJ/Robert Wood Johnson Medical School and
The Cancer Institute of New Jersey
New Brunswick, New Jersey

Bruce G. Haffty

Yale University School of Medicine
New Haven, Connecticut

MARCEL DEKKER, INC.   NEW YORK · BASEL

Library of Congress Cataloging-in-Publication Data

Expert consultations in breast cancer : critical pathways and clinical
   decision making / edited by William N. Hait, David A. August, Bruce
   G. Haffty.
       p.   cm.—(Basic and clinical oncology : 17)
   Includes bibliographical references and index.
   ISBN 0-8247-1954-9 (alk. paper)
   1. Breast—Cancer—Treatment—Decision making.   2. Critical path
analysis.   I. Hait, William N.   II. August, David A.
III. Haffty, Bruce G.   IV. Series.
   [DNLM: 1. Breast Neoplasms.   2. Critical Pathways.   W1 BA813W
v. 17   1999 / WP 870 E96 1999]
RC280.B8E86   1999
616.99′449—dc21
DNLM/DLC
for Library of Congress   99-11316
                                                                   CIP

This book is printed on acid-free paper.

Headquarters
Marcel Dekker, Inc.
270 Madison Avenue, New York, NY 10016
tel: 212-696-9000; fax: 212-685-4540

Eastern Hemisphere Distribution
Marcel Dekker AG
Hutgasse 4, Postfach 812, CH-4001 Basel, Switzerland
tel: 41-61-261-8482; fax: 41-61-261-8896

World Wide Web
http://www.dekker.com

The publisher offers discounts on this book when ordered in bulk quantities. For more information, write to Special Sales/Professional Marketing at the headquarters address above.

Current printing (last digit):
10 9 8 7 6 5 4 3 2 1

PRINTED IN THE UNITED STATES OF AMERICA

Series Introduction

The current volume, *Expert Consultations in Breast Cancer*, is Volume 17 in the Basic and Clinical Oncology series. Many of the advances in oncology have resulted from close interaction between the basic scientist and the clinical researcher. The current volume follows, expands on, and illustrates the success of this relationship as demonstrated by new therapies and promising areas for scientific research.

As editor of the series, my goal has been to recruit volume editors who not only have established reputations based on their outstanding contributions to oncology, but also have an appreciation for the dynamic interface between the laboratory and the clinic. To date, the series has consisted of monographs on topics such as chronic lymphocytic leukemia, nucleoside analogs in cancer therapy, therapeutic applications of interleukin-2, retinoids in oncology, gene therapy of cancer, and principles of antineoplastic drug development and pharmacology. *Expert Consultations in Breast Cancer* is certainly a most important addition to the series.

Volumes in progress include works on AIDS-related malignancies, secondary malignancies, chronic lymphoid leukemias, and controversies in gynecologic oncology. I anticipate that these volumes will provide a valuable contribution to the oncology literature.

Bruce D. Cheson, M.D.

Preface

Two overwhelming factors influence breast-cancer clinicians as the year 2000 approaches: dramatic advances in the clinical science of breast cancer and sweeping changes in the administrative and economic milieu within which care is provided. These forces may change the way in which evaluation and care of breast diseases are conducted.

Over the past 30 years, care of breast cancer patients has improved markedly. New diagnostic tools and a better understanding of breast physiology and endocrinology have refined the evaluation and treatment of breast diseases. Insights into the modes of spread of breast cancer and the recognition of breast cancer as a systemic disease have revolutionized treatment. Surgically, less is often better. Improvement in survival for many patients has been realized through the use of systemic chemotherapeutic and hormonal agents. The role of radiation therapy for breast cancer is being reconsidered and is likely to be expanded. Today, the majority of women with breast cancer are offered breast-conserving surgery, radiation therapy, and either chemotherapy or hormonal therapy. The patient who does *not* receive multimodality therapy is the exception.

Equally striking are changes in the health care environment. Over half of all Americans with health insurance are now participants in managed care programs. Even participants in Medicare and Medicaid are being encouraged to enroll in managed care plans. Market penetration of managed care has forced clinicians to be more aware of costs. It is no longer assumed that if no harm is done, a diagnostic study or therapeutic intervention is appropriate. All clinical decisions must now be evaluated not only with regard to medical effectiveness, but also with respect to cost-effectiveness.

   This book addresses both the clinical and process changes that are affecting the care of patients with breast cancer. The centerpiece of this book is the set of clinical pathways contained in Part II. The pathways were developed by the editors in consultation with more than 50 breast cancer experts representing all relevant disciplines. They offer a general approach to the evaluation and treatment of patients within the context of currently available data concerning medical and cost-effectiveness. Where the data are insufficient, expert consensus is offered along with the recommendation of enrollment in clinical trials. The pathways are neither specific patient care algorithms nor prescriptions for optimal care. Rather, they are a framework to guide the decision making that is required to formulate plans for care of individual patients.

   The pathways are preceded by a brief introduction, which summarizes data that form the foundation upon which the clinical pathways are built and a rationale for the application of those data. Unfortunately, many gaps remain in our knowledge. Whenever possible, we offer specific data to support the choices made in the creation of the pathways; when data are not available, we offer an explanation for the choices made.

   Finally, the pathways are followed by a set of case presentations with discussions by breast cancer experts. The purpose of Part III is to add vitality to the abstract pathways. The case presentations are keyed to the pathways. They are meant to amplify the telegraphic framework laid out in the pathways, to illuminate application of the pathways to patient care situations, and to broaden the clinical perspectives offered by enlisting the input of acknowledged clinical experts.

   The goal of this book is to improve the effectiveness and efficiency of clinicians' approaches to patients with breast cancer by offering a framework for clinical decision making and a data-based rationale for the decision pathway. We, the editors, have found the effort expended to develop, justify, and explain the clinical pathways enlightening, and it has influenced our approach to the practice of breast care. We hope that readers will be similarly rewarded.

William N. Hait
David A. August
Bruce G. Haffty

Contents

Contents ix

Contributors

Joseph Aisner, M.D.   Medical Oncology, UMDNJ/Robert Wood Johnson Medical School and The Cancer Institute of New Jersey, New Brunswick, New Jersey

David A. August, M.D.   Division of Surgical Oncology, UMDNJ/Robert Wood Johnson Medical School and The Cancer Institute of New Jersey, New Brunswick, New Jersey

Alan Axelrod, M.S.W., L.C.S.W.   The Cancer Institute of New Jersey, New Brunswick, New Jersey

Nicola Barnard, M.D.   UMDNJ/Robert Wood Johnson University Hospital, New Brunswick, New Jersey

Kirby I. Bland, M.D.   Department of Surgery, Brown University School of Medicine and Brown University Affiliated Hospitals, Providence, Rhode Island

Jean L. Bolognia, M.D.   Department of Dermatology, Yale University School of Medicine, New Haven, Connecticut

Thomas N. Byrne, M.D.   Neurology and Internal Medicine, Yale University School of Medicine, New Haven, Connecticut

Mihye Choi, M.D.   Institute of Reconstructive Plastic Surgery, New York University Medical Center, New York, New York

Robert S. DiPaola, M.D. Medical Oncology, UMDNJ/Robert Wood Johnson Medical School and The Cancer Institute of New Jersey, New Brunswick, New Jersey

Rosemary B. Duda, M.D., F.A.C.S. Department of Surgery, Beth Israel Deaconess Medical Center, Boston, Massachusetts

Kevin R. Fox, M.D. Department of Hematology, Oncology Division, University of Pennsylvania, Philadelphia, Pennsylvania

Judith E. Garber, M.D., M.P.H. Department of Adult Oncology, Dana-Farber Cancer Institute, Boston, and Harvard Medical School, Cambridge, Massachusetts

Teresa Gilewski, M.D. Department of Medicine, School of Solid Tumor Oncology, Breast Cancer Medicine Service, Memorial Sloan-Kettering Cancer Center, New York, New York

Susan Goodin, Pharm.D. The Cancer Institute of New Jersey, New Brunswick, New Jersey

Bruce G. Haffty, M.D. Department of Therapeutic Radiology, Yale University School of Medicine, New Haven, Connecticut

William N. Hait, M.D., Ph.D. Medical Oncology, UMDNJ/Robert Wood Johnson Medical School and The Cancer Institute of New Jersey, New Brunswick, New Jersey

Jay K. Harness, M.D., F.A.C.S. University of California, Davis—East Bay, Oakland, California

Daniel F. Hayes, M.D. Lombardi Cancer Center, Georgetown University Medical Center, Washington, D.C.

I. Craig Henderson, M.D. University of California at San Francisco, San Francisco, California

Susan A. Higgins, M.D. Department of Therapeutic Radiology, Yale University School of Medicine, New Haven, Connecticut

James F. Holland, M.D., Sc.D. Department of Medicine, Mount Sinai School of Medicine, New York, New York

Thomas J. Kearney, M.D. Division of Surgical Oncology, UMDNJ/ Robert Wood Johnson Medical School and The Cancer Institute of New Jersey, New Brunswick, New Jersey

Daniel S. Kim, M.D. Brown University School of Medicine, Providence, Rhode Island

Phyllis J. Kornguth, M.D., Ph.D. Department of Radiology, Duke University Medical Center, Durham, North Carolina

Robert R. Kuske, M.D. Ochsner Center for Radiation Oncology, New Orleans, Louisiana

Carol H. Lee, M.D. Department of Diagnostic Radiology, Yale University School of Medicine, New Haven, Connecticut

Allen S. Lichter, M.D. Department of Radiation Oncology, University of Michigan, Ann Arbor, Michigan

Monica L. Magee, M.S. Center for Human and Molecular Genetics, New Jersey Medical School, University of Medicine and Dentistry of New Jersey, Newark, New Jersey

Susan A. McManus, M.D. Robert Wood Johnson University Hospital, New Brunswick, New Jersey

Kiran Mehta, M.D. Department of Radiation Oncology, St. Francis Medical Center, Pittsburgh, Pennsylvania

Monica Morrow, M.D. Department of Surgery, Northwestern University Medical School, Northwestern Memorial Hospital, Chicago, Illinois

Larry Norton, M.D. Department of Medicine, Memorial Sloan-Kettering Cancer Center, New York, New York

Edward Obedian, M.D. Department of Therapeutic Radiology, Yale University School of Medicine, New Haven, Connecticut

William P. Peters, M.D., Ph.D. Barbara Ann Karmanos Cancer Institute, Detroit, Michigan

Michael Reiss, M.D. Section of Medical Oncology, Department of Medicine, Yale University School of Medicine, New Haven, Connecticut

Sandra F. Schnall, M.D.   Department of Hematology-Oncology, Temple University School of Medicine, Philadelphia, Pennsylvania

Lawrence J. Solin, M.D.   Department of Radiation Oncology, University of Pennsylvania, Philadelphia, Pennsylvania

Vernon K. Sondak, M.D.   Department of Surgery/Division of Surgical Oncology, University of Michigan Medical Center, Ann Arbor, Michigan

Deborah L. Toppmeyer, M.D.   Medical Oncology, UMDNJ/Robert Wood Johnson Medical School and The Cancer Institute of New Jersey, New Brunswick, New Jersey

Michael H. Torosian, M.D., F.A.C.S.   Department of Surgical Oncology, Fox Chase Cancer Center, Philadelphia, Pennsylvania

Barbara L. Weber, M.D.   University of Pennsylvania, Philadelphia, Pennsylvania

Christina Weltz, M.D.   Department of Surgery, Mount Sinai Medical Center, New York, New York

Philip D. Wey, M.D., F.A.C.S.   Department of Surgery, Division of Plastic Surgery, UMDNJ/Robert Wood Johnson Medical School, New Brunswick, New Jersey

Max S. Wicha, M.D.   Cancer Center, University of Michigan, Ann Arbor, Michigan

Julie A. Wolfe, M.D.   University of Michigan Medical Center, Department of Radiation Oncology, Ann Arbor, Michigan

I
THE MEDICAL BASIS FOR DECISION MAKING IN BREAST CANCER

1

The Natural History of Treated Breast Cancer
The Foundation of Clinical Decision Making

THOMAS J. KEARNEY and DAVID A. AUGUST
UMDNJ/Robert Wood Johnson Medical School and The Cancer Institute of New Jersey, New Brunswick, New Jersey

Appropriate decision making requires knowledge of the natural history of treated breast cancer. It is necessary to know the expected outcomes for the various presentations of breast cancer. This chapter outlines the overall results achieved with current standard-of-care therapy for invasive breast cancer (carcinoma in situ is discussed elsewhere). Although 5-year survival data are often used as a marker for outcome and will be referred to here, it must be recognized that breast cancer recurrences can appear two decades after initial treatment. Some authors even question whether cure of this disease is possible (1). The natural history of untreated breast cancer has been thoroughly reviewed (2).

Among the approximate 185,000 new cases of invasive breast cancer seen annually in the United States, the great majority are early stage, defined as AJCC stage I and II (Fig. 1) (3,4). These account for about 85% of all new patients. This does not include the 40,000 new cases of noninvasive breast cancer seen annually. Over the past decade, the average size of a newly diagnosed breast cancer has been decreasing, most likely due to the increased use of screening mammography. Currently the "average" breast cancer presents as a 2.1-cm mass (5); only about 15% of patients present with stage III and IV breast cancer. In unscreened populations, the percentage of patients with early disease is lower, so regional variations in screening can affect the stage distribution. The majority (75%) of new invasive breast cancers seen each year are invasive ductal carcinoma of no specific subtype.

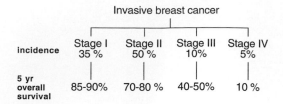

Figure 1   Stage breakdown of new breast cancer patients with 5 year overall survival. (From Ref. 3.)

Another 5–10% are infiltrating lobular carcinomas. Special subtypes such as medullary, mucinous, and tubular carcinomas compose the remainder. Most of these subtypes are associated with a better prognosis than invasive ductal carcinoma, the exception being metaplastic carcinoma, which confers a poor prognosis (6).

Patients with stage I disease (T1N0) have the best prognosis, with a 5-year overall survival of 85–90% (Fig. 2) (3). The best outcomes are seen in patients having tumors 1 cm or smaller. In areas where screening compliance is good, these patients can represent over 25% of the breast cancer population (7). Generally, the prognosis for stage I patients with tumors less then 1 cm (T1a, T1b) is so good that adjuvant systemic therapy is not indicated. Five-year overall survival exceeds 95% in some reports (8). Adjuvant therapy is generally recommended for stage I patients with tumors greater than 1 cm (T1c) (9). Approximately 30–35% of all node-negative patients with larger tumors (including those with stage I disease with tumors greater than 1 cm and some stage IIA and IIB patients) will develop metastatic disease after "curative" surgery alone. Virtually all patients with dis-

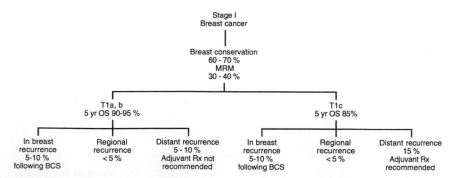

Figure 2   Expected outcome at 5 years for stage I breast cancer patients. (From Ref. 3.)

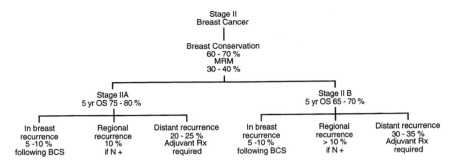

Figure 3 Expected outcome at 5 years for stage II breast cancer patients. (From Ref. 3.)

tant recurrences eventually die from their disease unless there is an unrelated intervening fatal event.

Women with stage II disease comprise the majority of breast cancer patients (10). Although mammographic screening helps detect smaller cancers, most breast cancers are still detected by palpation. Since breast masses cannot be reliably detected until they are 2 cm or greater, most tumors detected by palpation will be stage II (11). Stage II patients represent a heterogeneous population, from node-positive disease with small primary tumors to node-negative patients with tumors larger than 5 cm (Fig. 3). Overall 5-year survival for stage IIA patients approaches 80%; for stage IIB patients it is about 70% (3). Five-year overall survival underestimates the frequency of long-term recurrence of the disease, since patients can recur beyond the 5-year disease-free interval. The most significant prognostic indicators in early-stage patients are the number of positive lymph nodes and size of the tumor. Overall, 30–35% of node-negative patients with tumors greater than 2 cm will recur within 10–20 years of diagnosis (12). For all node-positive patients, between 50 and 70% will eventually develop distant recurrent disease (Fig. 4) (13). Certain subsets (T1 with only a single positive

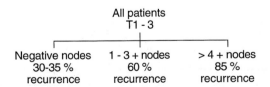

Figure 4 Long-term local-regional and distant recurrence of node-negative and node-positive patients (all tumor sizes). (From Ref. 13.)

node) can have excellent long-term disease-free survival (80% at 20 years) (14).

The presence of positive axillary nodes (particularly with large tumors) is also a marker for an increased risk of local-regional recurrence. Following mastectomy, patients with four or more positive nodes and tumors greater than 5 cm have a 20–30% chance of developing a local chest wall recurrence. This risk is markedly reduced by radiation therapy (15).

Stage III breast cancer may be divided into stage IIIA (technically operable) and stage IIIB (technically inoperable). Inoperability is usually due to extension of the tumor to the chest wall (T4a), skin ulceration or satellite nodules (T4b), chest wall extension combined with skin changes (T4c), or the presence of inflammatory carcinoma (T4d). Inflammatory breast cancer is a clinical syndrome characterized by warmth, tenderness, erythema, and edema. The edema often results in an orange-peel appearance of the skin (*peau d'orange*). An underlying breast mass or palpable axillary lymph nodes may or may not be present. Radiologically there may be a detectable mass and characteristic thickening of the skin over the breast. The histological hallmark of inflammatory breast cancer is dermal lymphatic invasion demonstrable on skin biopsy, although the clinical syndrome (with its attendant poor prognosis) may be present in the absence of this finding.

Stage IIIA breast cancer is usually treated with mastectomy followed by systemic adjuvant therapy and regional irradiation. The presence of stage IIIB disease mandates initial treatment with chemotherapy, usually followed by surgery, regional radiation, and additional systemic therapy (Fig. 5) (16). Overall 5-year survival for stage IIIA disease is 51% and for stage IIIB disease it is 41% (3). However, the overall poor prognosis is reflected in long-term survival rates of 30% or lower (16).

Virtually all patients with stage IV disease, either at presentation or secondary to recurrence, succumb to their disease. Median survival is 2 years, but 5-year survival is 13%, indicating that some patients with metastatic disease follow a more indolent course. Systemic treatment may delay the time to progression and provide good palliation but is not curative. Among the 185,000 new breast cancer cases diagnosed annually, 12,000 (5%) patients initially present with metastatic disease (4). About 23,000 node-negative patients and 47,000 stage II and III patients eventually develop systemic recurrence if followed for two decades (17). The death rate is currently about 46,000 women per year.

Distant recurrence of breast cancer must currently be considered a fatal form of the disease. The most common sites of distant recurrence of infiltrating ductal carcinoma are liver, lungs, and bone. Infiltrating lobular carcinoma has a tendency to recur with intra-abdominal disease. Other sites such as the ovaries and adrenals can also be involved. The time to recurrence

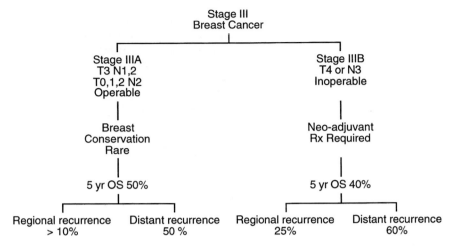

Figure 5 Expected outcome at 5 years for stage III breast cancer patients. (From Ref. 3.)

is related to the size of the original tumor, with larger tumors having a shorter time to recurrence (1).

Metastases can occur two decades or more after initial treatment. Because of the late recurrences seen with breast cancer, 5-year overall survival rates can be misleading. In addition, patients with recurrent disease can live for many years. Therefore, 10- and 20-year data are probably more reflective of the true success or failure of treatment. In general, 5-year overall survival rates are proportional to longer-term overall and disease-free survival. Therefore, 5-year overall survival can reliably be used to estimate the efficacy of new treatments.

The local recurrence rate following breast-conserving surgery relates to the use of radiation therapy. Numerous prospective studies of breast conserving-surgery (18) demonstrated an in-breast recurrence rate of approximately 10% at 10 years in patients receiving breast irradiation following lumpectomy. In unirradiated patients, the local recurrence rate is 30–40%. There may be favorable subsets of women who can safely omit radiation therapy after lumpectomy with negative margins (19). Two current trials, CALGB 9343 and NSABP B-21, are prospectively evaluating favorable patients (small tumors without palpable adenopathy, generally estrogen-receptor positive) with invasive cancer for breast-conserving surgery without radiation. The implications of local recurrence following breast-conserving surgery are less dismal than following mastectomy, with long-term disease-free survival seen in one-third to one-half of patients (20).

With a firm understanding of the natural course of treated breast cancer, clear information can be provided for patients. Clinical situations with expected poor outcomes can be readily identified and strong consideration should be given to enrolling such patients on clinical trials.

REFERENCES

1. Harris JR, Hellman S. Natural history of breast cancer. In: Harris JR, Lippmann ME, Morrow M, et al, eds. Diseases of the Breast. Philadelphia: Lippincott-Raven, 1996:375–392.
2. Bloom HJG, Richardson WW, Harries EJ. The natural history of untreated breast cancer. Br Med J 1962; 2:213–221.
3. American Joint Committee on Cancer: AJCC Cancer Staging Manual, 5th ed. Philadelphia: Lippincott-Raven, 1997.
4. Parker SL, Tong T, Bolden S, et al. Cancer statistics, 1996. CA Cancer J Clin 1996; 65:5–27.
5. Cady B, Stone MD, Schuler JG. The new era in breast cancer invasion, size and nodal involvement dramatically decreasing as a result of mammographic screening. Arch Surg 1996; 131:301.
6. Rosen PP. Breast Pathology. Philadelphia: Lippincott-Raven, 1997.
7. Cady B. New era in breast cancer: impact of screening on disease presentation. Surg Oncol Clin North Am 1997; 6:195–202.
8. Arnesson LG, Smeds S, Fagerberg G. Recurrence-free survival in patients with small breast cancers. Eur J Surg 1994; 160:271.
9. Early Breast Cancer Trialist's Collaborative Group. Systemic treatment of early breast cancer by hormonal, cytotoxic, or immune therapy. Lancet 1992; 339: 71.
10. Rosato FE, Rosenberg AL. Examination techniques: role of the physician and patient in evaluating breast diseases. In: Bland KI, Copeland EM, eds. The Breast: Comprehensive Management of Benign and Malignant Diseases. Philadelphia: WB Saunders, 1991:409.
11. Foster RS. Limitations of physical examination in the early diagnosis of breast cancer. Surg Oncol Clin North Am 1994; 3:55–65.
12. Quiet CA, Ferguson DJ, Weichselbaum RR, et al. Natural history of node-negative breast cancer: a study of 826 patients with long-term follow-up. J Clin Oncol 1995; 13:1144–1151.
13. Fisher B, Bauer M, Wickerham DL. Relation of the number of positive axillary nodes to the prognosis of patients with primary breast cancer: an NSABP update. Cancer 1983; 52:1551.
14. Quiet CA, Ferguson DJ, Weichselbaum RR, et al. Natural history of node-positive breast cancer: the curability of small cancers with a limited number of positive nodes. J Clin Oncol 1996; 14:3105–3111.
15. Fowble B, Gray R, Gilchrist K, et al. Identification of a subgroup of patients with breast cancer and histologically positive axillary nodes receiving adjuvant

chemotherapy who may benefit from postoperative radiotherapy. J Clin Oncol 1988; 6:1107–1117.

16. Buzdar AU, Singletary SE, Booser DJ, et al. Combined modality treatment of stage III and inflammatory breast cancer: M.D. Anderson cancer center experience. Surg Oncol Clin North Am 1995; 4:715–734.

17. Honig SF. Treatment of metastatic disease: hormonal therapy and chemotherapy. In: Harris JR, Lippmann ME, Morrow M, et al, eds. Diseases of the Breast. Philadelphia: Lippincott-Raven, 1996:669–734.

18. Fisher B, Redmond C, Poisson R. Eight year results of a randomized clinical trial comparing total mastectomy and lumpectomy with or without irradiation in the treatment of breast cancer. N Engl J Med 1989; 320:822–828.

19. Marks LB, Prosnitz LR. Lumpectomy with and without radiation for early-stage breast cancer and DCIS. Oncology 1997; 11:1361–1368.

20. Recht A, Hayes DF, Eberlein TJ, et al. Local-regional recurrence after mastectomy or breast conserving therapy. In: Harris JR, Lippmann ME, Morrow M, et al, eds. Diseases of the Breast. Philadelphia: Lippincott-Raven, 1996:649–667.

2

The Pathology of Breast Disease

NICOLA BARNARD
UMDNJ/Robert Wood Johnson University Hospital,
New Brunswick, New Jersey

The spectrum and management of breast cancer have changed significantly over the last 20 years, owing to widespread mammographic screening and evolving practices in surgery, radiotherapy, and chemotherapy. The pathologist is now required to provide ever-increasing amounts of information that may determine medical and surgical treatment as well as predict outcome.

The normal female breast is a glandular structure composed of lobules and ducts within variable amounts of adipose tissue. The acinar tissue is lobular in arrangement with a terminal ductule. This structure, termed the terminal duct-lobular unit (TDLU), is the secretory portion of the breast. It is supported by a zone of loose connective tissue. The TDLU drains into the subsegmental duct and thence to a collecting duct that finally empties to the nipple. Most of the changes seen in benign fibrocystic changes and most carcinomas originate in the TDLU (1). The large duct system gives rise to papillomas and only rarely to carcinoma.

Abnormalities of the breast may be detected by mammography or present as a palpable mass. Mammography is able to detect tumors as small as 1–2 mm, usually because of the presence of associated calcifications, which are seen in 50–60% of breast carcinoma and in over 90% of ductal carcinoma in situ (2,3). Up to 40% of nonpalpable carcinomas detected by mammography are in situ lesions. Prior to the widespread use of mammography, carcinoma of the breast usually presented as a palpable mass. Only about 5% of these cases were in situ carcinoma.

Tissue diagnosis of breast abnormalities may be obtained in a number of ways; fine-needle aspiration cytology, core-needle biopsy, and open biopsy. Cytology may be used to examine material from nipple discharge, cyst aspiration, and solid mass aspiration. Owing to the low yield of positive results, cytological examination of nipple discharge and cyst fluid is infrequently performed. Aspiration cytology from solid masses has proved to be a highly reliable (and inexpensive) method of diagnosis (4). False-positive results (mistaken diagnoses of carcinoma) have been reported, but are uncommon. These may occur due to the difficulty in interpreting the proliferative epithelium seen in fibroadenomas, in ductal hyperplasia, and in pregnancy and lactation (5). Cytological examination is unable to distinguish reliably between in situ carcinoma and invasive carcinoma. Core biopsies may be performed on palpable lesions and also on nonpalpable lesions using mammographically guided sterotactic needle biopsy. The sensitivity of this technique increases with the size of lesion and ranges from 75–90% (6).

Open biopsy for nonpalpable masses and microcalcifications requires that the lesion first be needle-localized. Once the localized area has been excised, specimen mammography is performed to establish that the entire lesion has been removed (7). The lesion can then be localized within the specimen using either a grid or additional markers so that the radiographically abnormal area is examined microscopically. Before the specimen is sectioned, the surface is usually coated with India ink to assist in evaluation of the surgical margins of the specimen. Samples for microscopy are taken from the abnormal designated area and also from all the fibrous breast tissue. Smaller specimens are embedded in their entirety. If the biopsy has been performed for microcalcifications and these are not seen microscopically, then the paraffin blocks are X-rayed and those containing microcalcifications are sectioned. Approximately 20% of biopsies performed for calcifications will demonstrate the presence of in situ or invasive carcinoma.

Frozen-section diagnosis of breast lesions is an accurate method of diagnosis and was widely used in the era of one-step breast surgery when a diagnosis of malignancy was immediately followed by mastectomy. Increasingly, with the diagnosis of smaller lesions and widespread use of breast-conserving surgery, the role of frozen-section diagnosis has diminished. Small lesions are more difficult to diagnose by frozen section, and if all the tissue is frozen, irretrievable artifact is introduced that may permanently impair the final diagnosis. Recently, the Association of Directors of Anatomic and Surgical Pathology has recommended that lesions less than 1 cm in diameter should not be frozen (8). Mammographically detected lesions are more likely to be in situ carcinoma and this entity is easier to diagnose on permanent sections. Therefore, breast tissue removed because of microcalcifications should not be frozen. Some benign proliferative lesions may resemble carcinoma grossly and are often a diagnostic challenge made even greater by superimposed freeze-artifact. Frozen sections of inflammatory lesions may closely resemble neoplastic proliferations. Frozen section is poorly suited to assessment of margins of resection as fatty tissue is technically difficult to process in this way and thus inadequate sections are usually obtained.

Benign breast diseases include fibroadenomas, the wide spectrum of fibrocystic changes, intraductal papillomas, and a few other conditions such as inflammatory lesions and unusual tumors, e.g, leiomyomas and granular cell tumors.

Inflammatory lesions of the breast (9) are often related to pregnancy and lactation. Rarely, tuberculosis may cause chronic mastitis. Noninfective granulomatous mastitis may occur, usually in older women, and is thought to be of autoimmune etiology. Mammary duct ectasia results in a mass, nipple discharge, and distortion. The lactiferous ducts are dilated with periductal fibrosis and chronic inflammation. Fat necrosis may follow trauma and may result in a firm, solid mass resembling carcinoma.

Fibroadenomas are benign stromal and epithelial tumors, which occur most commonly between the ages of 20 and 35 years. They appear grossly as well-circumscribed masses with a dense gray-white cut surface. Microscopically, fibroadenomas consist of epithelial and stromal elements in varying proportions. The epithelial component appears as either gland-like structures or small cleft-like spaces. The loose connective tissue stroma contains abundant mucopolysaccharides but may be densely fibrotic, especially in older patients. Areas of calcification may also occur. In less than 10% of fibroadenomas, fibrocystic-type changes may occur; these include cysts, sclerosing adenosis, and apocrine changes. These so-called complex fibroadenomas may be associated with a small long-term increased risk for developing breast cancer (10). Rarely, carcinoma may develop within a fibroadenoma; usually these are in situ lesions.

Fibrocystic changes (the term recommended by the College of American Pathologists) (11) are important because they are extremely common. They may simulate malignant lesions clinically, radiographically, grossly, and microscopically. In addition, some variants may confer increased risk for subsequent development of carcinoma. The most frequent features of fibrocystic disease include cysts, apocrine metaplasia, epithelial hyperplasia, and forms of adenosis including sclerosing adenosis, blunt duct adenosis, and microglandular adenosis. Adenosis is the term for a benign hyperplastic condition of the glandular tissue, which may result in the formation of mass lesions or stromal distortion. Microcalcifications that are detected radiologically are often seen in fibrocystic changes and are especially common in areas of sclerosing adenosis and blunt duct adenosis. Stromal fibrosis in fibrocystic disease is a common, but extremely variable feature. Occasionally, discrete sclerosing ductal lesions may be seen that consist of a central elastotic or fibrotic scar with radiating arms of proliferating epithelium, which may show hyperplastic change. This lesion, often referred to as a radial scar, may closely resemble carcinoma both mammographically and grossly.

Perhaps the most significant component of fibrocystic disease is the wide spectrum of epithelial hyperplasia that may involve both ductal and lobular structures. Many attempts have been made to correlate the degree of proliferation with risk of subsequent carcinoma. Dupont and Page (12) and Page et al. (13) identified atypical proliferative lesions with some features of in situ carcinoma and designated these as atypical ductal hyperplasia (ADH) and atypical lobular hyperplasia (ALH). In a retrospective study, they concluded that these patients had a four- to fivefold greater risk of developing invasive carcinoma. The risk is magnified when there is a family history of breast carcinoma. However, the histological criteria for the diagnosis of these atypical proliferative lesions are somewhat indistinct and there is considerable interobserver variability. A consensus meeting of the College of American Pathologists in 1985 (11) offered a statement of relative risk for development of carcinoma for the spectrum of epithelial lesions seen. It is evident, however, that patients with these proliferative lesions represent only a small subset of those developing carcinoma.

The majority of carcinomas of the breast can be classified as ductal carcinoma or lobular carcinoma. The distinction between lobular carcinoma and ductal carcinoma is based on the morphology of the tumor rather than the site of origin, as almost all breast carcinomas are thought to arise from the TDLU. In situ and invasive forms of both ductal and lobular carcinoma can be recognized. In situ carcinoma is a lesion in which malignant cells are confined within preexisting ductular and acinar structures and show no evidence of extension into the surrounding stroma. Invasive carcinoma consists of malignant cells extending into connective tissue.

Lobular carcinoma in situ (LCIS) is usually an incidental finding because it does not present as a mass lesion and is only infrequently associated with microcalcifications. It is usually associated with fibrocystic changes and occurs in approximately 3% of breast biopsies without other neoplastic lesions. The mean age at presentation is 53 years. Bilaterality can be demonstrated in up to 65% of cases. In addition, LCIS is frequently multifocal within the affected breast. When LCIS is diagnosed, the incidence of subsequent ipsilateral and contralateral breast cancer is equal, with ipsilateral disease developing slightly earlier. Of those women who do develop invasive cancers, 38% are diagnosed 20 or more years after the diagnosis of LCIS. The most common tumor histology seen in either breast is infiltrating ductal carcinoma (14,15).

Microscopically LCIS appears as a proliferation of the acinar cells with filling and distention of the lobules. The cells are usually uniform and lack cohesion; they occasionally extend into the terminal ductules. Atypical lobular hyperplasia is a lesion that does not quite fulfill the histological criteria for LCIS. The term "lobular neoplasia" has been used to encompass both conditions and to recognize that there is a spectrum of disease (16).

Ductal carcinoma in situ (DCIS) is increasingly diagnosed with the widespread use of mammography. Previously, DCIS presented as a mass lesion and comprised less than 5% of malignant diagnoses. Mammographically detected calcifications are found in up to 98% of DCIS. About 40% of carcinomas detected by initial mammographic screening are intraductal. In contrast to LCIS, DCIS is bilateral in less than 10% of cases. Multicentric, unilateral disease is found in approximately one-third of cases. Invasive carcinoma associated with DCIS is almost always ipsilateral and ductal in type.

Histologically, several different patterns of DCIS can be recognized—comedo, solid, papillary, micropapillary, and cribriform, along with a range of nuclear grades and presence or absence of necrosis (17). The most important aspect of the diagnosis of DCIS is exclusion of the presence of invasive carcinoma; tissue sampling must, therefore, be extensive.

The histological pattern of DCIS may predict the risk of local recurrence in those patients treated by local excision rather than mastectomy. The most significant features predicting relapse are high nuclear grade, the presence of necrosis, the size of the lesion, and the size of the margins of resection. Recent proposals for classification have emphasized these features and recognized three main subgroups of DCIS—low grade, intermediate grade, and high grade (18).

The risk of DCIS evolving into invasive carcinoma is uncertain. Small, low-grade lesions pose the least risk. High-grade and comedo-DCIS are more likely to progress to invasive carcinoma over a shorter period (19,20). The term "microinvasion" is poorly defined, but is generally reserved for lesions <2 mm or <10% of the total tumor mass. Up to 2% of cases thought to be entirely intraductal have metastatic carcinoma in regional lymph nodes. These cases probably represent instances where invasive carcinoma was not identified histologically owing to inadequate sampling.

Malignant tumors in the breast have a wide range of gross appearances. Typically, they have a stellate shape and a hard, gray-white, granular cut surface. Some tumors show areas of necrosis or hemorrhage. Less commonly, the tumor may appear circumscribed, particularly medullary and mucinous types. Infiltrating ductal carcinoma of the breast is the most common form of breast cancer, accounting for 75% of invasive carcinomas. Of the remainder, 5–10% are categorized separately as tubular, colloid, medullary

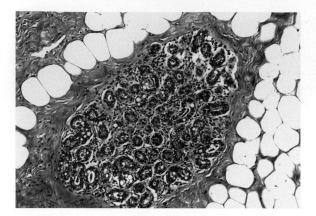

Figure 1   Normal lobule: clusters of two layered acini with supporting connective tisue stroma and surrounding adipose tissue (H&E × 60).

cribriform, and papillary and these types are considered to have a more favorable outcome.

Infiltrating lobular carcinoma (ILC) is relatively uncommon comprising 5–10% of all breast carcinoma. It usually appears as a poorly defined mass and may not be apparent mammographically. Several histological variants are recognized (21). The classic type has small cells, arranged in lines or so-called ''Indian file'' with a dense fibrotic stroma. These tumors are

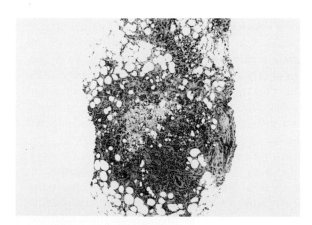

Figure 2   Core biopsy of breast: diagnostic tissue with infiltrating carcinoma obtained using core needle biopsy (H&E × 24).

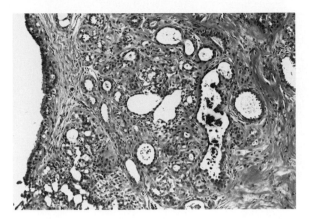

Figure 3 Fibrocystic change with microcalcification: biopsy performed for suspicious calcification seen on mammography (H&E × 60).

frequently estrogen-receptor positive. ILC tends to metastasize to serosal surfaces and also commonly to ovaries, uterus, and the gastrointestinal tract.

Infiltrating ductal carcinoma includes a wide spectrum of histological appearances. Many attempts have been made to recognize features that may be of prognostic significance. Tumor size, usually measured as gross maximum diameter, is one of the most important prognostic variables. In those lesions that microscopically contain extensive carcinoma in situ, it is the

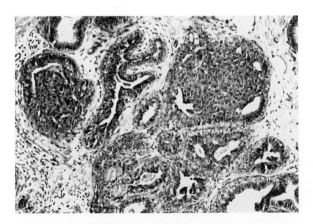

Figure 4 Proliferative fibrocystic change: area of ductal epithelial hyperplasia (H&E × 60).

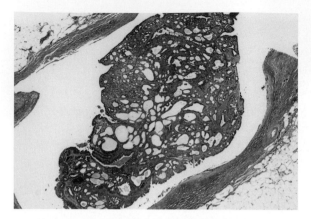

Figure 5 Intraductal papilloma: benign papilloma within dilated duct with fibrotic wall (H&E × 24).

size of the invasive component that predicts the likelihood of lymph node metastases (22).

Tumor grading was introduced to provide prognostic information about invasive carcinomas that fall into the same histological group. The most widely used grading system was introduced in the 1950s by Bloom and Richardson (23). This system scores three features of invasive ductal carcinomas—extent of duct formation, nuclear hyperchromasia, and mitotic activity, with 1–3 points assigned to each feature; these are added together

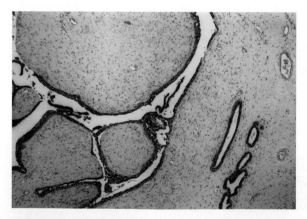

Figure 6 Fibroadenoma: cleft-like epithelial-lined spaces and loose connective tissue stroma (H&E × 24).

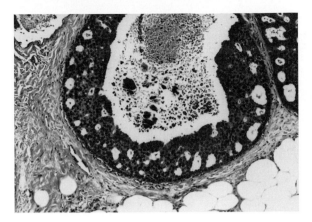

Figure 7 Ductal carcinoma in situ: cribriform pattern of monomorphic cell population with central necrosis and calcification (H&E × 60).

to produce a grade from 1 (low grade) to 3 (high grade). Many studies have demonstrated that high-grade invasive ductal carcinoma is more likely to be associated with lymph node metastasis, tumor recurrence, and death from metastatic disease than low-grade tumors (24).

The presence of tumor emboli within lymphatic spaces in the breast is an unfavorable finding, even in node-negative patients. Presence of lymphatic invasion may be difficult to confirm in tissue sections owing to frequent artifactual retraction of connective tissue around nests of tumor and

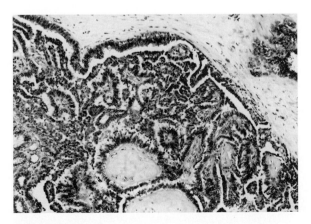

Figure 8 Papillary carcinoma in situ: fibrovascular cores covered by monomorphic cell population (H&E × 60).

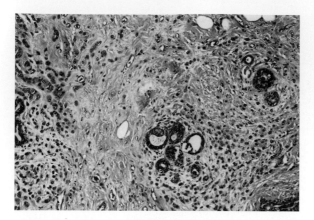

Figure 9 Infiltrating lobular carcinoma: single cells arranged in short cords infiltrate stroma and surround benign acinar structures (H&E × 60).

destruction of endothelium by tumor. Blood vessel invasion within the tumor is also associated with a slightly increased risk of tumor recurrence in patients with negative lymph nodes. A number of other histological findings have been examined for prognostic significance including tumor margins, tumor necrosis, inflammatory reaction, and stromal elastosis. Recently, it has been observed that the presence of increased numbers of microvessels occurring around the tumor correlates with more aggressive behavior of the tumor (25).

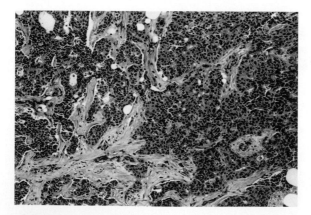

Figure 10 Infiltrating ductal carcinoma: sheets of tumor cells with some attempt at gland formation (H&E × 60).

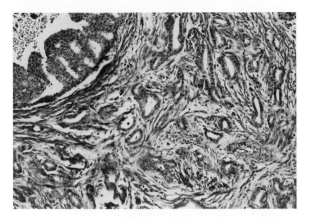

Figure 11   Well-differentiated ductal carcinoma: well-formed tubular structures. Focus of in situ ductal carcinoma present at top left of picture (H&E × 60).

The most important prognostic information is provided by the examination of axillary lymph nodes. Survival is correlated with the presence or absence of lymph-node metastasis and also by the absolute number of lymph nodes involved. The probability of finding metastatic tumor in a lymph node varies with the size of the lymph node and the size of the metastasis (26). At present, lymph nodes are usually examined on one section using routine staining. Additional sections and the use of immunohistochemical staining for epithelial markers increase the number of positive lymph nodes found.

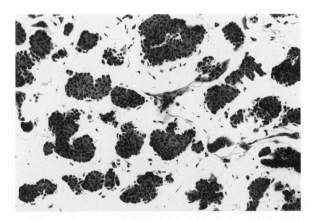

Figure 12   Colloid carcinoma: clusters of tumor cells float in lakes of mucin (H&E × 60).

This may be especially relevant in the evaluation of selective lymphadenectomy (sentinel lymph node biopsy) specimens in breast cancer patients.

A number of other studies should be performed on primary carcinomas to provide prognostic information. Evaluation of the presence of hormone (estrogen and progesterone) receptors may be performed using cytosolic methods or by immunohistochemistry (IHC). Currently, it appears that IHC may provide more accurate information. The presence of hormone receptors correlates with longer disease-free survival, although the difference in long-term prognosis is slight.

DNA and cell proliferation studies may be carried out using a number of methods. Information on S-phase fraction provided by flow cytometry appears most significant in node-negative patients. Tumor proliferation rates may also be assessed using mitotic counts or by immunostaining with antibodies such as Ki-67 (27). The prognostic significance of DNA ploidy is less clear and probably covaries with other tumor features such as size, grade, hormone receptor status, and lymph node status.

Amplification of the c-*erb* B-2 (Her-2-*neu*) oncogene can be detected by immunohistochemistry or by in situ hybridization of mRNA. Its presence, which correlates closely with tumor grade, is associated with a poorer prognosis, especially in node-positive patients.

Increased levels of the enzyme cathepsin D and the accumulation of p53 protein have been correlated with poorer patient survival. However, multivariate analyses indicate these findings are not independent of other morphological features previously mentioned. At present, most prognostic information for invasive breast carcinoma is derived from tumor stage, grade, and receptor status. Most other markers appear to contribute little independent information.

Paget's disease of the nipple is a lesion in which large, pale-staining cells are present within the epidermis of the nipple. It is almost invariably associated with an underlying carcinoma, which may be either in situ or invasive. The current belief is that Paget's disease represents spread of malignant cells from underlying carcinoma into the epidermis. Immunohistochemically, these cells stain with CEA, milk-fat globulin antigens, low-molecular-weight cytokeratins, estrogen receptors, and other antibodies, supporting their glandular origin. Paget's disease occurs in 1–2% of breast carcinoma patients; 50–60% of patients with Paget's disease have a palpable tumor. The underlying tumor is almost always of ductal type, but very rarely Paget's disease is associated with lobular carcinoma in situ extending into major ducts. The prognosis of Paget's disease is that of the associated carcinoma.

Cystosarcoma phyllodes, now usually referred to as phyllodes tumor, is a stromal neoplasm with an associated benign epithelial component. The behavior of this tumor ranges from benign but locally persistent to high-grade metastasizing tumors (28). These tumors occur predominantly in older women and often present as large masses. Grossly, the tumors are circumscribed and on cut section contain clefts and cysts. Microscopically, the clefts are elongated epithelial lined spaces. The stroma shows varying degrees of cellularity. A fully malignant phyllodes tumor has marked stromal overgrowth with >5 mitoses per 10 high-power fields with few epithelial elements. Since the major complication of phyllodes tumor is local recurrence, the main aim of surgical therapy is complete excision. This is especially important since recurrences tend to be of higher grade than the original tumor.

Breast disease in males is uncommon. The normal male breast consists of lactiferous ducts without lobular differentiation and a small amount of supporting stroma and fat. Gynecomastia in the most common abnormality seen. In this condition there is epithelial hyperplasia, which may be florid, with periductal edema and cellular stroma. Infrequently, lobular differentiation may occur. The result is breast enlargement, which may be unilateral.

Carcinoma of the male breast accounts for about 1% of breast carcinomas in the United States, but approaches 10% in other countries. The relationship between carcinoma and gynecomastia is unclear, but it appears that gynecomastia is rarely a predisposing factor. Most male breast carcinoma presents as a mass lesion at an average age of 60 years. The majority of male breast carcinomas seen are infiltrating ductal carcinoma. An intraductal component is often present. About 5% of cases show papillary carcinoma, often noninvasive. Lobular carcinoma is almost nonexistent. Male breast carcinoma is frequently estrogen-receptor positive. Prognosis depends on the stage of disease. When compared stage for stage with women with breast carcinoma, it appears that outcome is either similar or somewhat less favorable in men.

In summary, breast disease is associated with a wide spectrum of histological changes, many of which are complex and occasionally difficult to interpret. Careful handling of specimens and clinical-pathological correlation is essential to maximize the information that is gained. Microscopic examination of breast lesions not only establishes the diagnosis, but also provides much additional information vital to the management of the patient.

REFERENCES

1. Wellings SR, Jensen HM, Marcum RG. An atlas of subgross pathology of the human breast with special reference to possible precancerous lesions. J Natl Cancer Inst 1975; 55:231–273.

2. Ciatto S, Bonardi R, Cataliotti L, Cardona G. Intraductal breast carcinoma. Review of a multicenter series of 350 cases. Tumor 1990; 76:552–554.

3. Patchefsky AS, Shaber GS, Schwartz GF, Feig SA, Nerlinger RE. The pathology of breast cancer detected by mass population screening. Cancer 1977; 40: 1659–1670.

4. Fessia L, Botta G, Arisio R, Verga M, Aimone V. Fine-needle aspiration of breast lesions: role and accuracy in a review of 7495 cases. Diagn Cytopathol 1987; 3:121.

5. Kline TS, Joshi LP, Neal HS. Fine-needle aspiration of the breast: diagnosis and pitfalls. A review of 3545 cases. Cancer 1979; 44:1458–1464.

6. Minkowitz S, Moskowitz R, Khafif RA, Alderete MN. Trucut needle biopsy of the breast. An analysis of its specificity and sensitivity. Cancer 1986; 57: 320–323.

7. Gallagher HS. Breast specimen radiography. Obligatory, adjuvant and investigative. Am J Clin Pathol 1975; 64:749–755.

8. Fechner RE. Frozen section examination of breast biopsies: practice parameter. Am J Clin Pathol 1995; 103:6–7.

9. Rosen PP. Inflammatory and reactive tumors. Specific infections. In: Rosen PP. Rosen's Breast Pathology. Philadelphia: Lippincott-Raven, 1997:23–66.

10. Dupont WD, Page DL, Parl FF, Vnencak-Jones CL, Plummer WD Jr, Rados MS, Schuyler PA. Long term risk of breast cancer in women with fibroadenoma. N Engl J Med 1994; 331:10–15.

11. Consensus Meeting, Oct 3–5, 1985, New York, Cancer Committee of the College of American Pathologists. Is "fibrocystic disease" of the breast precancerous? Arch Pathol Lab Med 1986; 110:171–173.

12. Dupont WD, Page DL. Risk factors for breast cancer in women with proliferative breast disease. N Engl J Med 1985; 312:146–151.

13. Page DL, Dupont WD, Rogers LW, Rados MS. Atypical hyperplastic lesions of the female breast. A long-term follow-up study. Cancer 1985; 55:2698–2708.

14. Rosen PP, Senie R, Schottenfield D, Ashikari R. Noninvasive breast carcinoma: frequency of unsuspected invasion and implication for treatment. Ann Surg 1979; 189:98–103.

15. Hutter RVP. The management of patients with lobular carcinoma in-situ of the breast. Cancer 1984; 53:798–802.

16. Haagenen CD, Lane N, Lattes R, Bodian C. Lobular neoplasia (so-called lobular carcinoma in situ) of the breast. Cancer 1978; 42:737–769.

17. Patchefsky AS, Schwartz GF, Finkelstein SD, Prestipino A, Sohn SE, Singer JS, Feig SA. Heterogenicity of intraductal carcinoma of the breast cancer 1989; 63:731–741.

18. Silverstein MJ, Lagios MD, Craig PH, Waisman JR, Lewinsky BS, Colburn WJ, Poller DN. The Van Nuys Prognostic Index for ductal carcinoma in situ. Breast J 1996; 1:38–40.

19. Fisher ER, Constantino J, Fisher B, Palekar AS, Redmond C, Mamounas C, for the National Surgical Adjuvant Breast and Bowel Project Collaborating Investigators. Pathologic findings from the national surgical adjuvant breast

protocol (NSABP) protocol B-17. Intraductal carcinoma (ductal carcinoma in situ). Cancer 1995; 75:130–139.

20. Silverstein MJ, Waisman JR, Gamagami P, Gierson ED, Colburn WJ, Rosser RJ, Gordon RS, Lewinsky BS, Fingerhut A. Intraductal carcinoma of the breast (208 cases). Clinical factors influencing treatment choice. Cancer 1990; 66: 102–108.

21. DiConstanzo D, Rosen PP, Gareen I, Franklin S, Lesser M. Prognosis in infiltrating lobular carcinoma. An analysis of "clinical" and variant tumors. Am J Surg Pathol 1990; 14:12–23.

22. Seidman JD, Schnaper LA, Aisner SC. Relationship of the size of the invasive component of the primary breast carcinoma to axillary node metastasis. Cancer 1995; 75:65–71.

23. Bloom HJG, Richardson WW. Histological grading and prognosis in the prognosis of carcinoma of the breast. Br J Cancer 1957; 11:359–377.

24. Elston CW, Ellis IO. Pathological prognostic factors in breast cancer. I. The value of histological grade in breast cancer: experience from a large study with long-term follow-up. Histopathology 1991; 19:403–410.

25. Horak ER, Leek R, Klenk N, Lejeune S, Smith K, Stuart N, Greenall M, Stepniewska K, Harris AL. Angiogenesis assessed by platelet/endothelial cell adhesion molecule antibodies, as indicator of node metastases and survival in breast cancer. Lancet 1992; 340:1120–1124.

26. Wilkinson EJ, Hause S. Probability in lymph node sectioning. Cancer 1974; 33:1269.

27. Barnard NJ, Hall PA, Lemoine NR, Kadar N. Proliferative index in breast carcinoma determined in situ by ki67 immunostaining and its relationship to clinical and pathological variables. J Pathol 1987; 152:287–295.

28. Hart WR, Bauer RC, Oberman HA. Cystosarcoma phyllodes. A clinicopathological study of twenty-six hypercellular periductal tumors of the breast. Am J Clin Pathol 1978; 70:211–216.

3

Evaluation of Breast Abnormalities

DAVID A. AUGUST
UMDNJ/Robert Wood Johnson Medical School and The Cancer Institute of New Jersey, New Brunswick, New Jersey

Breast cancer generally presents in one of three ways: as a palpable abnormality; as a nonpalpable abnormality detected mammographically; or as a nipple discharge. Whatever the presentation, the initial focus must be on determining whether the lesion represents cancer or a benign problem. Within each of these symptom/sign categories, workup will be dictated both by the specific presentation and by the patient's age and menopausal status. Age and menopausal status are relevant because of the increasing cancer risk with age; because of the relative frequency of benign disease in premenopausal women; and because of the increased sensitivity of mammograms in older women as functional, radiographically dense glandular tissue is replaced by fat.

Often, an accurate diagnosis may only be accomplished by obtaining diagnostic tissue (Table 1). For a surgical biopsy, this requires histological examination of tissue that unequivocally contains the suspicious lesion. For a palpable lesion, palpation suffices to confirm removal of the lesion. For a radiographic abnormality, removal must be confirmed by images of the specimen that demonstrate the abnormality in the tissue removed (e.g., calcifications in a specimen mammogram). For X-ray-, ultrasound-, or palpation-guided fine-needle or core needle biopsies, a diagnostic biopsy is one that unequivocally reveals a specific benign entity or an unequivocal malignancy. A finding of normal epithelial or fat cells may mean that the biopsy needle missed the intended target; these findings should be interpreted as nondiagnostic. Readings such as acellular, fibrocystic, atypical, or suspicious are also nondiagnostic. Nondiagnostic readings mandate surgical biopsy (1–3).

Table 1 Breast Biopsy Techniques

Technique	Advantages	Disadvantages
Fine-needle aspirate	Minimally invasive Minimal discomfort Exam room procedure Results rapidly available Inexpensive	Cytology only Cannot distinguish carcinoma in-situ 10–20% false negatives
Core needle biopsy	Minimally invasive Exam room procedure Histological diagnosis Inexpensive	Patient discomfort Difficult with small lesions 5–15% false negatives
Incisional biopsy	Definitive Appropriate for large lesions	Postop bleeding more likely Invasive Anesthesia required Expensive
Excisional biopsy	The "gold standard" May be therapeutically definitive	Invasive Anesthesia required Expensive

X-ray guided	Good for nonpalpable
	  lesions
	Minimally invasive
	High sensitivity
		Moderately expensive
		Requires specialized
		  equipment

Diagnostic tissue should be obtained using the least invasive and most cost-effective technique possible. Formal surgical biopsy should be reserved for those situations when less invasive methods are not feasible or are ineffective; surgical biopsy is also appropriate when excision is likely to be necessary, whatever the biopsy results (e.g., when a benign lesion is growing, or when the suspicion of malignancy is so high by clinical or radiographic criteria that benign cytology or core biopsy results are not reliable). In other situations, fine-needle or core needle biopsy is indicated, guided by either palpation or radiographic findings. A recently developed technique, mammographically guided repetitive core (mammatome) biopsy, has significantly improved the yield of stereotactic tissue-sampling techniques. In our practice, this has dramatically increased our use of nonsurgical biopsy. The sensitivity and specificity of this technique exceed 90%.

I. PALPABLE ABNORMALITY

Although an increasing number of breast abnormalities are detected by screening mammography, most breast cancers still present as a palpable mass (4,5). In postmenopausal women, the replacement of glandular tissue by fat, the absence of hormone-related functional changes, and the high incidence of cancer make evaluation of breast masses straightforward. After bilateral mammograms are obtained to screen for concurrent, clinically unappreciated lesions, biopsy to obtain diagnostic tissue must be performed.

For women under the age of 30 years without major breast cancer risk factors, a well-circumscribed, discrete mass suggests the presence of a simple cyst, fibrocystic changes, or a fibroadenoma. Breast ultrasound can confirm the diagnosis of a simple cyst or, if a homogeneous, well-demarcated solid lesion is seen, support a diagnosis of fibroadenoma. Either lesion may be followed safely. Presumed fibroadenomas should be excised if they enlarge or change in consistency. Cysts may be aspirated if they are large, symptomatic, or recurrent. For any clinically atypical mass, even in this age group, tissue diagnosis should be pursued (6).

The presence of functional, cycling glandular tissue in premenopausal women, combined with an increasing incidence of cancer beyond the age of 30, makes evaluation of breast masses between age 30 and menopause problematic. Bilateral mammograms should be obtained to look for concurrent disease before a definitive diagnostic procedure is undertaken. Aspiration cytology may distinguish between benign and cancerous lesions without the need to resort to more invasive diagnostic methods.

II. NONPALPABLE ABNORMALITY

Nonpalpable lesions generally present as a mammographic abnormality, either a density or microcalcifications. The BI-RADS classification of mammograms, endorsed by the American College of Radiology (Table 2), is a helpful first step in formulating a strategy to evaluate mammographic findings (7). Class I (normal) and class II (unequivocally benign density or calcifications) mammograms require no further evaluation. Class IV (indeterminate finding, consistent with malignancy) and class V findings mandate acquisition of diagnostic tissue using the most appropriate biopsy technique.

Class III mammograms (probably benign, less than a 5% chance of malignancy) are more problematic. Old mammograms and, in the case of a discrete mass (as opposed to an asymmetrical density), a breast ultrasound should be obtained. Lesions stable over a 24-month period or found to be simple cysts ultrasonographically do not need to be further evaluated. Non-

Table 2 American College of Radiology: Breast Imaging Reporting and Data System (BI-RADS)

Class	Assessment	Clinical recommendation
I	Normal mammogram	No special follow-up; follow routine screening recommendations
II	Benign finding	Definitely benign; follow routine screening recommendations
III	Probably benign finding	Short-term mammographic follow-up (3–6 months) or biopsy
IV	Suspicious finding	Biopsy indicated
V	Likely malignancy	Biopsy/treatment necessary

cystic lesions (densities and microcalcifications) that have changed should be biopsied. New microcalcifications and new densities that are not simple cysts may be safely observed with follow-up mammography in 4–6 months; alternatively, patient preference may indicate tissue diagnosis using the least invasive technique likely to obtain a definitive diagnosis.

III. NIPPLE DISCHARGE

Nipple discharges are potentially pathological only if spontaneous. They may be classified as fibrocystic, bloody, or milky (galactorrhea). Fibrocystic discharges may be green, yellow, brown, blue, serous, or creamy. No specific evaluation is required.

A bloody or blood-tinged discharge is most often indicative of a benign intraductal papilloma, but should be evaluated to exclude carcinoma. Cytological examination of the discharge is sometimes employed, but false-negative and false-positive results are common. Bilateral mammograms should be obtained. If the duct from which the discharge is originating can be identified by inspection, duct excision for pathological evaluation is indicated. If the duct cannot be localized, close follow-up is necessary (8).

Galactorrhea is a bilateral milky white discharge that is not related to lactation or breast stimulation. Its presence more than two years after finishing lactation should prompt an evaluation for an underlying endocrinopathy resulting in hyperprolactinemia (often associated with amenorrhea). Nonphysiological causes of galactorrhea include hypothyroidism, medications (phenothiazines, metoclopramide, oral contraceptives, alpha-methyldopa, reserpine, tricyclic antidepressants), or a pituitary microadenoma-secreting prolactin. Galactorrhea that occurs without an underlying endocrinopathy may be safely followed (1–3).

REFERENCES

1. August DA, Sondak VK. Breast disease. In: Greenfield LJ, ed. Surgery: Scientific Principles and Practice, 2nd ed. Philadephia: Lippincott, 1996:1357–1415.
2. Burbank F, Parker SH, Fogarty TJ. Stereotactic breast biopsy: improved tissue harvesting with the mammatome. Am Surg 1996; 62:738–744.
3. Meyer JE, Smith DN, DiPiro PJ, Denison CM, Frenna TH, Harvey SC, Ko WD. Stereotactic breast biopsy of clustered microcalcifications with a directional, vacuum-assisted device. Radiology 1997; 204:575–576.
4. Donegan WL. Evaluation of a palpable breast mass. N Engl J Med 1992; 327:937–942.
5. Rosato FE, Rosenberg AL: Examination techniques: role of the physician and patient in evaluating breast diseases. In: Bland KI, Copeland EM, eds. The Breast: Comprehensive Management of Benign and Malignant Diseases. Philadelphia: W.B. Saunders, 1991:409–418.
6. Ferguson CM, Powell RW. Breast masses in young women. Arch Surg 1989; 124:1338.
7. Breast Imaging Reporting and Data System (BI-RADS). Reston, VA: American College of Radiology, 1993.
8. Winchester DP. Nipple discharge. In: Harris JR, Lippman ME, Morrow M, Hellman S, eds. Diseases of the Breast. Philadelphia: Lippincott-Raven, 1996:106–110.

4
Breast Cancer Staging

DAVID A. AUGUST
*UMDNJ/Robert Wood Johnson Medical School and The Cancer Institute
of New Jersey, New Brunswick, New Jersey*

Breast cancer staging permits meaningful prognostic and therapeutic distinctions. TNM (**T**umor size, **N**ode status, presence of **M**etastases) staging groups patients into prognostic categories. These groupings delineate treatment approaches; they identify those patients likely to benefit from adjuvant chemotherapy and radiation therapy; and they define those patients with locally advanced breast cancer in whom surgery plays only a secondary role (1).

Breast cancer staging involves a well-defined process by which the relevant information is obtained. Accurate staging is imperative for appropriate treatment. A thorough history and physical examination with accurate recording of the findings are the first elements of the staging process. Clinical staging should include notation of the size and mobility of the primary tumor and lymph nodes. Clinically enlarged axillary nodes are found to contain tumor in 75% of cases when examined histologically; similarly, the clinically normal axilla contains microscopic lymph node metastases 20–40% of the time (2).

Physicians must collaborate with pathologists to develop a standardized format for reporting pathology results. The pathology summary report should include tumor size, tumor histology, extent of nodal involvement, status of resection margins, receptor status, tumor grade, and other prognostic factors. Accurate staging also requires appropriate radiological evaluation, individualized for each patient according to signs, symptoms, and likelihood of the presence of metastatic disease.

The American Joint Committee on Cancer (AJCC) staging schema, based on TNM criteria, is widely accepted, and should be used for all breast

Table 1   TNM Classification for Staging of Cancer of the Breast

TNM DEFINITIONS

Primary tumor

TX	Primary tumor cannot be assessed
TO	No evidence of primary tumor
Tis	Carcinoma in situ
T1	Tumor 2 cm or less in greatest dimension
T2	Tumor more than 2 cm but not more than 5 cm in greatest dimension
T3	Tumor more than 5 cm in greatest dimension
T4	Tumor of any size with direct extension into chest wall (not including pectoral muscles) or skin edema or skin ulceration or satellite skin nodules confined to the same breast or inflammatory carcinoma

Regional lymph node involvement

NX	Regional lymph nodes cannot be assessed
N0	No regional lymph node involvement
N1	Metastasis to movable ipsilateral axillary lymph node(s)
N2	Metastasis to ipsilateral axillary lymph node(s) fixed to one another or to other structures
N3	Metastasis to ipsilateral internal mammary lymph nodes

Distant metastasis

MX	Presence of distant metastasis cannot be assessed
M0	No distant metastasis
M1	Distant metastasis present (including ipsilateral supraclavicular lymph nodes)

STAGE GROUPING

Stage 0	Tis, N0, M0
Stage I	T1, N0, M0
Stage IIA	T0–1, N1, M0
	T2, N0, M0
Stage IIB	T2, N1, M0
	T3, N0, M0
Stage IIIA	T0–2, N2, M0
	T3, N1–2, M0
Stage IIIB	T4, N1–2, M0
	Any T, N3, M0
Stage IV	Any T, any N, M1

Source: Ref. 1.

cancer patients. The AJCC schema for staging breast cancer is summarized in Table 1 (3). The schema is based on clinical data, including tumor size, tumor extension, and nodal status determined by clinical examination and operation. If information is obtained from pathological examination of biopsy or operative material, this should be specified.

The term "locally advanced breast cancer" defines a group of patients who have an especially poor prognosis because of the likely presence of micrometastatic disease. These patients have stage IIIB tumors in the AJCC schema. The clinical features of breast cancer that identify this subset of patients (Table 2) are based on Hagensen's "grave signs" and include edema of the skin of the breast, skin ulceration (not just dimpling), fixation of the tumor to the chest wall (not just to the pectoralis muscles), axillary nodes larger than 2.5 cm in diameter, and fixed axillary nodes (4). An even poorer prognosis is associated with the presence of extensive breast edema involving over one-third of the skin, satellite tumor nodules in the ipsilateral breast, or the presence of arm edema. The stigmata of inflammatory breast cancer, a distinctive presentation of locally advanced breast cancer, include breast

Table 2 Results of Radical Mastectomy in the Presence of Signs of Locally Advanced Breast Cancer

Clinical feature	Local recurrence (%)	5-Year disease-free survival rate (%)
GRAVE SIGNS		
Edema of less than one third of skin of breast	32	23
Skin ulceration	14	36
Solid fixation to chest wall beyond pectoralis muscles	40	5
Axillary lymph node larger than 2.5 cm	13	38
Fixed axillary nodes	13	13
OTHER SIGNS		
Edema of more than one third of skin of breast	61	0
Satellite tumor nodules in breast	57	0
Inflammatory carcinoma	60	0
Edema of arm	50	0

Source: Ref. 1.

warmth, tenderness, erythema, and edema. The edema often results in an orange-peel appearance of the overlying skin (*peau d'orange*). An underlying mass or palpable axillary lymph nodes may or may not be present.

The importance of recognizing the signs of locally advanced breast cancer relates to the dismal outcome associated with surgical therapy in these patients. Treatment generally involves initial chemotherapy, with surgery and/or radiation therapy deferred for subsequent consolidation of local tumor control.

REFERENCES

1. August DA, Sondak VK. Breast disease. In: Greenfield LJ, ed. Surgery: Scientific Principles and Practice, 2nd ed. Philadelphia: Lippincott, 1996:1357–1415.
2. Chevinsky AH, Ferrara J, James AG, Minton JP, Young D, Farrar WB. Prospective evaluation of clinical and pathologic detection of axillary metastases in patients with breast carcinoma. Surgery 1990; 108:612–618.
3. Beahrs OH, Henson DE, Hutter RVP, Kennedy RJ. Breast. In: Manual for Staging of Cancer, 4th ed. Philadelphia: Lippincott, 1992:149–154.
4. Haagensen CD. Clinical classification of the stage of advancement of breast carcinoma. In: Diseases of the Breast. Philadelphia: WB Saunders, 1986:851–863.

5
Carcinoma In Situ

DAVID A. AUGUST
UMDNJ/Robert Wood Johnson Medical School and The Cancer Institute of New Jersey, New Brunswick, New Jersey

Carcinoma in situ (noninvasive cancer) is a neoplastic entity confined entirely within its epithelium of origin and without invasion through the basement membrane. Noninvasive cancer has no access to lymphatic or vascular elements and hence should not metastasize. Therefore, issues concerning regional and distal spread are irrelevant when discussing carcinoma in situ of the breast. Although both are considered in situ malignancies of the breast, the significance and behavior of ductal carcinoma in situ (DCIS) and lobular carcinoma in-situ (LCIS) are quite different (Table 1).

DCIS may be considered a true precursor of invasive breast cancer. In some women with DCIS, time allows the noninvasive cancer cells to develop the ability to invade and metastasize, likely owing to the accumulation of somatic mutations. Eradication of DCIS cells before they acquire the ability to invade should mitigate the potentially life-threatening consequences of untreated DCIS. In contrast, LCIS may best be considered a marker lesion. The LCIS cells themselves are not a danger; they are not thought to have the ability to develop the capacity to invade and metastasize. Rather, the presence of LCIS is a marker for "influences" on the breast tissue that increase the likelihood of subsequent *de novo* invasive breast cancer development (1). Treatment of LCIS is best thought of within the context of the management of high-risk patients. This distinction between DCIS and LCIS marks the first branch point in the clinical decision pathway.

I. DUCTAL CARCINOMA IN SITU

Ductal carcinoma in situ refers to tumors that histologically show no evidence of invasion (cancer cells beyond the ductular basement membrane).

Table 1 Comparison of Ductal Carcinoma In Situ (DCIS) and Lobular Carcinoma In Situ (LCIS)

Feature	DCIS	LCIS
Menopausal status	Same as invasive cancer	Primarily premenopausal
Clinical findings	Usually microcalcifications	Clinically occult
Associated risk of invasive cancer	Same breast, ductal	Both breasts, lobular or ductal
Lifetime risk of invasive cancer	15–25%	15–30%
Biological behavior	Precursor lesion with potential to become invasive	Marker lesion

Invasive breast cancer can have a significant noninvasive component, either within or adjacent to the main tumor mass; the term DCIS excludes tumors with any microscopic evidence of invasion ("microinvasion").

A number of schemata have been developed to aid therapeutic decision making in patients with DCIS. They generally use features such as tumor size, histological and cytological grade, and presence of necrosis to guide therapy (2). Given the lack of long-term follow-up concerning the outcomes of various treatment approaches, the clinical pathway identifies tumor distribution (diffuse vs. focal) as the primary characteristic that determines therapeutic options. This approach is chosen because the largest, prospective, randomized trial performed to date in women with DCIS identified surgical margins as important when considering breast-conserving treatments (3).

Tumor distribution is the primary determinant of ability to achieve a negative-margin lumpectomy. Diffuse tumors are defined as those that mammographically (generally as determined by the extent of microcalcifications) extend over too broad an area to be encompassed in a discrete lumpectomy, or those tumors that on repeat excision yield positive resection margins. Focal tumors are those that can be encompassed within a negative margin lumpectomy.

Diffuse tumors are best treated with simple mastectomy. This results in cure in 97–99% of cases. In almost all women undergoing simple mastectomy, immediate breast reconstruction is an option. Axillary lymph node dissection is not indicated, because involved lymph nodes are found in fewer than 3% of patients (4). For focal tumors, lumpectomy with or without radiation therapy and simple mastectomy are appropriate options. Unfortunately, there are no direct comparisons (nor are there ever likely to be) of

Table 2 Lumpectomy With or Without Radiotherapy for Treatment of Focal Ductal Carcinoma In Situ of the Breast

	Annual incidence of recurrence according to treatment	
Type of recurrence	Lumpectomy	Lumpectomy and radiation therapy
DCIS	2.6%	1.5%
Invasive cancer	2.6%	0.6%

Source: Ref. 3.

these two approaches. Experience with the treatment of invasive breast cancer suggests that mastectomy will not offer a survival advantage over lumpectomy. It is clear, however, that event-free survival (absence of recurrence of either invasive or noninvasive cancer in either the breast or systemically) is better in women undergoing mastectomy. These facts must be discussed with patients when advising them on treatment options.

For patients choosing breast-conserving therapy, the role of radiation therapy after negative-margin lumpectomy is evolving. The results of National Surgical Adjuvant Breast Project trial B-17, which randomized women with DCIS to negative-margin lumpectomy with or without breast irradiation, are instructive (3). In all patients, radiation therapy reduced the incidence of in-breast occurrence of subsequent cancers and reduced the proportion of subsequent cancers that were invasive (Table 2). Data suggest, however, that in women with small (less than 2 cm) and well- or moderately differentiated tumors that may be widely excised (margins greater than 1 cm), the benefit of radiation therapy is marginal (3).

II. LOBULAR CARCINOMA IN SITU

Lobular carcinoma in situ accounts for about one-third of noninvasive breast cancers. LCIS is a marker of a susceptibility of the breasts to malignant change. All of the lobular and ductal elements of both breasts are marked ''at risk'' by the presence of LCIS anywhere in either breast. It seems clear that since both breasts are at equal risk, both breasts should be treated the same.

The prognosis of LCIS is solely related to the risk of subsequent development of invasive carcinoma. About one-fourth of patients with biopsy-demonstrated LCIS develop invasive cancer; half occur in the index breast and half in the contralateral breast (5). The subsequent breast cancers can be either lobular or ductal histology. The risk of invasive cancer may be influenced by family history (5). Therefore, although the LCIS treatment options in women with and without a family history of breast cancer include risk assessment and counseling followed by either observation or bilateral mastectomies (usually with immediate breast reconstruction), stratification according to family history seems prudent.

REFERENCES

1. August DA, Sondak VK. Breast disease. In: Greenfield LJ, ed. Surgery: Scientific Principles and Practice, 2nd ed. Philadelphia: Lippincott, 1996:1357–1415.
2. Silverstein MJ, Waisman JR, Gamagami P, et al. Intraductal carcinoma of the breast (208 cases): clinical factors influencing treatment choice. Cancer 1990; 66:102.
3. Fisher B, Constantino J, Redmond C, et al. Lumpectomy compared with lumpectomy and radiation therapy for the treatment of intraductal breast cancer. N Engl J Med 1993; 328:1581–1586.
4. Morrow M, Schnitt SJ, Harris J. Ductal carcinoma in situ. In: Harris JR, Lippman ME, Morrow M, Hellman S, eds. Diseases of the Breast. Philadelphia: Lippincott-Raven, 1996:355–368.
5. Haagensen CD. Lobular neoplasia (lobular carcinoma in situ. In: Diseases of the Breast. Philadelphia: WB Saunders, 1986:192–241.

6
Surgery for Breast Cancer

DAVID A. AUGUST
UMDNJ/Robert Wood Johnson Medical School and The Cancer Institute of New Jersey, New Brunswick, New Jersey

I. THE SCIENTIFIC BASIS OF BREAST CANCER SURGERY

The scientific basis of local/regional treatment for stage I and stage II breast cancer was established through studies conducted during the 1970s and 1980s. Two NSABP protocols were particularly influential.

NSABP protocol B-04 studied 1765 patients with primary operable breast cancer treated at 34 institutions between 1971 and 1974 (1). Women with clinically negative axillae were randomized to receive either radical mastectomy, total mastectomy followed by radiation to the chest wall and regional lymph nodes, or total mastectomy alone (without axillary lymph node dissection, ALND). In the latter group, women underwent subsequent ALND if they developed axillary recurrences. Women with clinically positive nodes were randomized to receive either radical mastectomy or total mastectomy followed by local-regional radiation therapy.

In clinically node-negative or node-positive patients, there were no significant differences at 10 years in disease-free or overall survival between the treatment groups (Table 1). These results suggested that radical mastectomy, because of its attendant disfigurement and disability, has no role in the treatment of primary operable breast cancer; lesser procedures are equally effective with less morbidity. Furthermore, they emphasized that axillary dissection in clinically node-negative patients has no therapeutic benefit if regional recurrences are detected and treated promptly. ALND is

Table 1   Radical Mastectomy (RM) versus Simple Mastectomy alone (SM) versus Simple Mastectomy with Regional Irradiation (SMRT) for Treatment of Primary Operable Invasive Breast Cancer: Ten-Year Results of NSABP B-04 trial

	10-year survival rate (%)	
	Disease-free survival	Overall survival
Node-negative		
RM	47	58
SM	42	54
SMRT	48	59
Node-positive		
RM	29	38
SMRT	25	39

indicated only when the staging information will influence subsequent therapeutic choices.

NSABP study B-06 investigated the role of lumpectomy and radiation therapy in the treatment of stage I and II breast cancer (2). Over 8 years, 1843 women with mobile tumors less than 4 cm in largest dimension were randomly assigned to receive either modified radical mastectomy (MRM), lumpectomy with ALND, or lumpectomy, ALND, and breast irradiation. Pathologically negative margins for the lumpectomy specimen were required.

The results of this study were definitive. MRM offered no advantage over the other treatments when analyzed by disease-free or overall survival in either node-negative or node-positive patients (Table 2). Breast irradiation after lumpectomy reduced the likelihood of in-breast tumor recurrence from 39% to 10% but did not affect overall survival when compared with lumpectomy alone. These results demonstrated the equivalence of breast-conserving surgery (with or without breast irradiation) to MRM for treatment of stage I and stage II breast cancer.

In most instances, patient preference should be the key factor in choosing between mastectomy and breast conservation. The addition of breast irradiation to lumpectomy improves local control but not overall survival. However, the average patient will have a sufficiently high risk of in-breast recurrence after lumpectomy alone to justify the routine use of postlumpectomy radiation in most cases of invasive cancer.

These and similar studies provide the scientific basis for simplifying and humanizing breast cancer treatment without compromising medical out-

Table 2 Simple Mastectomy (SM) versus Lumpectomy Alone (LPX) versus Lumpectomy and Breast Irradiation (LPXRT) for Treatment of Primary Operable Invasive Breast Cancer: Eight-Year Results of NSABP B-06 Trial

	8-year survival rate (%)		
	Disease-free in-breast	Disease-free survival	Overall survival
Node-negative			
SM	—	75	88
LPX	63	68	87
LPXRT	88	77	88
Node-positive			
SM	—	54	60
LPX	57	55	60
LPXRT	94	59	68

comes. They provide a firm foundation for the use of breast-conserving surgery in most situations.

The formulation of a surgical treatment plan for a woman with newly diagnosed primary operable (stage I or II) breast cancer may be simplified by separately considering three issues: staging; local control; and regional control.

II. THE ROLE OF SURGERY IN BREAST CANCER STAGING

Accurate pathological staging requires forethought to assure that appropriate tissues are acquired and sent to the pathology laboratory in a condition that permits complete analysis. What is appropriate may vary from patient to patient. Pathological staging begins with the initial biopsy. Adherence to a biopsy protocol ensures that all relevant staging information is obtained. The primary surgical procedure for the treatment of a breast cancer should be planned so that all necessary staging data are obtained.

The need to remove axillary nodes must be determined preoperatively. In most cases of invasive cancer, the prognostic and therapeutic information gained is compelling enough to recommend an axillary dissection. Axillary lymph node metastases will be found in approximately one-third of clinically negative axillae, but only if a proper axillary dissection is performed.

The axillary lymph nodes are surgically divided into three regions. The low, level I nodes are found lateral to the lateral border of the pectoralis minor muscle. The level II nodes are found deep to the pectoralis minor muscle. The level III axillary lymph nodes are found at the apex of the axilla, medial to the medial border of the pectoralis minor muscle, high on the chest wall. Removal of only level I nodes (so-called "axillary sampling") in a haphazard fashion increases the risk of injury to major axillary neurovascular structures and may understage up to 25% of women (3). Proper staging of axillary lymph nodes should include en bloc removal and examination of level I and level II nodes. When conducted for staging, axillary lymph node dissection should not include removal of level III axillary nodes; in fewer than 2% of cases are metastases present in level III nodes when the level I and level II nodes are negative (3). Removal of level III nodes, however, increases the incidence of postoperative arm lymphedema almost fivefold. Therapeutic (in contrast to staging) axillary lymph node dissection should include removal of level I, II, and III nodes as needed to clear all evident gross disease.

Recently, the technique of sentinel lymph node biopsy, initially developed to reduce the morbidity associated with surgical staging for melanoma, has been applied to axillary staging for breast cancer. The sentinel node hypothesis postulates that in most cases, breast cancer spreads to the axillary nodes along a pathway predetermined by the location of the tumor in the breast and the lymphatic anatomy. The technique involves injection of a visible dye and/or a radioactive tracer in the vicinity of the primary cancer. Shortly thereafter, limited exposure of the axilla is obtained, the dye/tracer is followed to the initial filtering node, and this sentinel node is removed for pathological examination. If it is free of metastatic tumor, it is assumed that no other nodal metastases are present. If tumor is found in the sentinel node, formal axillary dissection is performed. This technique has been demonstrated to be both specific and sensitive in those cases where a sentinel can be identified (70–90% of cases, depending upon the specific technique used and the experience of the surgeon with it); concordance between sentinel node histology and histology in the formally staged axilla exceeds 95% (4,5) It is not known, however, what the significance of demonstration of micrometastases in a sentinel node is in relation to the efficacy of adjuvant systemic therapy (5). Therefore, in the clinical pathway, we have chosen to exclude a role for sentinel node axillary staging. It is likely that clinical trials will ultimately establish a validated role for sentinel node biopsy in many women with breast cancer.

III.　THE ROLE OF SURGERY FOR LOCAL CONTROL

NSABP protocols B-04 and B-06 established that, in most situations, total mastectomy and lumpectomy with breast irradiation are equally effective at preventing local tumor recurrence. With either therapy, local control is achieved in about 90% of patients at 10 years. The presence of larger tumors (even 5 cm or larger) or clinically positive axillary nodes does not preclude achieving local control with breast conservation. A few factors, however, predict a higher likelihood of local failure after lumpectomy. Residual gross or microscopic tumor after lumpectomy is the most important; this may be unavoidable if the cancer is large, insidiously infiltrative, or multifocal. Additional factors include: (1) presence of multifocal tumor (separate foci in more than one quadrant of the breast not able to be encompassed in a single specimen); and (2) inability to administer adequate radiation therapy (because of prior breast or chest irradiation, pregnancy, presence of severe pulmonary disease, or presence of a collagen-vascular disorder). Furthermore, the expectation of an unfavorable aesthetic result because of the tumor size and location relative to the breast is a relative contraindication to breast conservation. In this situation, the patient should make an informed decision concerning what *she* believes would be aesthetically acceptable.

Factors favoring mastectomy include: patient preference for mastectomy; inability to achieve negative margin lumpectomy; tumor location and size not conducive to aesthetically acceptable breast-conserving surgery and radiation therapy; presence of multifocal tumor; and the presence of a contraindication to breast irradiation. Factors irrelevant to the decision between lumpectomy and mastectomy include: tumor size and breast size (except as they effect ability to achieve negative margins and impact upon the expected aesthetic result); axillary lymph node status; tumor histology; anticipated need for adjuvant chemotherapy; and patient age.

IV. THE ROLE OF SURGERY FOR REGIONAL CONTROL

Treatments to establish regional control focus on the axilla. Clinically significant internal mammary node recurrences are rare and prophylactic treatment does not improve survival; treatment of supraclavicular nodes is defined as an issue of distant, not regional, disease control. As demonstrated by NSABP protocol B-04, prophylactic treatment of the axilla with either radiation therapy or ALND does not improve survival, but ALND is often indicated for staging. Therapeutic ALND or irradiation is indicated in the presence of known regional lymph node metastases.

ALND performed to stage breast cancer should include removal of level I and level II nodes. This assures representative sampling while avoiding the additional morbidity associated with removal of level III nodes. However, all lymph nodes that are clinically abnormal, even in the level III region, should be removed at the time of ALND.

REFERENCES

1. Fisher B, Redmond C, Fisher ER, et al. Ten-year results of a randomized clinical trial comparing radical mastectomy and total mastectomy with or without radiation. N Engl J Med 1985; 312:674–681.
2. Fisher B, Redmond, Poisson R, et al. Eight-year results of a randomized clinical trial comparing total mastectomy and lumpectomy with or without irradiation in the treatment of breast cancer. N Engl J Med 1989; 320:822–828.
3. Chevinsky AH, Ferrara J, James AG, Minton JP, Young D, Farrar WB. Prospective evaluation of clinical and pathologic detection of axillary metastases in patients with breast carcinoma. Surgery 1990; 108:612–618.
4. Giuliano AE, Kirgan DM, Guenther JM, Morton DL. Lymphatic mapping and sentinel lymphadenectomy for breast cancer. Ann Surg 1994; 220:391–401.
5. Turner RR, Ollila DW, Krasne DL, Giuliano AE. Histopathologic validation of the sentinel lymph node hypothesis for breast cancer. Ann Surg 1996; 226: 271–278.

7

Radiation Therapy in the Management of Breast Cancer

SUSAN A. HIGGINS and BRUCE G. HAFFTY
Yale University School of Medicine, New Haven, Connecticut

I. BREAST-CONSERVING THERAPY

Breast-conserving therapy with lumpectomy followed by radiation therapy (RT) to the intact breast is widely embraced as an acceptable and preferable standard of care in the management of early-stage breast cancer (1–4). Although the majority of patients with operable breast cancer are candidates for conservative surgery followed by RT to the intact breast, there are a number of relative contraindications and a number of factors that may be predictive of an adverse outcome following breast conservation therapy (5–10). These factors may be used to identify patients who are not optimal candidates for breast conservation therapy based on either (1) a high risk of complication, (2) poor cosmetic result or (3) excessive risk of ipsilateral breast tumor recurrence (IBTR).

Optimally, the assessment of a patient with breast cancer is performed in a multidisciplinary setting with the involved specialists consulted prior to initiation of treatment. Following history and physical examination, as well as a thorough review of the mammograms and other diagnostic tests, the radiation oncologist should determine whether there are any contraindications to breast irradiation. Once eligibility for breast irradiation has been established, various tumor-, treatment-, and patient-related factors that influence the ultimate local control and cosmesis obtained with breast conservation therapy should be considered. While there are usually objective data to draw upon regarding the effect of various clinical and pathological factors and their relationship to long-term outcome and local control, cosmetic outcome is sometimes more difficult to predict and the anticipated results of therapy must be reconciled with the patient's expectations. Furthermore, there are important psychological issues regarding breast conservation versus mastectomy, which may need to be addressed so the physician can discuss the relevant advantages and disadvantages of these two approaches in relation to the patient's personal preferences.

Factors that have been identified as potential contraindications to breast conservation therapy based on increased risk of complications include, but are not limited to, pregnancy, history of prior irradiation, presence of collagen vascular disease, and technical and anatomical factors that may result in poor cosmetic outcome or increased complications (5–10).

A. Pregnancy

Due to the fact that treatment of the breast is inevitably associated with exposure of the fetus to irradiation, breast irradiation is generally contraindicated in a patient who is pregnant. When a patient is diagnosed with a presumed early-stage breast cancer during pregnancy, delaying breast irradiation until the postpartum period may be an option, depending on the clinical circumstances. For those patients who will not be able to delay breast irradiation, mastectomy may be considered. In selected cases, in the second or third trimester of pregnancy, systemic chemotherapy may be considered either following mastectomy or prior to surgery. Given the potential dangers of exposure of the fetus to irradiation, and the other options that are available, breast irradiation during pregnancy is contraindicated.

B. Prior Radiation

In patients with a history of previous radiation to the thorax, it is important to obtain a detailed history, including previous treatment records and/or simulation or port films, if they are available. Physical examination, with careful attention to skin changes and/or tattoos, may provide additional information regarding the location of previous treatment. In cases where there has been significant dose delivered to the breast, or a portion of the breast, mastectomy should be considered. If the patient gives a history consistent with a previous low dose of irradiation, i.e., diagnostic procedures or treatment of benign disease, and the skin shows minimal skin changes from prior radiation, breast preservation may be pursued.

C. Collagen Vascular Disease

Active or preexisting collagen vascular disease has been considered to be a relative contraindication to breast conservation therapy based on a number of reports that suggest that these patients have a significantly greater risk of complications. Fleck et al. (9) described exaggerated acute and late effects occurring within 2 years after definitive megavoltage RT for breast carcinoma in three of four women with preexisting collagen vascular disease. There have been additional case reports of exaggerated side effects in patients with collagen vascular disease following conventional doses of radiation to the breast or chest wall. The long-term effects include fibrosis and soft tissue or bone necrosis. Most of the reports, however, are anecdotal and the true incidence of complications secondary to RT in this group of patients is unclear. In a recent matched pair case-control study of patients with collagen vascular disease treated with radiation to various sites (including the breast and chest wall), there was only a slightly increased incidence of acute reactions and late complications in the group with collagen vascular disease. It is important, in patients with collagen vascular disease, to get an accurate history regarding the severity of the disease. Each case would be highly individualized and, depending on the extent of disase and the subtype of collagen vascular disease, the judicious use of radiation to the breast and/or chest wall may be considered.

D. Technical Considerations

There are a number of technical and anatomical factors that may result in suboptimal results in patients considering conservative surgery with lumpectomy and radiation. The standard technique of breast irradiation involves the use of tangential beams with the patient lying supine on a breast board with the ipsilateral arm extended. Some patients may be unable to assume or maintain this position due to physcial limitations (i.e., back pain or restricted mobility of the upper extremities). In patients with extremely large and/or pendulous breasts, the radiation oncologist should determine if it is technically feasible to deliver an adequate and homogeneous dose to the breast without irradiating an unacceptable amount of normal tissue. In patients with very pendulous breasts, special immobilization devices, such as an acquaplast or a breast ring, may be necessary. In morbidly obese patients, dimensions of the breast and/or chest wall may make it difficult to deliver homogeneous doses with standard beam energies and techniques. In this and in other situations, where there is a question as to whether the patient will be a candidate for breast irradiation due to anatomical and/or technical considerations, it is important that the radiation oncologist be involved in the decision-making process prior to definitive surgical procedure in an effort to determine whether breast irradiation can be accomplished with acceptable cosmesis and risk of side effects.

E. Prognostic Factors for IBTR

A number of studies have evaluated prognostic factors that may result in an increased risk of local recurrence. Gross multicentric or multifocal disease, detected either clinically or mammographically, generally is considered to be a contraindication to breast conservation. Although selected patients with two or more lesions may be considered candidates for breast conservation, patients with gross multicentric disease have been shown to have a high risk of local recurrence. The high incidence of breast recurrence may be secondary to the presence of significant residual tumor burden in the breast following conservative surgery. Another factor that must be considered in evaluating patients with gross multicentric disease is the cosmetic result, which may be significantly compromised by the surgical removal of two or more lesions from the same breast. Despite the relative contraindication of multicentric disease, there have been retrospective studies from several institutions of selected patients with two synchronous ipsilateral breast masses who underwent wide local excision of all gross disease and subsequently underwent RT. Although the local recurrence rate was slightly higher in this group of patients, selected patients with synchronous ipsilateral breast tumors may be considered for this approach provided they understand the potential of an increased risk of local recurrence (11).

Extensive intraductal component (EIC) is a pathological entity defined as having an invasive ductal carcinoma with an intraductal component comprising 25% or more of the primary invasive tumor with intraductal carcinoma in the surrounding normal breast tissue (12). A lesion composed of predominantly ductal carcinoma in situ with focal areas of invasion is also categorized as an EIC-positive tumor. Initial reports indicated that EIC was found to be a powerful predictor of local failure. It is important to note, however, that patients in these studies were treated at a time when microscopic assessment of the margins of resection was not routinely performed. In a recent update, the relationship between microscopic margins of resection, the presence of extensive intraductal component, and IBTR after breast-conserving therapy was evaluated. In that analysis, the 5-year rate of IBTR for all patients with negative margins was 2% and for all patients with focally positive margins was 9%. The authors recommended that breast conservation therapy be considered in patients with negative margins or focally involved margins whether or not EIC is present (7). In patients with greater than focally involved margins, the IBTR rate, particularly in patients with EIC-positive tumors, was high, and given these results, it is apparent that patients with extensive intraductal component with diffusely involved margins that cannot be cleared on reexcision are not optimal candidates for breast-conserving therapy.

A number of other clinical and/or pathological factors have been associated with high local recurrence rates. Although there have been some consistencies, there have also been a number of conflicting reports regarding clinical and/or pathological factors that may be predictive of IBTR. Factors typically predictive of a high rate of systemic metastasis, such as number of axillary lymph nodes involved, primary tumor size, lymphvascular invasion, DNA ploidy, and high S-phase fraction, have not been consistently shown to be predictive of IBTR. Although recently there have been a number of studies evaluating novel molecular markers such as Her-2-*neu*, p53, insulin-like growth factor receptor, and cyclin D as potential prognostic factors for local relapse, larger studies will be needed prior to the routine clinical use of molecular markers with respect to treatment decisions regarding breast-conserving therapy (13).

One prognostic factor for local recurrence that has been reported in several studies has been the association of young age with high local recurrence rates. Although a highly significant correlation with young age and local recurrence has been reported, there is no evidence that young patients electing breast-conserving therapy have a compromised survival and we continue to offer young patients lumpectomy followed by radiation therapy as an acceptable standard of care. To date, there is no evidence that patients with strong family history and/or hereditary forms of breast cancer have a high rate of local recurrence, although data regarding the risk of local recurrence in patients with BRCA1 and BRCA2 positivity are limited (14–16).

In summary, it is apparent that the vast majority of patients with operable breast cancer are acceptable candidates for breast conservation therapy, provided adequate excision of the tumor can be obtained with an acceptable cosmetic result.

F. Delivery of Radiation Therapy

Radiation therapy following breast conservation surgery should be employed using careful treatment-planning techniques that minimize treatment of the underlying heart and lung. To achieve the optimal cosmetic result, an effort should be made to obtain homogeneous dose distribution throughout the breast. Doses of 180–200 cGy/day to the intact breast to a total dose of 4500–5000 cGy are considered standard. Administration of a boost using an electron beam or interstitial implant to bring the tumor bed to a total dose of 6000–6600 cGy is frequently employed. Although the necessity of a boost is controversial, and has been the subject of debate, the majority of the radiation oncologists in the United States continue to use a boost. In a recently published randomized clinical trial, delivery of a boost of 10 Gy to the tumor bed after 50 Gy to the whole breast resulted in a statistically significant reduction in local recurrence, although the local recurrence rate in patients treated with or without the boost was quite acceptable.

In patients undergoing breast-conserving therapy who have had an axillary lymph node dissection, the role of regional nodal irradiation is controversial (17–19). In general, patients with pathologically negative axillary nodes would be treated to the breast only, eliminating radiation therapy to the internal mammary or supraclavicular fossa. In patients with node-positive disease, RT to the supraclavicular fossa and/or internal mammary chain may be considered, although the benefits are uncertain. Extrapolation from the results of recent randomized trials, indicating a survical benefit to regional nodal irradiation in the postmastectomy setting, indicates that regional nodal irradiation in node-positive, conservatively treated patients may be beneficial (20,21). Clearly, however, in conservatively treated patients, cosmesis must be considered and careful treatment planning techniques minimizing overlap between adjacent fields must be employed. In our own clinical practice, we do not routinely employ a separate internal mammary field for node-positive patients. In patients who have had an adequate axillary dissection, we do not routinely treat the axilla but do routinely treat the supraclavicular fossa in node-positive patients. For patients who do not undergo axillary dissection, or who have had an inadequate dissection, RT to the supraclavicular and axillary regions at the time of breast irradiation results in a high rate of regional nodal control with minimal morbidity.

G. Subsets of Patients in Whom Radiation Therapy May Be Avoided

Currently, for patients with invasive breast cancer, RT following lumpectomy remains the standard of care. A number of prospective randomized trials have addressed the issue of lumpectomy alone versus lumpectomy with radiation and have consistently been shown RT to significantly reduce the risk of IBTR (1–10). Although there has been no clearly established survival benefit from RT to the intact breast following lumpectomy, local recurrence rates in patients treated with lumpectomy alone have been shown to be as high as 40–50%, even with the use of systemic therapy. A recently reported prospective single-arm trial attempted to employ lumpectomy alone in a highly selected group of patients with small tumors, negative margins, and negative lymph nodes. Even in this select group of patients, the local recurrence rate approached 25% with relatively limited follow-up. Currently, there is an intergroup trial evaluating lumpectomy alone versus lumpectomy and RT in a select group of patients older than 70 years with estrogen-receptor tumors and negative margins. For patients with invasive carcinoma, the use of lumpectomy alone should currently be limited to prospective trials.

For patients with DCIS, lumpectomy alone versus lumpectomy with RT continues to be an active area of investigation and debate. The NSABP-17 trial, which randomized patients with DCIS to lumpectomy versus lumpectomy and RT, clearly showed a benefit to RT in reducing the risk of local recurrence (22). The benefit of RT was noted in all subsets of patients, including those with low-grade non-comedo-type DCIS. There have been a number of retrospective series with limited follow-up reporting acceptable local recurrence rates in selected patients with DCIS. These studies have employed careful treatment techniques with detailed attention to surgical margins. Currently, we continue to offer RT to the majority of patients with DCIS, although results of ongoing trials and longer follow-up of patients treated with lumpectomy alone with careful attention to surgical margins is likely to identify a subset of patients with DCIS who may be treated with excision alone.

H.   Sequencing of Chemo/Radiotherapy

The majority of patients undergoing lumpectomy followed by RT to the intact breast for invasive breast carcinoma will be receiving some form of systemic therapy, in the form of either cytotoxic chemotherapy or adjuvant hormonal treatment. For those patients undergoing cytotoxic chemotherapy, the optimal sequencing of radiation with chemotherapy remains an active area of investigation and an ongoing debate (23). There have been conflicting reports in the literature regarding the issue of whether a delay in RT compromises local control. Although initial reports indicated a high local recurrence rate in those patients in whom a course of definitive RT was delayed more than 16 weeks, a number of other series have failed to confirm these findings. Furthermore, a randomized clinical trial addressing the issue of the sequencing of chemotherapy and RT from the JCRT indicated that although delaying RT resulted in a slightly higher local recurrence rate, a delay in chemotherapy compromised distant metastasis. The vast majority of patients in this trial, however, were node-positive. Currently, in the majority of node-positive patients where systemic cytotoxic chemotherapy is being considered, initiation of chemotherapy prior to radiation appears reasonable. Concurrent chemo/radiotherapy, however, has also been employed, and although some have reported an increased risk of acute reactions and complications with this approach, others have not. Clearly, concomitant chemo/radiotherapy may be considered in selected patients provided radiation is not administered with concomitant adriamycin-based chemotherapy.

For patients with node-negative disease, the issue of the timing of chemotherapy with RT is more controversial. Currently, the decision regarding the timing of chemotherapy with RT is highly individualized, depending on risk factors for systemic and/or local disease, along with the patient's own preferences.

I.   Follow-up of the Conservatively Treated Patient

The follow-up program in the conservatively treated breast cancer patients serves several objectives. First, it provides an opportunity for the radiation oncologist to periodically assess the patient for local recurrence. Long-term follow-up of conservatively treated patients has consistently shown a local recurrence rate of 0.5–2%/year, plateauing at a long-term breast failure rate of 15–20% (5–10). It is important for the patient to continue with an adequate follow-up throughout her lifetime to allow for early detection of local recurrence with appropriate salvage management so as to not compromise her overall survival.

As with mastectomy, contralateral breast cancer is also a considerable risk in the conservatively treated breast cancer patient. Again, a risk of contralateral breast cancer approaching 1%/year has been reported and it is important for patients who carry the diagnosis of breast cancer to be followed not only for risk of recurrence in the ipsilateral breast, but so that contralateral breast carcinomas can also be detected at an earlier stage.

During the follow-up visit, the radiation oncologist should also assess the patient for cosmetic result, as well as short- and long-term treatment complications. The follow-up program provides the radiation oncologist an opportunity to assess the patient for treatment complications and cosmetic result and, if necessary, make appropriate changes in treatment policies.

Finally, the follow-up program provides the patient with a sense of reassurance and helps to diminish anxieties regarding the issue of local recurrence. While patient's needs in this regard will vary considerably, the value of an adequate follow-up program with respect to this issue should not be underestimated.

Patient history and physical examination complemented by mammography serve as the primary tools in the radiation oncologist's follow-up program. A history should be directed toward briefly surveying the patient for constitutional or localizing symptoms indicative of recurrent disease. Physical examination shoud include methodical survey of both breasts and lymph node regions. Careful attention to symmetry, postoperative surgical changes, skin thickening, edema, and radiation changes should be noted. In addition, attention should be directed toward short- and long-term complications, as well as cosmetic outcome. Following lumpectomy and radiation therapy, degree of skin thickening, edema, fibrosis, postoperative appearance of the surgical bed, and size of the breast may undergo significant changes. Examination in the majority of patients, however, will stabilize by 1 year following radiation. Close follow-up during the first few years following treatment will help the examiner distinguish the evolving postsurgical and radiation changes from more suspicious physical findings that may develop. Frequent follow-up during the first 2 years is also justified by the relatively aggressive clinical behavior that has been associated with early local relapses. At our own institution, our policy is to have follow-up visits at least every 6 months during the first 2–3 years post treatment, and then annually thereafter. Often, a patient is also seeing a surgeon and/or medical oncologist in conjunction with the radiation oncologist. After the first few years, annual visits should continue indefinitely, if not with a radiation oncologist, at least with one of the patient's treating physicians. A protracted clinical course of local recurrence, as well as the long-term risk of cancer in the contralateral breast, mandates a continued follow-up program.

Mammography is an essential complement to the physical examination in following the conservatively treated breast cancer patient. Those patients with nonpalpable mammographically detected IBTRs have an excellent prognosis. As with physical examination, interpretation of mammography can be difficult owing to breast retraction, changes in density, skin thickening, and other postsurgical and postradiation changes. The majority of these changes will stabilize by 3–6 months following treatment. Although the optimal timing and frequency of mammography following conservative surgery is controversial, our own practice is to obtain a post-RT baseline mammogram approximately six months following treatment. Annual mammography thereafter is generally recommended unless there are persistent changes or suspicious findings, in which case more frequent mammography and/or other diagnostic intervention may be indicated.

Even in patients whose original breast cancer was not visualized on mammogram, follow-up mammography is helpful. In our own experience, we have noted that four or six local recurrences in a group of patients whose original mammogram was negative had their recurrence detected on follow-up mammography.

The combination of physical examination and mammography will inevitably yield suspicious findings in some patients. Recent studies have reported an overall positive biopsy rate on suspicious findings in the conservatively treated breast cancer patient of just over 50%. The importance of early detection and intervention, coupled with the low complication rate associated with biopsy of the conservatively treated breast, justifies a policy of early biopsy of suspicious findings on physical examination, mammography, or both.

II. POSTMASTECTOMY RADIATION

A number of prospective and retrospective series in patients treated with mastectomy have demonstrated that patients with primary tumors greater than 5 cm and/or involvement of four or more lymph nodes have a high risk of locoregional failure following mastectomy. These patients as well as those with positive margins should also be considered for postmastectomy radiation in an effort to minimize the risk of local regional recurrence. Even in patients who have undergone high-dose chemotherapy with or without stem cell rescue, locoregional failure is a significant problem in this group of patients without the use of postmastectomy radiation. Most current on-going clinical trials evaluating dose-intensive chemotherapy with or without bone marrow stem cells transplantation routinely include postmastectomy RT to the chest wall and/or regional lymph nodes to minimize locoregional recurrence in patients with locally advanced cancer and multiple positive nodes.

The use of postmastectomy RT in patients with earlier stages of disease is more controversial. Two recently conducted randomized clinical trials, however, demonstrated a disease-free survival and overall survival advantage with postmastectomy radiation in node-positive patients (20,21). In both of these trials, patients were treated with mastectomy and cytotoxic chemotherapy and were randomized to receive or not receive postmastectomy radiation to the chest wall and regional lymph nodes. Long-term follow-up of these trials has shown an improvement in distant metastasis and overall survival, not only in patients with four or more nodes, but also in premenopausal patients with one to three nodes. Thus, these trials have resurrected the issue of postmastectomy RT in patients with earlier stages of disease and limited nodal involvement. Although there are a number of controversies regarding the extent of axillary lymph node dissection in these patients, subset analysis, as well as RT techniques employed, these trials have brought forward the issue of considering postmastectomy radiation in patients with earlier stages of disease. Currently, we strongly recommend postmastectomy radiation in patients with four or more positive nodes and/or T3 primary tumors. In premenopausal patients with one to three nodes, we would also consider postmastectomy radiation and discuss the risks and benefits of postmastectomy radiation with each patient on an individualized basis.

In those patients in whom postmastectomy RT is employed, careful treatment techniques and field arrangements that minimize overlap between adjacent fields and minimize the dose to underlying cardiac and pulmonary structures are required. Whether to include the internal mammary (IM) chain, supraclavicular fossa, and/or axilla remains controversial. Although both randomized trials employed techniques treating the internal mammary and axillary nodes, the risk/benefit of the extent of nodal irradiation is unclear. A current ongoing trial in Europe randomizing patients to tangential fields alone compared to tangential fields with IM and supraclavicular radiation is ongoing, although the results of that trial will not be available for several years. Our own policy in patients undergoing postmastectomy RT is to treat the chest wall with tangential fields. A separate supraclavicular field half beam-blocked and matched to the tangential field in an effort to avoid overlap between the adjacent fields is routinely employed. In patients with an adequately dissected axilla, we do not extend the supraclavicular field to treat the axillary contents. We have not been routinely treating the IM chain, although in those selected patients in whom treatment of the IM chain is warranted, we would obtain a treatment-planning computed-tomography (CT) scan and attempt to include the IM chain in the tangential fields when possible. Alternatively, a separate IM field using electrons or a combination of photon/electrons carefully matched to the tangential field and minimizing the dose to the underlying heart may be employed.

III. LOCAL REGIONAL RECURRENCE OF DISEASE

Local regional recurrence of disease remains a major clinical problem for patients carrying the diagnosis of breast cancer. Depending on patient's initial presentation and subsequent management, local regional recurrence rates as high as 50% have been reported. Obviously, appropriate use of surgery, systemic therapy, and radiation should be employed, as outlined in previous sections, in an effort to minimize the chance of local regional recurrence in patients carrying the diagnosis of breast cancer. Despite adequate and appropriate local regional and systemic therapy, however, between 5 and 20% of patients will experience local regional recurrence of disease. With over 150,000 new cases of breast cancer per year, local regional recurrence obviously remains a major problem that the clinical oncologist faces. Since up to 30% of patients presenting with local regional relapse may have simultaneous distant metastasis, a systemic disease evaluation should be carried out at the time of local regional relapse. CT scanning of the chest will not only rule out pulmonary metastasis, but aids in evaluating the extent of local regional disease. For those patients with clinically evident systemic metastasis, the reader is referred to the pathways for systemic disease. It should be noted, however, that even with systemic metastasis, local control may be a significant issue and should be addressed. Local regional recurrences can be divided into the following categories: tumors in the ipsilateral breast following conservative surgery, postmastectomy chest wall recurrences, and regional nodal recurrences following conservative surgery or mastectomy.

A. IBTRs following Lumpectomy With or Without Radiation

For those patients who develop a local failure after breast-conserving surgery for invasive breast cancer or DCIS, tumor usually develops in the region of the initial primary tumor. Although the prognosis following IBTR is more favorable than for other local regional relapses, early IBTRs following lumpectomy and RT have been associated with a relatively high rate of systemic metastasis (24). For those patients who have undergone lumpectomy alone without radiation, reexcision at the time of local recurrence followed by RT may be an option, although there are limited data on this approach.

For patients experiencing an IBTR following lumpectomy with RT, mastectomy is the most commonly employed and standard treatment modality. Although there have been some studies reporting acceptable results with repeat wide local excision, or repeat wide local excision with additional radiation, selection criteria for this approach are unclear and long-term follow-up regarding this management option is lacking. Studies from the University of Pennsylvania evaluating salvage mastectomy specimens of patients who sustained an IBTR failed to identify a subgroup of patients in whom local excision of the tumor bed would provide adequate local treatment. There is a subgroup of patients, however, who are unwilling to consider salvage mastectomy who, based on available data, may be managed by wide local excision with or without the addition of limited field reirradiation provided these patients are willing to accept some uncertainty regarding this treatment approach.

Following definitive surgical treatment with salvage mastectomy for those patients experiencing an IBTR, reconstruction with autologous tissue using a TRAM flap may be considered. Acceptable long-term results in previously irradiated patients have been reported using these surgical techniques. Reconstruction with saline or silicon implants following radiation have been associated with a high rate of complications and should generally be avoided.

There are limited data regarding the role of systemic therapy following salvage mastectomy for IBTR. Although patients with early IBTRs have a relatively high rate of subsequent systemic metastasis, the benefit of adjuvant systemic therapy in this setting is unclear. Given the high rate of metastasis in more agressive IBTRs, however, some patients and/or their oncologists may consider the use of adjuvant systemic therapy in those patients with aggressive early local recurrences based on extrapolation of data regarding the potential benefits of systemic therapy in those patients likely to be harboring subclinical and micrometastatic disease. In those patients not previously on hormonal therapy with estrogen-receptor-positive recurrences, adjuvant tamoxifen may also be considered, although there are no available data on this subject. For patients with late local recurrences, which may represent new primary tumors and may be distinctly removed from the original tumor bed, evaluation of the tumor for prognostic factors such as tumor size, ER status, DNA ploidy, S-phase fraction, and other prognostic factors may aid the clinician in making a decision regarding the use of adjuvant systemic therapy, assuming this is the development of a new primary tumor. Owing to the lack of available data on adjuvant systemic therapy in the setting of an IBTR, the approach to these patients is, by necessity, highly individualized.

B.   Chest Wall Recurrences After Mastectomy

Patients who develop a postmastectomy chest wall recurrence have a relatively high rate of subsequent systemic metastasis. Many of these patients will experience long disease-free intervals, and for those patients with isolated chest wall recurrences, long-term 5–10-year disease-free survivals of >50% have been reported (25). It is therefore important to attempt to obtain adequate local regional control in these patients who may experience a relatively long survival following chest wall recurrence. In patients suspected of having a chest wall recurrence, biopsy is clearly indicated. When feasible, excision of the mass should be attempted followed by comprehensive RT to involve the chest wall and/or regional lymph nodes. Radiation treatment techniques are generally similar to those employed with standard postmastectomy radiation therapy and consist of photon and/or electron beam directed at the chest wall and adjacent lymph nodes. Treatment planning should strive for homogeneous dose distributions throughout the target area while minimizing the dose to the underlying cardiac and pulmonary structures. Conventional fractionation of 180–200 cGy/day to the area of local regional recurrence and immediately adjacent areas at risk to a total dose of 4500–5000 cGy with a boost to the area of recurrence or gross residual disease to a dose of 6000–6500 cGy results in acceptable long-term local regional control.

In patients who experienced a chest wall recurrence and had previously undergone RT, additional limited-field RT may be considered. Reirradiation to the chest wall with limited fields has been associated with acceptable long-term complications. Several reports regarding the use of hyperthermia with concomitant RT in this setting have also shown acceptable local control and complication rates.

Clearly, patients with chest wall recurrences following mastectomy have a relatively high rate of systemic metastasis. There are limited data, however, regarding the use of adjuvant systemic therapy in this setting. A recently reported randomized trial demonstrated disease-free survival benefit with the use of adjuvant tamoxifen following RT at the time of postmastectomy chest wall recurrence in patients with ER-positive tumors. Patients with ER-negative tumors and aggressive local regional recurrences may be considered for cytotoxic chemotherapy given their relatively poor prognosis and high rate of distant metastasis, although prospective randomized trials addressing the use of adjuvant systemic therapy in this setting are nonexistent.

C. Treatment of Regional Nodal Recurrences

Regional nodal relapses following mastectomy or conservative surgery with RT carry a relatively poor prognosis. Although patients initially treated with a simple mastectomy experiencing an axillary recurrence had a favorable prognosis, the majority of patients sustaining recurrences in the IM chain, supraclavicular fossa, or axilla following dissection and/or RT have a high rate of systemic metastasis. Nonetheless, adequate local regional control in these patients at the time of regional relapse is an important goal. Following biopsy and/or surgical resection, when feasible, RT can provide adequate long-term local regional control. Depending on the location of the regional relapse, RT to the nodal relapse and adjacent areas at risk can be accomplished using treatment techniques as previously described. Conventional doses of 180–200 cGy/fraction to total doses of 4500–5000 cGy with cone-down to the area of residual disease to doses of 5000–6000 cGy should result in adequate long-term local regional control. These patients have an extremely high risk of systemic metastasis, but as with postmastectomy chest wall recurrences and IBTRs, there are limited data regarding the role of adjuvant systemic therapy in this setting. Again, owing to the lack of available data, adjuvant systemic therapy can be employed on an individualized basis. For those patients who have not previously been on hormonal therapy and are receptor positive, it would be reasonable to consider tamoxifen in addition to any other systemic therapy.

Clearly, the role of systemic therapy at the time of local regional relapse has not been well defined. Given the significant numbers of patients who experience local regional relapse, along with the relatively high rate of subsequent systemic disease in these patients, consideration of systemic therapy is reasonable. This area is clearly in need of well-designed multi-institutional trials to address the issue of adjuvant systemic therapy at the time of local relapse.

REFERENCES

1. Haffty BG, Ward BA. Is breast-conserving surgery with radiation superior to mastectomy in selected patients? Cancer J Sci Am 1997; 3:2–3.

2. Fisher B, Redmond C, Poisson R, et al. Eight-year results of a randomized clinical trial comparing total mastectomy and lumpectomy with or without irradiation in the treatment of breast cancer. N Engl J Med 1989; 320:822–828.

3. Veronesi U, Sacozzi R, Del Vecchio M, et al. Comparing radical mastectomy with quadrantectomy, axillary dissection and radiotherapy in patients with small cancers of the breast. N Engl J Med 1981; 305:6–11.

4. Fowble B, Solin LJ, Schultz DJ. Conservative surgery and radiation for early stage breast cancer. In: Fowble B, Goodman RL, Glick JH, et al, eds. Breast Cancer Treatment. A Comprehensive Guide to Management. St. Louis, MO: CV Mosby, 1991:3–88.

5. Haffty BG, Fischer D, Rose M, et al. Prognostic factors for local recurrence in the conservatively treated breast cancer patient: a cautious interpretation of the data. J Clin Oncol 1991; 9:997–1003.

6. Harris J, Recht A, Almaric R, et al. Time course and prognosis of local recurrence following primary radiation therapy for early breast cancer. J Clin Oncol 1984; 2:37–41.

7. Gage I, Schnitt SJ, Nixon AJ, et al. Pathologic margin involvement and the risk of recurrence in patients treated with breast-conserving therapy. Cancer 1996; 78:1921–1928.

8. Smitt MC, Nowels JW, Zdeblich MJ, et al. The importance of the lumpectomy surgical margin status in long term results of breast conservation. Cancer 1995; 76:259–267.

9. Fleck R, McNeese MD, Ellerbroek NA, et al. Consequences of breast irradiation in patients with pre-existing collagen vascular diseases. Int J Radiat Oncol Biol Phys 1989; 17:829–833.

10. DiPaola RS, Orel SG, Fowble BL. Ipsilateral breast tumor recurrence following conservative surgery and radiation therapy. Oncology 1994; 8:59–68.

11. Wilson LD, Beinfield M, McKhann CF, Haffty BG. Conservative surgery and radiation in the treatment of synchronous ipsilateral breast cancers. Cancer 1993; 72:137–142.

12. Schnitt SJ, Connolly JL, Harris JR, et al. Pathologic predictors of early local recurrence in stage I and II breast cancer treated by primary radiation therapy. Cancer 1984; 53:1049.

13. Turner BC, Haffty BG, Narayanan L, et al. Insulin-like growth factor-I receptor overexpression mediates cellular radioresistance and local breast cancer recurrence after lumpectomy and radiation. Cancer Res 1997; 57:3079–3083.

14. Fowble BL, Schultz DJ, Overmoyer B, et al. The influence of young age on outcome in early stage breast cancer. Int J Radiat Oncol Biol Phys 1994; 30:23–33.

15. Chabner E, Nixon AJ, Garber J, et al. Family history suggestive of an inherited susceptibility to breast cancer and treatment outcome in young women after breast-conserving therapy. Int J Radiat Oncol Biol Phys 1997; 39:137.

16. Peterson M, Fowble B, Solin LJ, et al. Family history status as a prognostic factor for breast cancer patients treated with conservative surgery and irradiation. Breast J 1995; 1:202–209.

17.   Haffty BG, Ward B, Pathare P, et al. Reappraisal of the role of axillary lymph node dissection in the conservative treatment of breast cancer. J Clin Oncol 1997; 15:691–700.

18.   Recht A, Pierce SM, Abner A, et al. Regional nodal failure after conservative surgery and radiotherapy for early-stage breast carcinoma. J Clin Oncol 1991; 9:988–996.

19.   Haffty BG, Fischer D, Fischer JJ. Regional nodal irradiation in the conservative treatment of breast cancer. Int J Radiat Oncol Biol Phys 1990; 19:859–865.

20.   Overgaard M, Hansen PS, Overgaard J, et al. Postoperative radiotherapy in high-risk premenopausal women with breast cancer who receive adjuvant chemotherapy. N Engl J Med 1997; 337:949–955.

21.   Ragaz J, Jackson SM, Le N, et al. Adjuvant radiotherapy and chemotherapy in node-positive premenopausal women with breast cancer. N Engl J Med 1997; 337:956–962.

22.   Fisher B, Costintino J, Redmond C, et al. Lumpectomy compared with lumpectomy and radiation therapy for the treatment of intraductal breast cancer. N Engl J Med 1993; 328:1581–1586.

23.   Recht A, Come SE, Henderson C, et al. The sequencing of chemotherapy and radiation therapy after conservative surgery for early-stage breast cancer. N Engl J Med 1996; 334:1356–1399.

24.   Haffty BG, Reiss M, Beinfield M, et al. Ipsilateral breast tumor recurrence as a predictor of distant disease: implications for systemic therapy at the time of local relapse. J Clin Oncol 1996; 13:52–57.

25.   Borner M, Bacchi M, Goldhirsch A, et al. First isolated loco-regional recurrence following mastectomy for breast cancer: results of a phase III multicenter study comparing systemic treatment with observation after excision and radiation. J Clin Oncol 1994; 12:2071–2077.

8
Breast Reconstruction

PHILIP D. WEY
*UMDNJ/Robert Wood Johnson Medical School,
New Brunswick, New Jersey*

The option to restore a woman's breast after mastectomy is an important component of multidisciplinary breast cancer care. Safe, effective breast reconstruction is available to most women undergoing mastectomy because advances in breast cancer therapy have improved coordination between medical oncologists, surgeons, radiation therapists, and other care providers. Improvements in surgical techniques as well as advances in technology allow a customized approach to reconstruction. Plastic surgery of the breast has advanced beyond merely restoring a breast mound; current techniques routinely achieve a natural-appearing reconstructed breast and nipple that matches the opposite side. The end result is a symmetrical, harmonious, and proportionate reconstruction.

Although the availability of breast reconstruction may ease the emotional distress encountered when facing loss of the breast, the decision for mastectomy should be made independent of the decision for reconstruction. In the unlikely event of complications resulting in loss of the reconstruction, it would be unfortunate for a woman to regret her decision for mastectomy (vs. conservation surgery) because of the inability to complete the reconstruction process.

To develop a treatment plan for the individual patient, a rational decision-making process should be followed (Fig. 1) (1). No single reconstructive pathway is clearly superior in all circumstances and a variety of options can often produce a satisfactory outcome. The initial consideration is whether an immediate or delayed procedure is desired. With proper patient selection, reconstruction can be safely performed either immediately or in a delayed fashion with high patient satisfaction and acceptable morbidity (2).

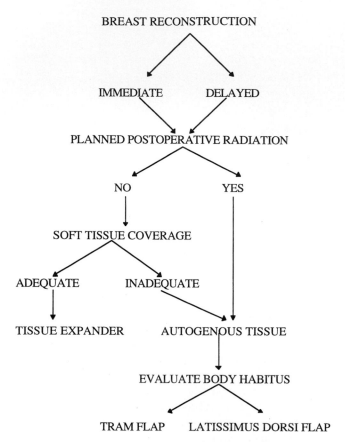

Figure 1   Decision-making in breast reconstruction.

Immediate breast reconstruction following mastectomy for early-stage breast cancer (stage I and II) is well established (3). Administration of conventional adjuvant chemotherapy on schedule and without an increased frequency of wound complications is readily accomplished (4).

The second question is the choice of material to be used to recreate the breast. Should a prosthetic implant be used, or is an autogenous tissue reconstruction better for the individual circumstances?

The technology of implantable devices has evolved dramatically. The availability of tissue expanders and implants in a variety of sizes and shapes permits the plastic surgeon greater accuracy and flexibility in reconstruction. Prosthetic reconstruction usually involves placement of either an expander or an implant deep to the pectoralis major muscle to recreate the breast mound. When there is adequate skin to cover a full-sized implant, the definitive prosthesis may be considered at the time of mastectomy, avoiding the need for a major subsequent operative procedure. In most situations, however, the amount of skin sacrificed to perform an appropriate mastectomy, or the size of the implant required to match the opposite breast, makes closure of the skin over the definitive prosthesis impossible. In these circumstances, a deflated expander is placed in the subpectoral position at the time of reconstruction. The expander is essentially a contoured, deflated sac attached to a subcutaneous reservoir. The sac is gradually filled with saline (introduced percutaneously through the port) over a period of weeks to months following surgery, until the overlying skin is adequately stretched to accommodate exchange of the expander for the definitive, permanent prosthesis. Generally, prosthetic reconstruction can be performed using simpler and shorter operative techniques. Additionally, there is no donor site morbidity, because autogenous tissue is not harvested.

Autogenous reconstruction involves harvest of tissue from a donor site, with transposition of the tissue to the chest wall defect created by the mastectomy. The donor tissue is then sculpted and contoured to recreate the breast. Blood supply to the transposed tissue is maintained either through a vascular pedicle left attached at the donor site, or by microsurgical anastomosis of a donor artery and vein to vessels at the mastectomy site (generally the thoracodorsal vessels in the axilla). Patients who select autogenous tissue reconstruction have several donor site options. The most suitable choice depends on general health and body habitus and upon the size and shape of the contralateral breast. Latissimus dorsi flaps often have inadequate volume to provide a sizable reconstructed breast and usually require the supplemental use of an implant. The transverse rectus abdominis myocutaneous (TRAM) flap site in the lower abdominal wall usually has substantial soft tissue available for reconstruction and is used without prosthetic supplementation.

Donor site morbidity is an important consideration when evaluating the abdomen for breast reconstruction. In obese patients, in patients with multiple surgical scars, or in those with other unfavorable risk factors, the search for alternative sites is indicated. In the properly selected patient however, TRAM flaps are the first choice among many plastic surgeons performing autogenous tissue breast reconstruction (6–8).

Reconstruction with autogenous tissue has fewer complications than reconstruction with prosthetic devices (Table 1) (5). Implant reconstructions may change over time as a result of scarring, leading to poorer long-term aesthetic results and the potential for capsular contracture (formation of a thick, fibrous peel around the prosthesis, resulting in contour deformity and abnormal texture). In contrast, autogenous reconstructions, especially TRAM

Table 1   A Comparison of Breast Reconstruction
Complications

Reconstructive method	Complication rate
Tissue expander/implant	21%
Latissimus flap	9%
TRAM flap	3%

Source: Ref. 5.

flaps, are usually quite stable over time. The impact of donor site morbidity, however, should not be underestimated. Implant reconstruction may add minimally to the recuperation from a mastectomy, whereas autogenous reconstruction involves a more prolonged rehabilitation.

Breast reconstruction, whether prosthetic or autogenous, is often a staged procedure. When an expander is used as part of an implant procedure, a second operative intervention is always required for exchange of the expander for a permanent implant. Even primary implants and autogenous reconstructions may require a secondary procedure to achieve an optimal final result. These procedures, often performed in an ambulatory setting, may involve creation of a nipple-areolar complex, recontouring of the reconstruction, and "adjustment" (mastopexy, reduction, or augmentation) of the contralateral breast to achieve symmetry.

What does the future hold? Implant technology continues to evolve. The molecular basis of flap physiology continues to be studied (9). Advanced-stage breast cancer (stage III and IV) remains problematic. Indications for reconstruction in this setting are still undetermined, and there may even be a limited role for breast conservation (10–12). Outcome data are needed to support treatment decisions. It is hoped that as survival among women with primary breast cancer continues to increase, the opportunity for breast reconstruction after mastectomy in a variety of settings will increase even further.

REFERENCES

1. Nemecek JR, Young VL. Postmastectomy reconstruction. In: Marsh JL, ed. Decision Making in Plastic Surgery. St. Louis, MO: Mosby–Year Book, 1993.
2. Noda S, Eberlein TJ, Eriksson E. Breast reconstruction. Cancer 1994.
3. Yule GJ, Concannon MJ, Croll G, Puckett CL. Is there liability with chemotherapy following immediate breast reconstruction? Plast Reconstr Surg 1996; 97:969.

4. Furey PC, Macgillivray DC, Castiglione CL, Allen L. Wound complications in patients receiving adjuvant chemotherapy after mastectomy and immediate breast reconstruction for breast cancer. J Surg Oncol 1994; 55:194.

5. Kroll SS, Baldwin B. A comparison of outcomes using three different methods of breast reconstruction. Plast Reconstr Surg 1992; 90:455.

6. Beasley ME. The pedicled TRAM as preference for immediate autogenous tissue breast reconstruction. Clin Plast Surg 1994; 21:191.

7. Elliott LF, Eskenazi L, Beegle PJ, Podres PE, Drazan L. Immediate TRAM flap breast reconstruction: 128 consecutive cases. Plast Reconstr Surg 1993; 92:217.

8. King GM, Rademaker AW, Mustoe TA. Abdominal-wall recovery following TRAM flap: a functional outcome study. Plast Reconstr Surg 1997; 99:417.

9. Restifo RJ, Ward BA, Scoutt LM, Broen JM, Taylor KJ. Timing, magnitude, and utility of surgical delay in the TRAM flap. I. Animal studies. Plast Reconstr Surg 1997; 99:1211.

10. Wey PD, Highstein JB, Borah GL. Immediate breast reconstruction in the high-risk adjuvant setting. Ann Plast Surg 1997; 38:342.

11. Sultan MR, Smith ML, Esatbrook A, Schnabel F, Singh D. Immediate breast reconstruction in patients with locally advanced disease. Ann Plast Surg 1997; 38:345.

12. Slavin SA, Love SM, Sadowsky NL. Reconstruction of the radiated partial mastectomy defect with autogenous tissues. Plast Reconstr Surg 1992; 90:854.

9
Medical Treatment of Breast Cancer

WILLIAM N. HAIT, DEBORAH L. TOPPMEYER, and ROBERT S. DIPAOLA
UMDNJ/Robert Wood Johnson Medical School and The Cancer Institute of New Jersey, New Brunswick, New Jersey

The medical treatment of breast cancer encompasses the use of hormonal and chemotherapies, coordinated with surgery and radiation. This coordinated approach is designed to provide patients with individualized treatment for their particular breast cancer and their potentially unique manifestations of disease. Providing individualized, cost-efficient care, while incorporating clinical trials into every aspect of patient management, is the challenge of modern medical oncology in academic centers and in the community.

I. HORMONAL THERAPY

First shown to be effective by Beatson in 1896 (1), hormonal therapy is effective in the treatment of all stages of breast cancer and offers the advantage of low toxicity compared to chemotherapy. Response rates are proportional to expression of estrogen and progesterone receptors (2; Table 1).

Tamoxifen is the most commonly used hormonal therapy and has been shown to be effective in patients with metastatic disease and in the adjuvant setting (3). The major mechanism of action of tamoxifen is competitive inhibition of estrogen binding to the estrogen receptor, which prevents transcriptional activation of genes having estrogen-response elements (4). However, the overall effect of tamoxifen is more complex and may involve increased production of TGF-β (5), antibody production, and natural killer cell activity, as well as decreased suppressor-T-cell activity, IGF-1, protein kinase C, and calmodulin-dependent protein kinase activities (5–9).

Table 1 Influence of Hormone
Receptor Status on Response to
Hormonal Therapy in Patients with
Metastatic Disease

Receptor status	Response rate
ER+/PR−	25–35%
ER−/PR+	30–40%
ER+/PR+	60–70%
ER−/PR−	<10%

We do not recommend the routine use of tamoxifen in patients with hormone-receptor (HR)-negative disease. Response rates in HR− patients with metastatic disease have been reported to be <10% (2); a few trials demonstrated a benefit from tamoxifen in HR− patients in the adjuvant setting (10–13). However, a critical review of the literature reveals a direct correlation between the quantity of HR expression and response to hormonal therapy (10,13). Therefore, in patients with HR < 10 fmol/mg protein or its equivalent, whatever benefit exists must be very small.*

Tamoxifen is well tolerated. The most common side effects are hot flashes, mild nausea, menorrhagia, and weight gain (4). Far less common are thromboembolic events, retinopathy (rare at currently used doses), and hepatic tumors. Endometrial cancer is an uncommon side effect. A thorough review reveals that the risk of endometrial cancer is <3 cases/1000 individuals and that greater than half of these cases are early stage (14). In addition, it appears that a certain number of these cases were present at the time of initiation of tamoxifen therapy and that careful medical observation led to detection bias on the part of the reporting physicians (14). Nonetheless, endometrial cancer is a complication of tamoxifen therapy and all patients should be counseled about the risks and benefits.

A common practice in the United States is to monitor patients on tamoxifen by yearly vaginal examinations, PAP smears, and vaginal ultrasound to measure the thickness of the endometrium (15). It is now appreciated that tamoxifen produces thickening of the endometrium by several mechanisms including stromal hyperplasia and edema and that the upper limits of normal may have to be increased. Whether or not vaginal ultrasound is a useful surveillance for tamoxifen-induced endometrial cancer re-

---

*Recent evidence suggests that overexpression of Her-2-*neu/erb*-B may render tumors particularly resistant to tamoxifen.

mains unproven; rather its use represents a reaction by a responsible medical community to a potential complication of therapy.

When discussing the potential adverse side effects of tamoxifen with patients it is important to point out the potential beneficial effects as well, which include a decrease in second breast primaries, a lower HDL cholesterol, the potential to lower cardiovascular mortality, and an increase in bone mineral density (4).

We recommend second-line hormonal therapies such as anastrazole or megesterol acetate in HR+ patients who experienced a measurable response to tamoxifen and whose disease is non-life-threatening, e.g., does not include major involvement of lung, liver, or nervous system. Several consultants prefer anastrazole because of ease of administration and lack of serious side effects. Because a thorough review of all the possible endocrine approaches is beyond the scope of this introduction, the reader is referred to several excellent discussions (16–18).

A.   Adjuvant Use of Hormonal Therapy

Hormonal therapy can reduce recurrences from breast cancer when used in the adjuvant setting (10). Hormonal therapy was shown to prolong disease-free survival (DFS) in most trials and improve overall survival (OS) in some trials in premenopausal patients with node-negative disease (19). The overall changes predicted from the meta-analysis of all patients treated with tamoxifen (with or without chemotherapy) was a 25% reduction in the odds of recurrence and a 16% reduction in the odds of death (10).

In our decision-making pathways, we have chosen age rather than menopausal status to distinguish between the use of hormonal therapy and chemotherapy for HR+ tumors in the adjuvant setting. This decision was based on the overview analysis, where age was more strongly correlated with benefit from hormonal therapy. For example, patients $\geq$ 50 treated with adjuvant tamoxifen with or without chemotherapy achieved a reduction in the annual odds of recurrence and OS of 29 $\pm$ 2% (10). Patients < 50 treated with adjuvant tamoxifen also achieved a reduction in the annual odds of recurrence, but no significant benefit in overall survival. In patients < 50, oophorectomy reduced the annual odds of recurrence by 26 $\pm$ 6%. The relative value of oophorectomy versus tamoxifen in premenopausal patients in the adjuvant setting is under investigation. We have chosen to treat only HR+ disease with adjuvant hormonal therapy since the overview analysis demonstrated a far greater benefit in these patients (10).

The appropriate duration of treatment with tamoxifen in the adjuvant setting is uncertain, although 5 years has become a common practice. Early studies demonstrated a significant advantage to 5 years of treatment over 3 years. A recent NSABP trial compared 10 years to 5 years of treatment with tamoxifen in postmenopausal, node-negative, ER+ patients (12). The trial was terminated when no statistical benefit could be shown in the group of women who received tamoxifen beyond 5 years; there was a non–statistically significant increase in breast cancer recurrences in women taking tamoxifen for longer than 5 years. These results have been challenged based on statistical considerations. Suffice it to say that this is the only prospective randomized trial comparing 5 years of tamoxifen therapy to a longer duration and that it applies to postmenopausal, node-negative women, whose tumors are ER+. The meta-analysis, which included five randomized trials comparing 3–5 years of tamoxifen with 1–2 years of treatment, showed a reduction in recurrence (22 ± 8%) but no significant reduction in mortality (7 ± 11%) with 3–5 years of use compared to 1–2 years (10).

II. CHEMOTHERAPY

Chemotherapy is effective treatment of breast cancer in all stages of disease. There are many drugs with proven activity in phase II trials and several active combinations. A discussion of the individual agents and combinations is beyond the scope of this introduction and readers are referred to several excellent reviews (21–23).

Response rates for single drugs range from 0 to 71%; most currently used drugs have a single-agent overall response rate of approximately 50%, with a complete response rate of less than 25% (22). Whereas hormone-receptor status can guide the use of hormonal therapies, no similar marker exists for predicting responsiveness to chemotherapy, although the overexpression of the Her-2-*neu/erb*-B oncogene may predict the need for full-dose anthracycline treatment in the adjuvant setting.

Combination chemotherapy is believed to be superior to the use of single agents in the adjuvant setting (10); the data are less clear in metastatic disease (23–26). Firm conclusions are hampered by the lack of studies comparing optimal dose and schedule for the most active agents to the best current combinations. The current standard for adjuvant therapy consists of combination therapy for less than 1 year. This is supported by a SWOG trial showing that 1 year of CMFVP was superior to 2 years of melphalan (27), and an NSABP trial showing that melphalan plus fluorouracil was superior to melphalan alone (28). The meta-analysis also compared combination chemotherapy to single-agent therapy. Combination therapy achieved a 12 ± 5% reduction in the annual odds of recurrence and a 17 ± 5% reduction in the annual odds of death, figures that were marginally superior to the results obtained in single-agent studies; however, none of the trials investigated single-agent anthracyclines (10).

The superiority of combination therapy to single agents in metastatic disease is more controversial. For example, numerous attempts at demonstrating superiority of doxorubicin-containing combinations to doxorubicin alone have been performed with conflicting results (22). Recently, doxorubicin alone was compared to paclitaxel alone or to the combination of paclitaxel plus doxorubicin (26). Paclitaxel and doxorubicin had equal activity. Although the combination produced higher response rates, the effect on survival was not appreciably greater than the results obtained with either drug alone (26).

The choice of individual agents for treatment of metastatic disease is based on limited data. For example, the taxanes, paclitaxel and docetaxel, have been approved for use in breast cancer and a recent comparison suggests that docetaxol may be more active (29). However, until larger, more definitive trials are completed, we view the taxanes to be equivalent. A new vinca alkaloid, vinorelbine, has recently been approved for the treatment of breast cancer (30,31). In general, it is as active as other drugs, but offers no clear superiority as a single agent.

A. Adjuvant use of Chemotherapy

Adjuvant chemotherapy improves DFS and OS in both node-positive and node-negative disease (10; Table 2). The benefits from adjuvant chemotherapy are greater in patients < 50 years old (10).

Combination therapies appear superior to single agents (10,27,28). CMF-based regimens appear as active as doxorubicin-containing regimens (10), although many physicians feel that the addition of doxorubicin is advantageous.

The optimum adjuvant chemotherapy regimen is unknown. We have included cyclophosphamide plus doxorubicin (600 mg/m^2 cyclophosphamide and 60 mg/m^2 doxorubicin every 21 days times 4 cycles) as a reference adjuvant treatment in patients < 50 years of age and cyclophosphamide,

Table 2 Effects of Adjuvant Chemotherapy as Calculated by Meta-Analysis

	Reduction in annual odds	
	Recurrence (%)	Death (%)
Node-negative	26	18
Node-positive	30	18

Source: Ref. 10.

methotrexate, fluorouracil (100 mg/m^2 days 1–14 cyclophosphamide p.o.; 40 mg/m^2 methotrexate days 1 and 8 i.v., and 600 mg/m^2 days 1 and 8 fluorouracil i.v. every 28 days time 6 cycles) as the reference in older women. This subjective decision was based on NSABP B15, which demonstrated four cycles of AC to be equivalent to six cycles of CMF in node-positive, ER− patients; in this study, there were several advantages to AC including shorter time to completion (approximately 3 months), fewer physician visits, and less nausea (32). Cardiac toxicity from AC was not demonstrable; alopecia was more severe. A recent Intergroup trial in node-positive patients demonstrated a significant improvement in DFS and OS when paclitaxel was given after the completion of four cycles of AC compared to AC alone.[32a] Therefore, incorporation of taxanes into adjuvant chemotherapy regimens may prove superior to current standard regimens.

III. COMBINATION HORMONAL AND CHEMOTHERAPY

We recommend that women < 50 years old receive adjuvant chemotherapy and women > 50 years old (with HR+ tumors) receive adjuvant hormonal therapy as the cornerstone of their treatment. We recommend considering combination hormonal and chemotherapy in all high-risk patients with HR+ tumors; this approach may prove most effective in women 45–55 years old. This is based on data showing that younger women experience a superior result from chemotherapy whereas older women do better with hormonal treatment (10); therefore, it may become progressively more difficult to demonstrate a clear advantage to adding tamoxifen to chemotherapy in very young women and equally difficult to show an advantage for adding chemotherapy to tamoxifen in very old women. Several clinical trials have attempted to clarify this issue. NSABP 09 compared melphalan plus 5-fluorouracil to melphalan, 5-fluorouracil, plus tamoxifen in 1858 patients, approximately half of whom were <50 years old (11). An advantage for the tamoxifen arm was seen only in postmenopausal patients. NSABP B16 compared tamoxifen alone to tamoxifen plus four cycles of AC chemotherapy in postmenopausal, node-positive, ER+ patients. This study demonstrated an increased DFS and OS for chemotherapy plus tamoxifen versus tamoxifen alone (33). In contrast, a SWOG trial found no benefit to the addition of CMFVP to tamoxifen in postmenopausal, node-positive patients (34). Two recently published studies also produced conflicting results (35,36). One, a study conducted by NCI Canada, found no benefit to the addition of CMF to tamoxifen in node-positive, HR+ patients (36). In contrast, the study conducted by the International Breast Cancer Study Group found that CMF added to tamoxifen improved DFS in node-positive, postmenopausal women (35).

A recent SWOG/Intergroup trial compared tamoxifen, to CAF plus tamoxifen, to CAF followed by tamoxifen, in 1470 postmenopausal women with N1 and N2 disease; all patients were ER+ (37). The early analysis of this trial revealed a benefit in terms of DFS for the CAF + T groups, and the benefit was more striking in women with more than four positive nodes and age < 65. No data are yet available to compare the concomitant to the sequential use of CAF + T. NSABP B20 has recently compared tamoxifen, to sequential methotrexate/5-fluorouracil + tamoxifen, to concomitant CMF + tamoxifen in 2363 ER+, node-negative patients (38). At first analysis, the chemotherapy plus tamoxifen arms are superior to tamoxifen alone in terms of DFS (20–25% reduction in relapse rate). As in the previous SWOG/ Intergroup study, the benefit was greater in the younger (<50 years) patients. However, these studies must be interpreted with caution as they lack a chemotherapy-alone arm, which might have shown that chemotherapy was as effective as chemotherapy plus tamoxifen in the <50-years-old population. Finally, the inclusion of oophorectomy with chemotherapy in premenopausal patients with HR+ disease remains of unproven advantage (39,40).

In summary, the effects of adding chemotherapy to tamoxifen in postmenopausal women or tamoxifen to chemotherapy in premenopausal women with HR+, node + breast cancer are inconclusive. It is the authors' opinion that the group who may benefit the most from this approach are women in the perimenopausal period, aged 45–55, although this remains untested. Therefore, all patients at high risk for relapse should be offered enrollment on clinical research trials attempting to clarify this approach.

IV. NEOADJUVANT THERAPY

Neoadjuvant therapy is based on the concept that systemic treatment given before definitive local treatment will make tumors more resectable, decrease the spread of disease, and treat existing micrometastases at a time when fewer drug-resistance mechanisms are present. Several nonrandomized trials suggested a high response rate and low rate of recurrence with this approach (41,42). However, NSABP B18 highlighted the benefits and limitations of neoadjuvant chemotherapy (43). In this trial, 1523 patients matched for age, size of tumor, number of lymph nodes, and operability were randomly assigned to receive either preoperative AC or postoperative AC for four cycles; all patients received tamoxifen for 5 years. An overall response rate of 80% was achieved (36% complete response, 43% partial response); many patients who may not have been good candidates for breast conservation were made potentially eligible for this approach. However, at a median follow-up of 6 years, there was no difference between the two groups in terms of DFS, OS, or site of first recurrence. Therefore, outside of a clinical trial, we do not recommend the use of neoadjuvant chemotherapy in patients with resectable disease, but reserve this approach for patients who desire breast conservation but present with lesions requiring mastectomy. Furthermore, failure to respond to neoadjuvant chemotherapy is an ominous sign; these patients should be considered for investigational approaches.

V. HIGH-DOSE CHEMOTHERAPY

The initial results in patients with metastatic disease using high-dose chemotherapy with autologous bone marrow rescue were mixed. Whereas the overall response rates were high, the durations of response were brief (44,45). In a recent analysis comparing median and overall 3-year survival in trials of high-dose chemotherapy with autologus bone marrow rescue to historical controls, an advantage to transplantation was suggested. In this analysis, the median duration of response was 1.8–2.06 years versus 1–1.2 years, and the 3-year OS rate was 33–37% versus 5–8% (46). While these and other analyses suffer from the usual problems inherent in nonprospective trials, the data appropriately suggest that randomized trials are warranted.

It was a logical extension to apply the principles of high-dose chemotherapy to women at extremely high risk of recurrence following definitive local therapy. Peters and colleagues at Duke University carried out some of the earliest studies in women with >10 involved lymph nodes at the time of surgery (47). Although their results were far superior to historical controls, this approach has not yet been confirmed in a randomized clinical trial. A recent report from the Netherlands failed to demonstrate a benefit for high-dose chemotherapy with stem cell rescue in high-risk, node-positive patients (48). However, the sample size in this study was not large enough to detect small differences.

A pivotal trial is being conducted jointly by the Cancer and Leukemia Group B, the South West Oncology Group, and the National Cancer Institute of Canada to compare high-dose chemotherapy after four cycles of CAF with either high doses of cyclophosphamide, carboplatin, and BCNU with the use of autologous cellular support or cyclophosphamide, carboplatin, and BCNU at the highest achievable doses without the use of cellular and cytokine support. Both groups will subsequently receive local regional radiation therapy; patients who are hormone-receptor positive will receive tamoxifen. More than 900 patients have been enrolled and accrual should be nearing completion. The results of this trial will not be available until the year 2000. Therefore, high-dose chemotherapy remains an investigational approach and should not be performed outside of carefully controlled clinical trials.

VI. TREATMENT GUIDELINES

A. Systemic Adjuvant Therapy

1. Node-Negative Disease

We divided our approach to node-negative disease by age, number of involved lymph nodes, and HR status. We recommend entering eligible patients with node-negative disease on clinical trials to help define the optimum regimens in this setting.

Although chemotherapy was first shown to be effective for patients with breast cancer involving axillary lymph nodes, it was subsequently shown to be as least as effective for women with disease confined to the breast (10). For example, Bonnadona and colleagues demonstrated a remarkable improvement in DFS in node-negative patients treated with CMF in a pilot study (49). This study also highlighted the overall risk of recurrence in a high-risk subset of patients with node-negative disease; over 30% of the untreated group relapsed within 3 years of follow-up. These data were later confirmed in larger studies carried out by the NSABP B13 (50), the ECOG/SWOG Intergroup (51), and the Ludwig consortium (52). The improvement in disease-free survival for women included in these trials is shown in Table 3.

Outside of a clinical trial, we recommend observation for patients with node-negative disease and tumors < 1 cm. Since approximately 10% of these patients relapse, and adjuvant therapy to date has produced no better than a 30% decrease in recurrence, the maximum expected benefit would be to decrease recurrence by 2–3%.

We recommend the use of adjuvant chemotherapy (HR−) or chemotherapy followed by tamoxifen (HR+) in patients ≤ 50 years old with node-negative disease and tumors > 1 cm. We have chosen size as the first variable

Table 3 Effect of Adjuvant Chemotherapy in Node-Negative Patients

	Disease-free survival		
	Milan (CMF)	NSABP (M-F)	Intergroup (CMFP)
Control	39%	67%	61%
	$p = 0.0002$	$p = 0.007$	$p < 0.0001$
Treatment	80%	76%	83%

Source: Modified from Harris JR, Morrow M, Lippman ME, Hellman S, eds. Diseases of the Breast. Philadelphia: Lippincott-Raven, 1996.

as it is a widely available and relatively accurate measurement with strong prognostic implications. For example, tumors < 1 cm have a 10–15% chance of recurrence; in contrast, tumors > 3 cm recur approximately 50% of the time (53).

   a. <50 Years Old   We recommend treating HR− patients with adjuvant chemotherapy. The studies of adjuvant tamoxifen in young, HR+ patients demonstrate a prolongation of DFS and OS, but the results are not as favorable as those seen with chemotherapy (10). Many oncologists add hormonal therapy to chemotherapy in <50-year-old patients whose tumors are HR+. However, as described above, the magnitude of the advantage from adding tamoxifen to chemotherapy in younger patients remains to be defined but is likely to be low. The meta-analysis suggests that younger patients may do better with oophorectomy than with tamoxifen, but this has not yet been confirmed in a randomized clinical trial.

   b. >50 Years Old; HR− Disease   We recommend treating patients with adjuvant chemotherapy who have HR− disease and are able to tolerate the side effects. Although adjuvant chemotherapy is less effective in postmenopausal women, improvements in DFS and OS have been reported in several well-designed trials (50,54). The meta-analysis implies that for women > 50 years old, chemotherapy produces a 23% reduction in recurrence and 13% reduction in deaths, a third to one-half as great an effect as that seen in the <50-year-old group (10). Benefits from chemotherapy in the postmenopausal group are age related; the closer to 50 years old, the greater the anticipated effect. The effects of chemotherapy are independent of menopausal status.

   c. >50 Years Old; HR+ Disease   We recommend the use of adjuvant hormonal therapy in patients ≥50 with HR+, node-negative disease. The addition of chemotherapy in this group should be reserved for women whose tumor characteristics significantly worsen overall prognosis. Tamoxifen is the hormonal treatment of choice in the adjuvant setting. The benefits appear to be related to age and to the expression of hormone receptors; i.e., the older the patient and the greater the expression of hormone receptors, the greater the response. NSABP B14, which compared 5 years of tamoxifen to placebo in node-negative, HR+ patients of all ages demonstrated the following: (1) benefits to women in all age groups; (2) decreased recurrence of breast cancer in the ipsilateral and contralateral breast, and; (3) excellent compliance and tolerability (19). The demonstration of decreased in-breast recurrences and tumors in the contralateral breast in a small subset of patients led to a large trial designed to determine the worth of tamoxifen as a preventive in women at ''high risk.'' The results of this trial have not yet

Table 4 Preliminary Results of Breast Cancer Prevention Trial in 13,388 High-Risk Women

	Tamoxifen	Placebo
	(number of patients)	
Breast cancer	85	154
Endometrial cancer	33 (0.25%)	14 (0.1%)
Pulmonary emboli	17 (0.13%)	6 (0.04%)
Deep venous thromboses	30 (0.22%)	19 (0.14%)

been published. However, the results of a preliminary analysis were announced and these data are summarized in Table 4.*

2. Node-Positive Disease

We divided our approach to node-positive disease by age, number of positive lymph nodes, and HR status. We recommend entering eligible patients with node-positive disease on clinical trials to help define the optimum regimens in this setting. The meta-analysis suggests that at 10 years, in node-positive patients, chemotherapy will produce a 30% reduction in the odds of recurrence and an 18% reduction in the odds of death (10). To date, tamoxifen remains the mainstay of treatment in the HR+ patient > 50 years old and chemotherapy the mainstay in HR− patients regardless of age.

   a. <50 Years Old; 1–3 Positive Nodes/HR− We recommend chemotherapy for patients < 50 years old with HR−, node-positive disease. The landmark trials of Bonnadona and colleagues and the NSABP demonstrated a survival advantage for premenopausal women with one to three lymph nodes who received 12 cycles of CMF or 2 years of melphalan, respectively (56,57).

   b. <50 Years Old; 1–3 Positive Nodes/HR+ We recommend chemotherapy for women in this group. The benefits to adding tamoxifen or oophorectomy to chemotherapy in younger patients have not been clearly established (see above).

   c. <50 Years Old; 4–9 Positive Nodes/HR+ or HR− We subdivided our pathways according to number of nodes, realizing that this is somewhat artificial as risk of recurrence appears to be linearly related to this

---

*Tamoxifen has been recently approved by the FDA for the prevention of breast cancer in high-risk patients.

variable. We recommend entering on a clinical trial for any patient with more than three positive lymph nodes. This recommendation is based on a relapse rate of >50% despite standard adjuvant therapy. A recent clinical trial carried out by Buzzoni et al. compared doxorubicin plus CMF given in sequence (doxorubicin × 4, CMF × 8) to an alternating regimen of CMF × 2, doxorubicin × 1 for a total of 12 courses. There was a significant improvement in DFS and OS for the sequential over the alternating approach in women with four or more positive lymph nodes (58). In many practices, this has become a standard for women with greater than three positive lymph nodes. However, this small trial should be viewed with caution, and results from larger randomized trials are necessary to help define the optimum treatment for these patients. As a general rule, we recommend the inclusion of hormonal therapy in high-risk patients with HR + tumors.

We recommend enrolling patients <50 with four to nine nodes and HR− disease on clinical trials evaluating new combinations of active compounds or dose-intensification regimens. In addition, in patients with more than four positive lymph nodes, we recommend radiation therapy after mastectomy.

d. <50 Years Old; ≥10 Positive Nodes/HR− or HR+ The prognosis of this group is sufficiently grim as to recommend experimental therapies using new active compounds or clinical trials exploring dose intensification with or without stem cell rescue. A major challenge to traditional treatment came from the work of Peters and colleagues, who reported a highly favorable DFS in women undergoing high-dose chemotherapy with autologous bone marrow transplantation compared to historical controls (47). However, these studies must be viewed as preliminary since no large randomized trial has been reported to show a benefit from this approach. Variables such as selection bias must be accounted for before this approach becomes standard (52). Once again, in women at high risk for relapse and HR+ disease, we would consider including hormonal therapy as part of any treatment regimen.

e. >50 Years Old; 1–3 Positive Nodes/HR− We recommend adjuvant chemotherapy for this group of patients. Since the >50-year-old population will include those with a variety of complicating medical problems, clinical judgment will dictate the proper use of chemotherapy in individual patients.

Five-year follow-up of the original study of Bonadonna and colleagues failed to show a benefit of adjuvant CMF in postmenopausal, node-positive patients. A subset analysis of these data published in 1981 suggested that older women who received greater than 85% of the prescribed dose of drugs would theoretically benefit in terms of DFS (60). What followed was a trial that compared six cycles to 12 cycles of adjuvant CMF in node-positive, postmenopausal patients, with chemotherapy given intravenously every 21 days to avoid issues of noncompliance with oral cyclophosphamide (61). The results of this trial were far better than those obtained even in the premenopausal women in the original CMF trial (62). Although these data should have been viewed with caution because of the use of historical controls rather than a no-treatment arm, adjuvant chemotherapy became a widely accepted approach in postmenopausal women.

   f.   >50 Years Old; 1–3 Positive Nodes/HR+   We recommend tamoxifen as the cornerstone of treatment in this group. We feel that the addition of chemotherapy should be considered as part of a clinical trial or in patients who have no significant complicating medical problems.

   g.   >50 Years Old; >3 Positive Nodes/ HR– or HR+   Our recommendations for this group of patients are similar to those for the less-than-50-year-old group discussed above, with the same precautions raised for patients with confounding medical problems.

B.   Locally Advanced Breast Cancer (LABC)

We divided LABC patients into either operable (stage IIIA) or inoperable (stage IIIB) categories. The operable patients are managed like those with other forms of early breast cancer, i.e., surgery followed by adjuvant chemotherapy and radiation. The inoperable patient presents significant challenges to the team of physicians, nurses, and social workers involved. A coordinated approach between medical, surgical, and radiation oncologist should be presented to the patient, so that she may be assured that her treatment is logical and carefully conceived. The current approach to this problem is to use up-front chemotherapy for three cycles or to "best response," a term that is loosely interpreted as a clinical impression that additional cycles of chemotherapy will produce little additional result. This approach was popularized by Lippman et al., who used a mechanistic-based sequence of chemotherapy and careful measurements of rates of response and achieved response rates of 90% (63). Following chemotherapy the asymptomatic patient should undergo a limited search for metastatic disease guided by the presence of symptoms or signs, e.g., liver function tests, computed-tomography scans of chest and abdomen. If these are negative, surgery (usually modified radical mastectomy) should be performed. Additional chemotherapy with a "non-cross-resistant regimen" for at least three cycles should be followed by radiation to achieve maximum local control. This approach produces 30–50% DFS at 5 years (64).

   Inflammatory carcinoma of the breast (IBC) is seen in 1–3% of breast cancer patients. It is a clinical diagnosis based on the rapid appearance of erythema and edema (*peau d'orange*) of the skin of the breast and may often be associated with invasion of dermal lymphatics by tumor cells. For this reason, in patients suspected of having IBC, a biopsy that includes a full thickness of the skin is preferred. The treatment of IBC does not differ substantially from that of other forms of inoperable LABC. The mainstays of treatment include induction chemotherapy, followed by mastectomy, chemotherapy, and radiation. Breast conservation is rarely recommended and should be reserved for those patients who present with a defined breast mass (uncommon) and who achieve a complete clinical response to chemotherapy and are strongly opposed to mastectomy. The results of treatment have improved dramatically from the prechemotherapy era, where the disease was uniformly fatal (5-year survival rate < 5%). Today, with the use of a triple-modality approach, response rates over 80% are not uncommon and up to a third of patients remain alive after 10 years (65).

The optimal chemotherapy regimen for LABC is unknown. Many oncologists begin with an anthracycline-containing regimen such as CAF and choose either CMF or a taxane for adjuvant treatment after mastectomy. The dose and fractionation of radiation therapy after mastectomy should be standard. Because of the infiltrative nature of IBC, those patients chosen for breast conservation may need to receive more dose-intense radiation therapy with the potential for a higher rate of postradiation complications.

C. Metastatic Disease

1. Hormonal Therapy

We recommend hormonal therapy for patients with HR+ tumors without life-threatening manifestations of metastatic disease. Patients who experience a >1-year disease-free interval from the time of diagnosis may experience a better response. Response rates are directly related to the expression of hormone receptors and to previous hormonal treatments. Response rates to second-line treatments are, in general, 50% less than observed for first-line therapies. Duration of response is related to the duration of initial response. For example, a patient who enjoyed an 18-month response from first-line therapy is likely to enjoy a 50% shorter duration of response, or 9 months, from second-line therapy. This "50% rule" holds up fairly well for subsequent relapses (66,67).

2. Chemotherapy

We recommend chemotherapy for patients with HR− disease or for those with life-threatening manifestations of metastatic disease. Metastatic breast cancer remains a treatable, but incurable problem. Therefore, we have yet to determine the proper chemotherapeutic approach. Nonetheless, several generalizations can be drawn. First, for women who present with stage IV disease or those who relapse at a distant site, several highly active drugs and/or drug regimens are available. Perhaps the most widely used are CMF and CAF. Doxorubicin is active, well tolerated, and can be used alone in this setting. The recent introduction of the taxanes has given the oncologist another effective class of drugs. Whether taxane-based combinations will produce meaningful improvements in outcome remains to be determined. The overall response rate to chemotherapy in this setting ranges from 40 to 80%, with wide enough confidence limits to make a definitive recommendation impossible.

We recommend that chemotherapy be continued in responding patients as long as disease is present. Results from several carefully designed trials indicate that in responding patients, continuation of therapy until disease progression improves both time to progression (68) and quality of life (69). Of course, the latter must be judged individually by the patient and physician. Usually, several rate-limiting events occur, including the achievement of a cumulative dose of doxorubicin that threatens to compromise cardiac ejection fraction (>500 mg/m^2), or development of intolerable neurological complications from paclitaxel.

The choice of chemotherapy following relapse becomes more difficult since the response rate and overall duration of response are far lower than with previously untreated patients. A good rule of thumb is that the duration of a second response will be half as long as the first and toxicities will be worse. Therefore, in this setting, we recommend that all eligible patients be enrolled onto approved clinical trials. We prefer this approach because it offers a patient the chance, while healthy enough to be eligible, to experience the potential benefit of new and promising treatments.

REFERENCES

1. Ravdin RG, Lewison EF, Slack NH, et al. Results of a clinical trial concerning the worth of prophylactic oophorectomy for breast carcinoma. Surg Gynecol Obstet 1970; 31:1055.
2. Witliff JL. Steroid-hormone receptors in breast cancer. Cancer 1984; 53:638.
3. Cole MP, Jones CTA, Todd IDH. A new antiestrogenic agent in late breast cancer: an early clinical appraisal with ICI 46474. Br J Cancer 1971; 25:270.
4. Furr JA, Jordan VC. The pharmacology and clinical use of tamoxifen. Pharmacol Ther 1984; 25:127.
5. Butta A, Maclenan D, Flanders KC, et al. Induction of transforming growth factor beta-1 in human breast cancer in vivo following tamoxifen treatment. Cancer Res 1992; 52:4261.
6. Epstein RJ. The clinical biology of hormone-responsive breast cancer. Cancer Treat Rev 1988; 15:33.

7. Gulino A, Santoni A, Screpanti A, et al. Antitumoral antiestrogen stimulates natural killer (NK) activity in C3M mouse. J Leukoc Biol 1985; 38:159.

8. Colletti RB, Roberts JD, Devlin JT, et al. Effects of tamoxifen on plasma insulin-like growth factor I in patients with breast cancer. Cancer Res 1989; 49:1882.

9. O'Brian CA, Liskamp RM, Solomon, et al. Inhibition of protein kinase C by tamoxifen. Cancer Res 1985; 45:2462.

10. Early Breast Cancer Trialists' Collaborative Group. Systemic treatment of early breast cancer by hormonal, cytotoxic, or immune therapy. Lancet 1992; 339:1.

11. Fisher B, Redmond C, Brown A, et al. Adjuvant chemotherapy with and without tamoxifen in the treatment of primary breast cancer: 5 years' results for the National Surgical Adjuvant Breast and Bowel Project Trial. J Clin Oncol 1986; 4:459.

12. NATO Steering Committee. Controlled trial of tamoxifen as a single adjuvant agent in the management of early breast cancer. Br J Cancer 1988; 57:608.

13. Report from the Breast Cancer Trials Committee, Scottish Cancer Trials Office, Edinburgh. Adjuvant tamoxifen in the management of operable breast cancer: the Scottish Trial. Lancet 1987; 8552.

14. Fisher B, Costantino JP, Redmond CK, et al. Endometrial cancer in tamoxifen-treated breast cancer patients: findings from the NSABP B-14. J Natl Cancer Inst 1994; 86:527.

15. Kedar RP, Bourne TH, Powles TJ, et al. Effects of tamoxifen on uterus and ovaries of postmenopausal women in a randomised breast cancer prevention trial. Lancet 1994; 343:1318.

16. Goss PE, Gwyn KMEH. Current perspectives on aromatase inhibitors in breast cancer. J Clin Oncol 1994; 11:2460.

17. Gale KE, Anderson JW, Tormey DC, et al. Hormonal treatment for metastatic breast cancer. Cancer 1994; 73:354.

18. Buzdar A, Jonat W, Howell A, Jones S, Blomqvist C, Vogel C, et al. Anastrozole, a potent and selective aromatase inhibitor, versus megestrol acetate in postmenopausal women with advanced breast cancer: results of overview analysis of two phase III trials. J Clin Oncol 1996; 14:2000.

19. Fisher B, Constantino J, Redmond C et al. A randomized clinical trial evaluating tamoxifen in the treatment of patients with node-negative breast cancer who have estrogen-receptor positive tumors. N Engl J Med 1989; 320:479–484.

20. Fisher B, Dignam J, Bryant J, et al: Five versus more than five years of tamoxifen therapy for breast cancer patients with negative lymph nodes and estrogen receptor-positive tumors. J Natl Cancer Inst 1996; 88:1529–1542.

21. Honig SF. Treatment of metastatic disease: hormonal therapy and chemotherapy. In: Harris JR, Lippman ME, Morrow M, Zhellman S, eds. Diseases of the Breast. Philadelphia: Lippincott-Raven, 1996.

22. Hayes DF, Henderson IC, Shapiro CL. Treatment of metastatic breast cancer: present and future prospects. Semin Oncol 1995; 22:5.

23. Bezwoda WR, De Moor NG, Derman D, et al. Combination chemotherapy of metastatic breast cancer. Cancer 1979; 44:392.

24. Smally RV, Carpenter J, Bartolucci A, et al. A comparison of cyclophosphamide, adriamycin, 5-fluorouracil (CAF) and cyclophosphamide, methotrexate, 5-fluorouracil, vincristine, prednisone (CMFVP) in patients with metastatic breast cancer. Cancer 1977; 40:625.

25. Mouridsen HT, Palshof T, Brahm M, et al. Evaluation of single-drug versus multiple-drug chemotherapy in the treatment of advanced breast cancer. Cancer Treat Rep 1977; 61:47.

26. Sledge G, Neuberg D, Ingle J, Martino S, Wood W. Phase III trial of doxorubicin vs. paclitaxel vs doxorubicin + paclitaxel as first line therapy for metastatic breast cancer: An Intergroup trial. Proc Am Soc Clin Oncol 1997; 16:1a.

27. Rivkin SE, Green S, Metch B, et al. Adjuvant CMFVP versus melphalan for operable breast cancer with positive axillary nodes: 10 year results of a Southwest Oncology Group study. J Clin Oncol 1989; 7:1229.

28. Fisher B, Redmond C, Fisher ER, Wolmark N. Systemic adjuvant therapy in the treatment of primary operable breast cancer: NSABP experience. NCI Monogr 1986; 1:35.

29. Valero V, Burris HA III, Jones SE, et al. Multicenter pilot study of taxotere in paclitaxel-resistant metastatic breast cancer. Proc Am Soc Clin Oncol 1996; 15:95.

30. Gasparini G, Caffo O, Barni S, et al. Vinorelbine is an active antiproliferative agent in pretreated advanced breast cancer patients: a phase II study. J Clin Oncol 1993; 11:1245.

31. Weber BL, Vogel C, Jones S, Harvey H, Hutchins L, Bigley J, Hohneker J. Intravenous vinorelbine as first-line and second-line therapy in advanced breast cancer. J Clin Oncol 1995; 13:2722.

32. Fisher B, Brown AM, Dimitrov NV, et al. Two months of doxorubicin-cyclophosphamide with and without interval reinduction therapy compared with 6 months of cyclophosphamide, methotrexate, and fluorouracil in positive-node breast cancer patients with tamoxifen-nonresponsive tumors: results from the NSABP B-15. J Clin Oncol 1990; 8:1483–1496.

32a. Henderson IC, et al. Proc Am Soc Clin Oncol 1998; 17:101a.

33. Fisher B, Redmond C, Legault-Poiisson S, et al. Postoperative chemotherapy and tamoxifen compared with tamoxifen alone in the treatment of positive-node breast cancer patients aged 50 year and older with tumors responsive to tamoxifen: results for the National Surgical Adjuvant Breast and Bowel Project B-16. J Clin Oncol 1990; 8:1005.

34. Rivkin SE, Green S, Metch B, et al. Adjuvant CMFVP versus tamoxifen versus concurrent CMFVP and tamoxifen for post-menopausal, node-positive and estrogen receptor-positive breast cancer patients: a Southwest Oncology Group Study. J Clin Oncol 1994; 12:2078.

35. International Breast Cancer Study Group. Effectiveness of adjuvant chemotherapy in combination with tamoxifen for node-positive postmenopausal breast cancer patients. J Clin Oncol 1997; 15:1385–1394.

36. Pritchard KI, Paterson AHG, Fine S, et al. Randomized trial of cyclophos-
     phamide, methotrexate, and fluorouracil chemotherapy added to tamoxifen as
     adjuvant therapy in postmenopausal women with node-positive estrogen
     and/or progesterone receptor-positive breast cancer: a report of the Na-
     tional Cancer Institute of Canada Clinical Trials Group. J Clin Oncol 1997;
     15:2302.
37. Albain K, Green S, Osborne K, et al. Tamoxifen versus cyclophosphamide
     adriamycin and 5-FU plus either concurrent or sequential tamoxifen in post-
     menopausal receptor +, node + breast cancer: a Southwest Oncology Group
     Phase III Intergroup trial (SWOG-8814, INT-0100). Proc Am Soc Clin Oncol
     1997; 16:128a.
38. Fisher B, Dignam J, DeCillis DL, et al. The worth of chemotherapy and
     tamoxifen over tamoxifen alone in node-negative with estrogen receptor pos-
     itive invasive breast cancer: first results from NSABP B20. Proc Am Soc of
     Clin Oncol 1997; 16:1a.
39. The International Breast Cancer Study Group. Late effects of adjuvant oo-
     phorectomy and chemotherapy upon premenopausal breast cancer patients.
     Ann Oncol 1990; 1:30.
40. Rivkin S, Green S, Metch B, et al. Adjuvant combination chemotherapy
     (CMFVP) vs oophorectomy followed by CMFVP (OCMFVP) for premeno-
     pausal women with ER+ operable breast cancer with positive axillary lymph
     nodes: an Intergroup study. Proc Am Soc Clin Oncol 1991; 10:47.
41. Jacquillat C, Weil M, Baillet F, et al. Results of neoadjuvant chemotherapy
     and radiation therapy in the breast-conserving treatment of 250 patients with
     all stages of infiltrative breast cancer. Cancer 1990; 66:119–129.
42. Mauriac L, Durand M, Avril A, et al. Effects of primary chemotherapy in
     conservative treatment of breast cancer patients with operable tumors larger
     than 3 cm: results of a randomized trial in a single center. Ann Oncol 1991;
     2:347.
43. Fisher B, Brown A, Mamounas E, et al. Effect of preoperative chemotherapy
     on local-regional disease in women with operable breast cancer: findings from
     National Surgical Adjuvant Breast and Bowel Project B-18. J Clin Oncol
     1997; 15:2483–2493.
44. Bezwoda W, Seymour L, Dansey R. High-dose chemotherapy with hemato-
     poietic rescue as primary treatment for metastatic breast cancer: a randomized
     trial. J Clin Oncol 1995; 13:2483–2489.
45. Peters W, Jones R, Vredengburgh J, Shpall E, Hussein A, Elkordy M, et al.
     A large prospective randomized trial of high-dose combination alkylating
     agents with autologous cellular support as consolidation for patients with met-
     astatic breast cancer achieving complete remission after intensive doxorubi-
     cin-based induction therapy. Proc Am Soc Clin Oncol 1996; 15:121a.
46. Peters WP. High-dose chemotherapy for breast cancer. In: Harris JR, Lippman
     ME, Morrow M, Zhellman S, eds. Diseases of the Breast. Philadelphia: Lip-
     pincott-Raven, 1996.
47. Peters WP, Ross M, Vrendenburgh JJ, et al. High dose chemotherapy and
     autologous bone marrow support as consolidation after standard-dose adjuvant
     therapy for high risk primary breast cancer. J Clin Oncol 1993; 11:1132.

48. Rodenhuis S, Richel DJ, Baars JW, et al. A randomized single-institution study of high-dose chemotherapy with cyclophosphamide, thiotepa and carboplatin in high-risk breast cancer. Proc Am Assoc Cancer Res 1997; 38:438.

49. Zambetti M, Bonadonna G, Valagussa P, et al. Adjuvant CMF for node-negative and estrogen receptor negative breast cancer patients. J Natl Cancer Inst Monogr 1992; 11:77.

50. Fisher B, Redmond C, Dimitrov N, et al. A randomized clinical trial evaluating sequential methotrexate and fluorouracil in the treatment of patients with node-negative breast cancer who have estrogen-receptor negative tumors. N Engl J Med 1989; 320:473.

51. Mansour EG, Gray R, Shatila AH, et al. Efficacy of adjuvant chemotherapy in high-risk node-negative breast cancer. N Engl J Med 1989; 320:485–490.

52. Ludwig Breast Cancer Study Group. Prolonged disease-free survival after one course of perioperative adjuvant chemotherapy for node-negative breast cancer. N Engl J Med 1989; 320:491–496.

53. McGuire WL, Clark GM. Prognostic factors for recurrence and survival in axillary node-negative breast cancer. J Steroid Biochem 1989; 34:145.

54. Bonadonna G, Valagussa P, Rossi A, et al. Ten year experience with CMF-based adjuvant chemotherapy in resectable breast cancer. Breast Cancer Res Treat 1985; 5:95.

55. Fisher B, Fisher ER, Redmond C, et al. Ten year results from the NSABP clinical trial evaluating the use of L-phenylalanine mustard in the management of primary breast cancer. J Clin Oncol 1986; 4:929.

56. Bonadonna G, Brusamolino E, Valagussa P, et al. Combination chemotherapy as an adjuvant treatment in operable breast cancer. N Engl J Med 1976; 284: 405–410.

57. Kaufmann M, Janor W, Abel U, et al. Adjuvant randomized trials of doxorubicin/cyclophosphamide versus doxorubicin/cyclophosphamide tamoxifen and CMF chemotherapy versus tamoxifen in women with node-positive breast cancer. J Clin Oncol 1993; 11:454.

58. Buzzoni R, Bonadonna G, Valagussa P, Zambetti M. Adjuvant chemotherapy with doxorubicin plus cyclophosphamide, methotrexate, and fluorouracil in the treatment of resectable breast cancer with more than three positive axillary nodes. J Clin Oncol 1991; 9:2134–2140.

59. Crump M, Goss PE, Prince M, et al. Outcome of extensive evaluation before adjuvant therapy in women with breast cancer and 10 or more positive axillary lymph nodes. J Clin Oncol 1996; 14:66–69.

60. Bonadonna G, Valagussa P. Dose-response effect of adjuvant chemotherapy in breast cancer. N Engl J Med 1981; 304:10–15.

61. Tancini G, Bonadonna G, Valagussa P, et al. Adjuvant CMF in breast cancer: comparative five year results of 12 versus six cycles. J Clin Oncol 1983; 1: 2.

62. Bonadonna G, Moliterni A, et al. Adjuvant cyclophosphamide, methotrexate, and fluorouracil in node-positive breast cancer; the results of 20 years of follow-up. N Engl J Med 1995; 332:901–906.

63. Lippman ME, Sorace RA, Bagley CS, et al. Treatment of locally advanced breast cancer using primary induction chemotherapy with hormonal synchro-

nization followed by radiation with or without debulking surgery. Natl Cancer Inst Monogr 1986; 1:153.

64. Hortobagyi GN, Buzdar AU. Locally advanced breast cancer: a review including the MD Anderson experience: In: Ragaz J, Ariel IM, eds. High Risk Breast Cancer. Berlin: Springer-Verlag, 1991:382.

65. Jaiyesimi IA, Buzdar AU, Hortobagyi G. Inflammatory breast cancer: a review. J Clin Oncol 1992; 10:1014–1024.

66. Kennedy BJ. Hormonal therapies in breast cancer. Semin Oncol 1974; 1:119.

67. Garcia-Giralt E, Ayme Y, Carton M, et al. Second and third line hormonal therapy in advanced post-menopausal breast cancer: a multicenter randomized trial comparing medroxyprogesterone acetate with aminoglutethimide in patients who have become resistant to tamoxifen. Breast Cancer Res Treat 1993; 24:139.

68. Muss HB, Case LD, Richards F, et al. Interrupted versus continuous chemotherapy in patients with metastatic breast cancer. N Engl J Med 1991; 325: 1342.

69. Coates A, Gebski V, Stat M, et al. Improving the quality of life during chemotherapy for advanced breast cancer: a comparison of intermittent and continuous treatment strategies. N Engl J Med 1987; 317:1490.

10
Familial Breast Cancer

DEBORAH L. TOPPMEYER
UMDNJ/Robert Wood Johnson Medical School and The Cancer Institute of New Jersey, New Brunswick, New Jersey

JUDITH E. GARBER
Dana-Farber Cancer Institute, Boston, and Harvard Medical School, Cambridge, Massachusetts

I. BACKGROUND

Identifying patients at increased risk of developing breast cancer serves several purposes: improved understanding of the pathogenesis of breast cancer; enhanced opportunities for appropriate surveillance programs; increased participation in prevention trials; improved use of genetic screening for cancer susceptibility (e.g., DNA-based testing for mutations in breast cancer susceptibility genes); development of registries and research protocols to generate a database from which better surveillance and prevention recommendations can be made.

Clinicians must understand how risk factors impact on an individual's risk assessment so that counseling and recommendations can be tailored appropriately. Family history is the most important determinant of breast cancer risk. Therefore, an accurate and detailed family history must be obtained. The percentage of breast cancer patients who present with a positive family history varies from 6% to 17% (1,2). Genetic factors contribute to ~5–10% of all cases of breast cancer and to ~25% of cases diagnosed before age 30.

For risk assessment, women are typically classified as belonging to a moderate- or high-risk family. The distinction between these two groups lies in the risk for individual family members, the method used to quantitate risk, and the underlying molecular basis for cancer susceptibility. Moderate-risk families are characterized by less-striking family histories, older average age at the time of diagnosis (i.e., postmenopausal breast cancer), and absence of other tumors such as ovarian cancer. In the moderate-risk family, the molecular contribution to breast cancer risk is less clear, but is less likely due to a mutation in a single, dominant, breast-cancer-susceptibility gene.

In contrast, the high-risk family has multiple relatives (generally at least three) affected with breast cancer at an early age (<45), a higher incidence of bilateral disease, and a family history of ovarian cancer. The high-risk family has a high likelihood of harboring a mutation in a single, highly penetrant, autosomal dominant susceptibility gene such as *BRCA1* or *BRCA2*.

The high- and moderate-risk groups differ with respect to the models used to determine individual risk as well as to how they are counseled. For women classified as members of a moderate-risk family, one of two risk prediction models is used. The Claus model best predicts risk for women with a family history of breast cancer. Claus et al. analyzed data from the Cancer and Steroid Hormone (CASH) study of breast cancer incidence in a population that was not extensively screened. Risk was estimated on the basis of the number of relatives with breast cancer, their relationship to the proband, and the age of onset of breast cancer in affected relatives. In contrast, the Gail model best predicts risk in women without a strong family history. This model estimates breast cancer risk by a formula that incorporates age at menarche, age at first live birth, number of first-degree relatives with breast cancer, number of previous breast biopsies, and patient age. This model was derived from a population of primarily white women undergoing annual screening mammography, and like the Claus model, is most accurate when used to predict risk for women without a striking family history of breast cancer. Use of these models in clinical practice may help to broadly classify women into low- and moderate-risk categories and is best performed by specialists in settings specifically structured for appropriate counseling.

For the high-risk patient (early age of onset, bilateral or multifocal disease, two or more first-degree relatives with breast or ovarian cancer, and the presence of ovarian cancer) neither the Claus nor the Gail model is applicable. These families have a high probability of carrying a mutation in a dominant breast-cancer-susceptibility gene. The inheritance of the mutated gene follows a classic Mendelian pattern of autosomal dominant transmission, with each child of the carriers having a 50% chance of inheriting the mutation.

At least eight candidate breast-cancer-susceptibility genes exist. *BRCA1* and *BRCA2*, cloned in 1994 and 1995, respectively, account for 75–80% of hereditary breast cancer and 5–6% of all breast cancers. The estimated prevalence of *BRCA1* mutations in the general population is 1 in 833.

The incidence in Ashkenazi Jews, a genetically distinct population of central European origin known to be affected with various inherited diseases, is significantly higher. After it was recognized that one mutation in *BRCA1*, specifically, 185delAG, occurred with a very high frequency among Ashkenazim, the frequency of the mutation was sought in 858 healthy Ashkenazi men and women who had participated in a genetic testing program for cystic fibrosis and Tay-Sachs disease. Remarkably, 0.9% of Ashkenazi Jews without cancer carried this mutation (3), which is a 10-fold higher rate than in the general population. The 185delAG mutation and a specific mutation in *BRCA2* (617delT) together may account for greater than 25% of all early-onset breast cancer cases and for 66% of early-onset breast cancer in hereditary breast and breast/ovarian families of Ashkenazi Jewish heritage. Prospective studies should provide a better estimate of the penetrance of these specific mutations.

Epidemiological studies suggest that carriers of *BRCA1* and *BRCA2* mutations have an 87% cumulative lifetime risk of developing breast cancer. This risk is 50% by age 45 and 87% by age 70. Furthermore, 65% of these women who live to age 70 will develop a second primary breast tumor. Women with either a *BRCA1* or *BRCA2* mutation have a 40–60% and 15–20% lifetime risk of ovarian cancer, respectively. Although *BRCA2* mutations are associated with an increased risk of male breast cancer, there is no increased risk of male breast cancer with mutations in *BRCA1*. Other tumor types associated with *BRCA1* and *BRCA2* mutations include colon, prostate, melanoma, laryngeal, and pancreatic cancer.

Having identified an individual from a family at high risk for harboring a *BRCA1* or *BRCA2* mutation, consideration of DNA-based predictive testing is appropriate. The determination of when and to whom to offer testing is complex with far-reaching consequences. Most academic, professional, and government organizations that addressed this issue concluded that offering *BRCA1* and *BRCA2* testing as a routine clinical service is premature (3). Although the ability to identify a patient at risk holds potential promise with regard to early detection or prevention, it is also fraught with pitfalls, such as risk of insurance or employer discrimination; these issues need to be addressed in the context of informed consent prior to performing predictive testing. The many scientific, technical, socioeconomic, psychosocial, medical, ethical, and legal issues that accompany genetic testing must be considered and explained to the patient. A position paper published by the American Society of Clinical Oncology (ASCO) (4) addressed many of these issues. They concluded that genetic testing for cancer susceptibility should be performed in the setting of clinical trials designed to assess long-term outcomes. Long-term outcome studies are necessary to confirm predicted age-specific risks (penetrance) of mutations and to document the effectiveness of interventions such as counseling, surveillance, and prevention. Ge-

Table 1 Indications for Referral for Breast Cancer Risk Assessment and Possible Genetic Testing

Breast cancer before age 30
Breast or ovarian cancer before 50 in the subject and a first-degree relative
Breast cancer (any age) and a family history of two or more breast cancers and one or more ovarian cancers
An affected first-degree relative of someone with a known *BRCA1* or *BRCA2* mutation
Askenazi women with breast cancer before age 40 or ovarian cancer at any age

netic testing should be made available to selected patients as part of the preventive oncological care of families in conjunction with appropriate patient education, informed consent, support, and pre- and posttest counseling. The ASCO paper concludes that the medical benefit of identifying a *BRCA1* carrier is "presumed but not established" and emphasizes that the commercial availability of a new genetic test does not ensure that the test is indicated for clinical use (3,4). A summary of who should be referred for breast cancer risk assessment and possible predictive testing is shown in Table 1.

If a family is deemed appropriate and has consented to have genetic testing, an affected family member would be selected for screening. If a *BRCA1* mutation is identified and is predicted to be of functional significance, then individual testing for the presence of that specific mutation can be initiated for interested family members. Given that greater than 500 and 300 mutations have been identified in the coding regions *BRCA1* and *BRCA2*, respectively, it is not yet possible to offer genetic testing in the absence of an affected living relative. In this setting, the significance of a negative or even positive test in an unaffected individual is not interpretable.

Once a person is identified as being at high risk, management options include increased surveillance, prophylactic surgery (mastectomy and oophorectomy), as well as participation in prevention trials. Yet, none of these options is proven to prevent the development of cancer in high-risk individuals. Only after studying these strategies in a prospective manner will we be able to determine the efficacy of any one intervention.

II. FUTURE TRENDS AND CONTROVERSIES

The Cancer Genetics Studies Consortium recently published recommendations for follow-up care of carriers of *BRCA1* and *BRCA2* mutations or those at high risk based on family pedigree. They recommended that women perform monthly breast self-examination (BSE) by age 18–21 and undergo an annual or semiannual clinician breast examination (CBE) beginning at age 25–35 (see Table 2). There is conflicting data regarding the benefit of these interventions in patients of average risk; no data are available for women with an autosomal dominant predisposition to cancer. Given the lower sensitivity of mammograms in younger women and the higher incidence of breast cancer in this population, BSE and CBE may be of greater value than mammography in carriers of a susceptibility gene.

Annual mammography is suggested beginning at age 25–35 and tailored according to the youngest age of cancer diagnosis in an affected relative. In general, screening mammograms are recommended for women at high risk beginning 5–10 years earlier than the age of the youngest affected relative. The role of mammography in women < 40 years of age is controversial; the benefit in high-risk women is unknown. Furthermore, no data are available on radiation risk in *BRCA1* or *BRCA2* mutation carriers. Increased risk could derive either from increased radiation sensitivity or from the cumulative effect of increased imaging beginning at an early age (5). Despite the potential limitations of screening mammography in this population, it will continue to be a component of the surveillance program until well-designed, prospective studies show otherwise.

The consortium recommends annual or semiannual screening for ovarian cancer beginning at age 25–35 using transvaginal ultrasound, serum CA125, and pelvic examinations for carriers of *BRCA1* mutations. (Despite the lack of proven value for detecting early lesions.) Carriers of *BRCA2* mutations should be counseled that their risk of ovarian cancer appears to be lower than their risk of breast cancer, although increased above that of the general population; ovarian cancer surveillance is an option.

With regard to preventive surgery, it is recommended that prophylactic mastectomy be discussed as one option for managing breast-cancer risk for women with known inherited cancer susceptibility or woman deemed to be at high risk by virtue of histological markers such a LCIS. Women should be told that there are currently no data with which to estimate the efficacy

Table 2 Cancer Genetics Studies Consortium Recommendations for Follow-up of Individuals with *BRCA1* or *BRCA2* Mutations

1. Monthly breast self-examination starting at age 18–21
2. Annual or semiannual clinical examination at age 25–35
3. Annual or semiannual screening for ovarian cancer beginning at age 25–35 using transvaginal ultrasound and serum CA125
4. Discussion of prophylactic mastectomy
5. Discussion of prophylactic oophorectomy

of the procedure; it is known that current surgical approaches do not completely eliminate the risk of subsequent breast cancer. This is due, in part, to the inability to surgically remove breast tissue completely; residual breast tissue has been found in the chest wall, axilla, and abdomen following mastectomy. Any residual cell of breast origin remains at risk for mutagenesis and transformation to breast cancer. We prefer simple mastectomy for prophylactic procedures, with or without reconstruction. Women should be counseled that cancer risk is distributed over time; thus, the decision to undergo prophylactic mastectomy should not be made in haste, but deliberately and thoughtfully.

Similarly, prophylactic oophorectomy should be discussed as an intervention for carriers of *BRCA1* mutations and for carriers of *BRCA2* mutations from families in which ovarian cancer has occurred. Once again, women should be counseled regarding the limitations of surgery, based on documented cases of peritoneal carcinomatosis occurring following oophorectomy. The optimum age for the procedure has not been established; however, the mean age for ovarian cancer in hereditary breast/ovarian families is the midforties. A recent National Institutes of Health consensus conference recommended that women with two or more first-degree relatives with ovarian cancer be offered prophylactic oophorectomy after completion of childbearing, or at age 35 years based on two series of high-risk families demonstrating a mean age of ovarian cancer ranging from 45 to 52 years. The decision to undergo prophylactic oophorectomy must be weighed against the known side effects of surgical ablation. These include typical vasomotor menopausal symptoms as well as more significant long-term effects such as osteoporosis and cardiovascular disease. The use of hormone replacement in this high-risk population is controversial given the associated breast cancer risk; however, there are limited data available to recommend for or against hormone replacement therapy (5). A small, retrospective study suggests that use of oral contraceptives may increase the risk of breast cancer to a greater degree in mutation carriers than in noncarriers (6). These data underscore the need for additional well-designed studies examining the influence of exogenous exposures on mutation carriers.

These recommendations may also be applicable to (1) individuals whose mutation status is unknown but who have a substantial likelihood of being mutation carriers, i.e., individuals from families in which a mutation is a breast cancer susceptibility gene is present, who have not been tested for a variety of reasons, and (2) individuals from families segregating along an autosomal dominant pattern of predisposition to breast or ovarian cancer when molecular studies have not been done or have failed to identify a specific mutation.

In summary, exciting developments in genetic epidemiology and molecular biology may revolutionize our present thinking about the role of hereditary factors in breast cancer and provide new tools for the diagnosis and treatment of breast cancer in women affected with either the inherited or sporadic form of this disease.

REFERENCES

1. Colditz GA, Willett WC, Hunter DJ, et al. Family history, age, and risk of breast cancer. JAMA 1993; 270:338–343.
2. Slattery ML, Kerber RA. A comprehensive evaluation of family history and breast cancer risk. JAMA 1993; 270:1563–1568.
3. Greene MH. Genetics of breast cancer. Mayo Clin Proc 1997; 72:54–65.
4. American Society of Clinical Oncology. Statement of the American Society of Clinical Oncology: genetic testing for cancer susceptibility. J Clin Oncol 1996; 14(5):1730–1736.
5. Burke W, Daly M, Garber J, Botkin J, Kahn MJ, Lynch P, Mctiernan A, Offit K, Perlman J, Petersen G, Thomson E, Varricchio C. Recommendations for follow-up care of individuals with an inherited predisposition to cancer. JAMA 1997; 277(12):997–1003.
6. Ursin G. Does oral contraceptive use increase the risk of breast cancer in women with *BRCA1/BRCA2* mutations more than in other women? Cancer Res 1997; 57(17):3678–3681.

II
CRITICAL PATHWAYS

The decision-making required to care for patients with breast cancer is based on principles that were developed over many years of experience and through the accumulation of data from several sources, including well-designed randomized clinical trials. In the introductory chapters, we attempted to present succinctly these data where they exist and point out where they don't, and to present what we hope is a logical approach to problems as they arise. Based on this work, we have constructed Clinical Decision Pathways *that summarize these data and provide the scaffolding on which the subsequent case presentations were organized. The pathways are not meant to be specific guidelines for the management of individual patients, but rather, general approaches to decision making based on our best formulation of the current state of care for breast cancer patients.*

Clinical Decision Pathways

Overview

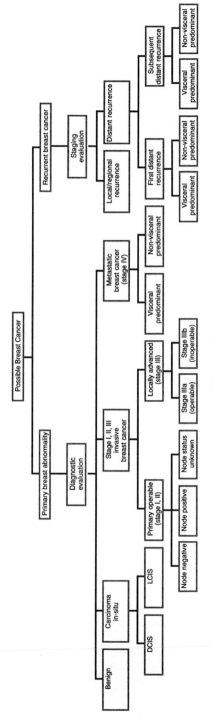

Figure 1

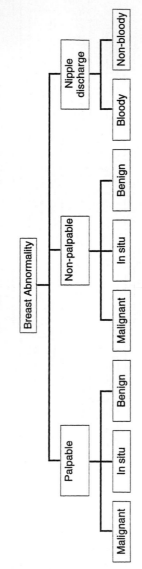

Figure 2

Non-Palpable Abnormality

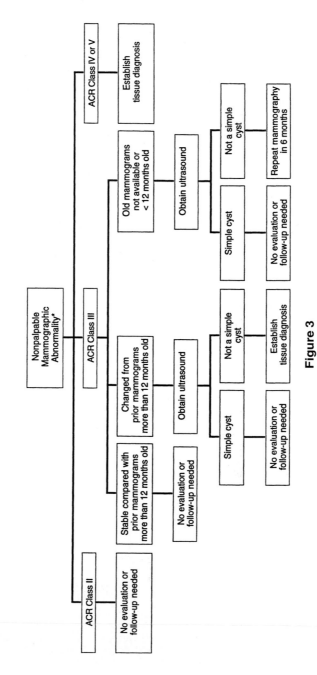

Figure 3

Palpable Abnormality

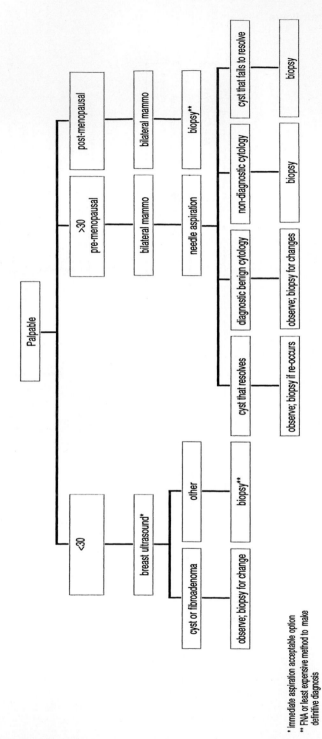

Figure 4

* immediate aspiration acceptable option
** FNA or least expensive method to make
   definitive diagnosis

Nipple Discharge

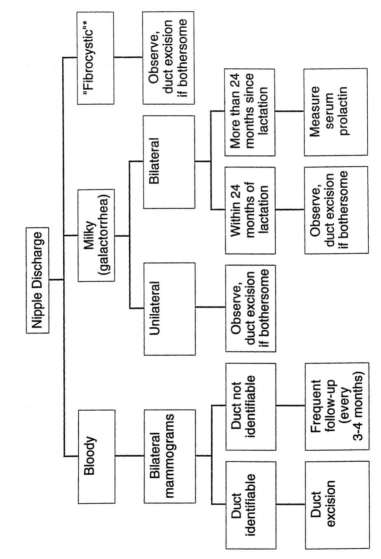

Nipple Discharge

- Bloody
  - Bilateral mammograms
    - Duct identifiable
      - Duct excision
    - Duct not identifiable
      - Frequent follow-up (every 3-4 months)
- Milky (galactorrhea)
  - Unilateral
    - Observe, duct excision if bothersome
  - Bilateral
    - Within 24 months of lactation
      - Observe, duct excision if bothersome
    - More than 24 months since lactation
      - Measure serum prolactin
- "Fibrocystic"*
  - Observe, duct excision if bothersome

*Green, blue, brown, creamy, or serous discharge

Figure 5

LCIS

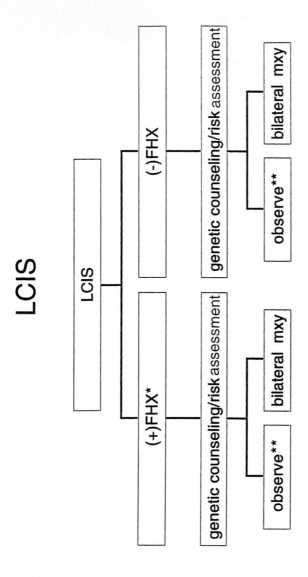

* candidates for approved clinical trials for high risk patients
** yearly evaluation including bilateral mammography

Figure 6

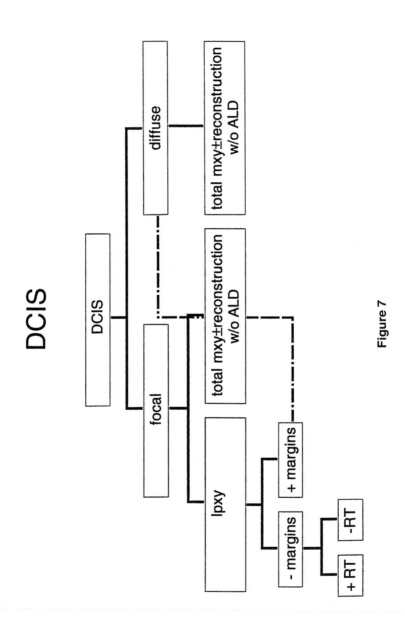

Figure 7

INVASIVE BREAST CANCER

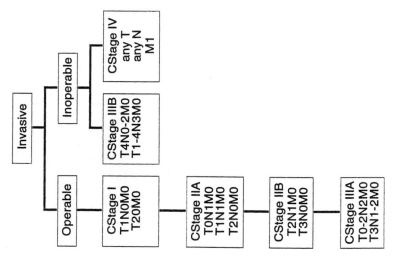

Figure 8

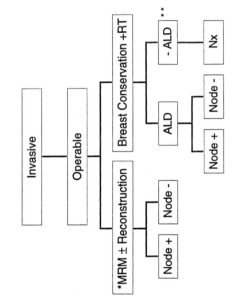

Invasive Operable

Invasive — Operable

*MRM ± Reconstruction

Breast Conservation +RT

Node + | Node -

ALD | - ALD **

Node + | Node - | Nx

* Add radiation
therapy if T≥5cm
N≥4+LN

** Axilllary lymph node dissection

Figure 9

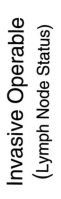

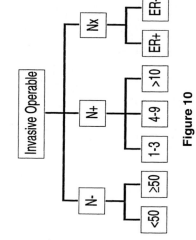

Figure 10

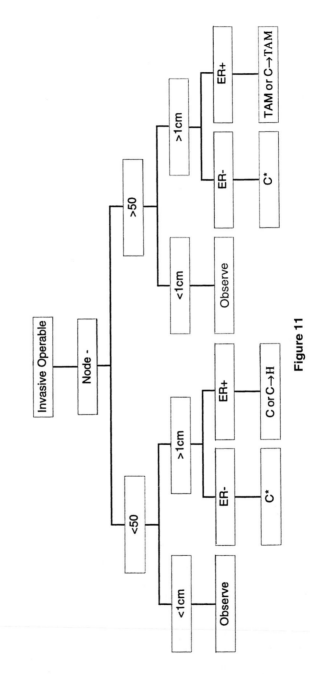

Node-Negative Disease

Figure 11

Node-Positive Disease

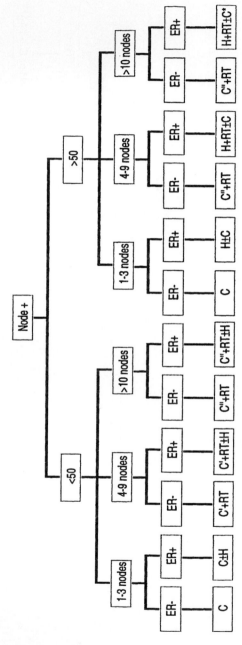

C=e.g. Cyclophosphamide (C)/Adriamycin (A) (CA), or Cyclophosphamide, Methotrexate, Fluorouracil, or equivalent

C'=e.g. A → CMF, or clinical trials evaluating dose intensification ±stem cell rescue

C''=clinical trials evaluating dose intensification ±stem cell rescue

H=hormonal therapy

*Use of dose-intensification chemotherapy in >50 yo must be highly selected and ideally part of a clinical trial.

Figure 12

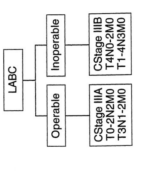

LOCALLY ADVANCED BREAST CANCER

Figure 13

LOCALLY ADVANCED BREAST CANCER

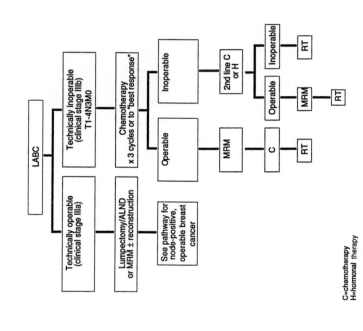

LABC

Technically operable (clinical stage IIIa)

Technically inoperable (clinical stage IIIb) T1-4N3M0

Lumpectomy/ALND or MRM ± reconstruction

See pathway for node-positive, operable breast cancer

Chemotherapy x 3 cycles or to "best response"

Operable

Inoperable

MRM

2nd line C or H

C

Operable

Inoperable

RT

MRM

Inoperable

RT

RT

C=chemotherapy
H=hormonal therapy

Figure 14

Local/Regional Recurrences

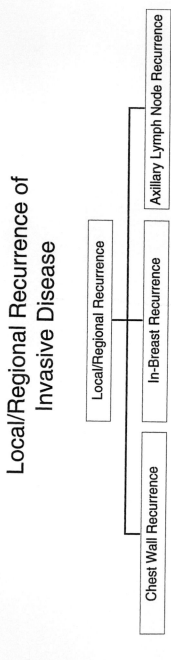

Local/Regional Recurrence of Invasive Disease

Local/Regional Recurrence

Chest Wall Recurrence

In-Breast Recurrence

Axillary Lymph Node Recurrence

Figure 15

Chest Wall Recurrence

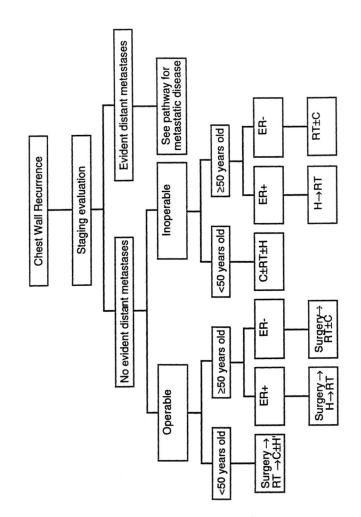

Figure 16

C=chemotherapy
H=hormonal therapy
RT=radiation therapy

In-Breast Recurrence

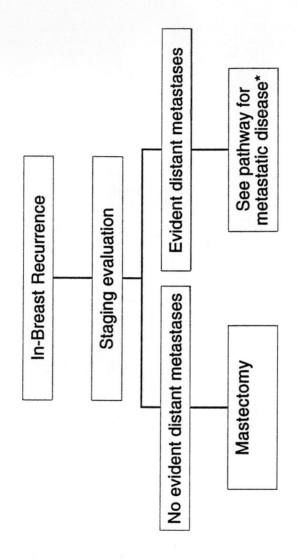

In-Breast Recurrence

Staging evaluation

Evident distant metastases

See pathway for metastatic disease*

No evident distant metastases

Mastectomy

* Mastectomy may be indicated for palliation

Figure 17

Recurrent/Metastatic Disease

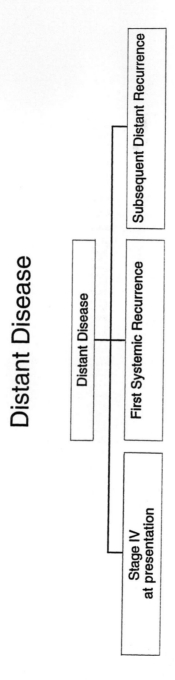

Distant Disease

Figure 18

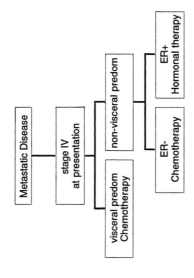

Stage IV at Presentation

Metastatic Disease

stage IV
at presentation

visceral predom
Chemotherapy

non-visceral predom

ER-
Chemotherapy

ER+
Hormonal therapy

*all patients with metastatic disease should be considered for
clinical trials

Figure 19

First Systemic Recurrence

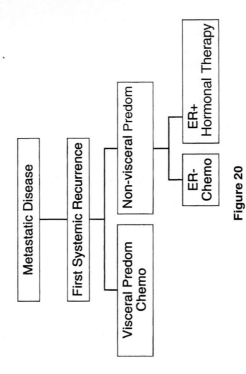

Figure 20

Subsequent Relapse

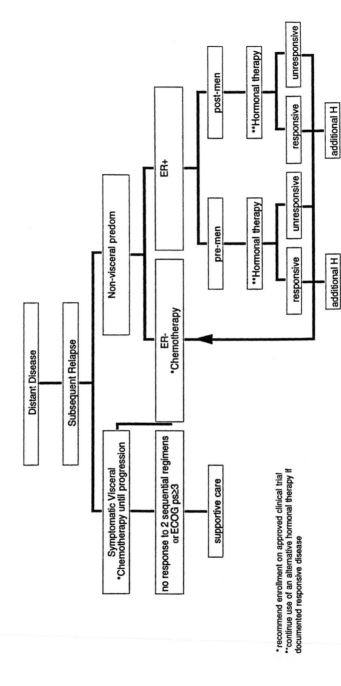

Figure 21

III
CASES ALONG THE
CRITICAL PATHWAYS

A. Diagnosis of Breast Cancer

A.1. PALPABLE BREAST LESIONS

Introduction

The goal of the cases to be presented along this pathway is to address the options available to clinicians and their patients when presented with an abnormality in the breast. We have chosen to make the fundamental division at this starting point be the difference between a palpable versus a nonpalpable lesion. The key to successful and efficient management of these patients is a familiarity with the key pieces of data underlying a relatively few fundamental decisions. These include: (1) indicators of malignancy; (2) risks and benefits of procedural options.

Case #A.1.1
Goal: Evaluation of young women with multiple breast masses

THOMAS J. KEARNEY

A 23-year-old woman who had breast biopsies at ages 12 and 14 revealing fibroadenomas presents with six breast masses. One enlarged significantly over the past 6 months (now 5 cm in diameter); the other five are distributed bilaterally and are stable, ranging from 1 to 4 cm in diameter. All are smooth, firm, mobile, and nontender on examination. Ultrasonographically all are solid, homogeneous, and well marginated.

For women under 30 years of age without major risk factors for breast cancer, a well-circumscribed, discrete breast mass suggests the presence of a simple cyst, fibroadenoma, or fibrocystic changes. Mammography may not be helpful in young women with dense breasts; breast ultrasound is preferred and can confirm the diagnosis of a simple cyst. If a homogeneous, well-demarcated solid lesion is seen on ultrasound, the clinical diagnosis of fibroadenoma may be supported. Further support for this diagnosis can be obtained by fine-needle aspiration (FNA) or core biopsy of the lesion. It is imperative, however, that a specific appointment for reevaluation at regular intervals be planned. In 10–15% of women, multiple fibroadenomas are present. Attempts at multiple excisions would be unwise. However, in the setting of multiple fibroadenomas, it is prudent to obtain a tissue diagnosis of at least one of the lesions. The remainder can be followed clinically. In the current case, a tissue diagnosis had been obtained many years earlier. Cancer can develop in or next to a fibroadenoma. However, this is a rare event and does not warrant routine removal of fibroadenomas.

Excision is indicated if a mass suspected of being a fibroadenoma changes significantly. Because of the occasional phylloides tumor or fibrosarcoma of the breast, it is prudent to excise lesions that are growing and I would recommend that the large, changing lesion in this patient be excised. Excisions must be conservative in adolescent women owing to the concern of affecting the developing breast bud. Even in a young woman, a dominant mass not typical of either a cyst or a fibroadenoma should undergo biopsy. In a study of 951 breast biopsies performed in young women, no patients under age 21 were found to have breast cancer, but 1.3% of biopsies in women aged 21–25 and 4.0% in women aged 26–30 were positive for malignancy. Thus, young age alone cannot be used to reliably exclude malignancy.

BIBLIOGRAPHY

August DA, Sondak VK. Breast disease. In: Greenfield LJ, ed. Surgery: Scientific
       Principles and Practice, 2nd ed. Philadelphia: Lippincott, 1996; 1357–1415.
Dent DM, Cant PF. Fibroadenoma. World J Surg 1989; 13:706–710.
Ferguson CM, Powell RW. Breast masses in young women. Arch Surg 1989; 124:
       1338.

Case #A.1.2
Goal: To discuss the management of "benign"-appearing lesions in young women

ROSEMARY B. DUDA

A 24-year-old woman presents with a 2.5-cm palpable, smooth-edged, freely movable mass that developed over the last 3 months. How would you recommend evaluating this patient?

The appearance of a new palpable breast lesion in a woman of any age mandates immediate attention. In this case, the differential encompasses solid and cystic lesions. Simple cysts are benign, fluid-filled lesions. Cysts are derived from the terminal duct lobular unit and consist of two layers, the luminal epithelial layer and the outer myoepithelial layer. The epithelium may be markedly attenuated or absent. Cysts are often smooth and mobile to palpation.

The most common solid, discrete mass in a young woman is a fibroadenoma. Fibroadenomas are smooth, rounded, or lobulated masses that are frequently described as mobile. They are pseudoencapsulated and can be sharply delineated from the surrounding breast tissue. These lesions represent a hyperplastic process that involves a single terminal duct lobular unit and the surrounding connective tissue. They usually present as a solitary mass, but multiple lesions are seen in 10–15% of cases.

There are other solitary lesions that may present as a discrete mass in a young woman. Cancer is rare in this age group and is unlikely to be described as smooth and mobile. Nonetheless, malignancies must be included in the differential. Tubular or mucinous cancers may present as a discrete, firm mass. Other lesions that may present as a smooth, mobile mass include hamartomas, juvenile fibroadenomas, lactational fibroadenomas, cystosarcoma phylloides, fibrosis, lipomas, and less commonly, trauma and fat necrosis.

There are several approaches to differentiate between a solid mass and a cyst. A fine-needle aspirate (FNA) can be performed in the office at the initial visit. A return of gray, green, or yellowish fluid, with complete disappearance of the mass, confirms the diagnosis of a simple cyst and the fluid may be discarded. Return of bloody fluid raises the possibility of a cyst with an associated intracystic carcinoma. Any bloody fluid aspirate should be submitted for a cytological evaluation. If the FNA reveals a solid lesion, cells aspirated from the lesion should be submitted for cytological evaluation. If the lesion is clinically benign and consistent with a fibroadenoma, and the cytology report reveals cells consistent with a fibroadenoma, no further evaluation is necessary. Any equivocal cytology findings or a report suggesting an atypical finding or malignancy must be further pursued with excision of the mass.

For the patient who declines an FNA, as is common for some young women, ultrasound can determine whether a lesion is cystic or solid. If the lesion is a simple cyst, observation is appropriate. If the ultrasound reveals a well-defined, well-demarcated lesion consistent with a fibroadenoma, observation is also appropriate. FNA or excision should be recommended if the lesion increases in size. If the lesion appears to have irregular borders or appears to be a cyst with debris, an FNA or excision should be performed.

Excisional biopsy is also appropriate for any solid, discrete, palpable lesion. FNA or ultrasound, however, may eliminate the need for surgical intervention for many women with clearly benign lesions. If observation is chosen following nonsurgical evaluation, a baseline ultrasound should be performed to accurately document the dimensions of the lesion. Accurate clinical dimensions and characteristics should also be carefully recorded for future comparisons. A clinical examination every 6 months with an ultrasound evaluation is also recommended for at least 1 year. If the lesion remains stable, the mass can be followed yearly.

The most important pitfall in observing a solid mass in any woman is the risk of missing a cancer. Any change in the size or character of the mass mandates an excisional biopsy. In summary, while it is uncommon for a 24-year-old woman to have breast cancer, it is a real possibility that should not be overlooked.

BIBLIOGRAPHY

Azzopardi JG, Ahmed A, Millis RR. Problems in breast pathology. Major Prob
    Pathol 1979; 11:39.
Dent DM, Cant PF. Fibroadenoma. World J Surg 1989; 13:706–710.
Ferguson CM, Powell RW. Breast masses in young women. Arch Surg 1989; 124:
    1338.
Haagensen CD. In: Diseases of the Breast, 3rd ed. Philadelphia: WB Saunders, 1986.

Case #A.1.3
Goal: To discuss an approach to fibrocystic disease

VERNON K. SONDAK and JULIE A. WOLFE

*A 42-year-old woman presents to her gynecologist with a complaint of
waxing and waning breast masses and cyclical tenderness. Breast
examination reveals diffuse "lumpiness" without a dominant mass. What
features of her evaluation would allow you to make a diagnosis of
fibrocystic breast disease without subjecting the patient to a surgical
procedure?*

When is a disease *really* a disease? With fibrocystic "disease," this
question is more than rhetorical. Histological changes compatible with fibrocystic disease can be found in breast biopsy specimens from nearly all
premenopausal women—clearly *all* of these women don't have a true disease. What we call fibrocystic disease is a common group of related symptoms, clinical and radiological findings, and histological changes that are
often normal, but sometimes exaggerated, reactions to the cyclical development and involution of the female breast during the phases of the menstrual cycle. When these reactions cause "dis-ease"—breast pain or tenderness beyond the typical discomfort experienced as "normal" by most
women just before the onset of menses; a palpable mass or thickening that
must be differentiated from cancer; or other abnormal manifestations like a
nipple discharge—the patient seeks medical attention and can truly be considered to be suffering from a disease.

This case presentation illustrates that patients sometimes present to
their primary health care provider (for many women of reproductive age,
their gynecologist) for evaluation of complaints that may not fully meet the
criteria of a "disease." Many, if not most, women note cyclical tenderness
and breast nodularity in the week or so just prior to their menses, which
generally resolves nearly completely after the menstrual period begins. Occasionally, as appears to be the case here, something has changed enough
from the typical pattern for the patient, so she seeks medical evaluation. We

most often see this occurring in women in their late twenties and early thirties, but there is another peak in the early to midforties.

The evaluation should begin with a thorough history that documents the patient's normal pattern of cyclical breast-related changes and how the current situation differs from that norm. The history should also include an assessment of the recognized risk factors for breast cancer, including a reproductive history and family and personal history of breast disease. Also relevant is the timing of the last menstrual period and the next expected period, and any history of current or past hormone usage (including oral contraceptives and postmenopausal replacement hormones). Next, the physical examination should document the overall degree of breast nodularity as well as any areas of thickening or asymmetry, the presence or absence of a dominant mass, the presence or absence of skin or nipple changes or nipple discharge, and the status of the regional lymph nodes. Ideally, the examination should be conducted at a point in the patient's menstrual cycle when her breasts are least nodular and tender. Rarely, an examination may need to be rescheduled if significant premenstrual tenderness or nodularity makes a thorough examination difficult.

Management of the symptomatic patient requires exclusion of malignancy and treatment of the specific symptom complex. The physical examination combined with mammography and/or ultrasonography as appropriate (mammography generally restricted to symptomatic women 30–35 years of age or older; ultrasonography used selectively to assess specific palpable findings or areas of particular tenderness) is sufficient to exclude cancer in most cases. Occasionally, an area of fibrocystic disease presents as a mass clinically indistinguishable from cancer, and a tissue diagnosis must be established.

If the examination reveals a palpable lesion suspected of being a cyst (smoothly marginated and soft or fluctuant), fine-needle aspiration is indicated. Physical examination is not highly accurate at distinguishing cystic from solid lesions, but if needle aspiration yields clear, yellow, or green fluid without blood and the mass completely disappears, no further evaluation is required and the patient should be followed for recurrence of the cyst. Cytological analysis is *not* routinely performed on fluid aspirated from breast cysts and excision of the cyst is not required. If the lesion proves solid or only partially cystic on aspiration (i.e., there is residual palpable mass despite removal of some fluid), or if the aspirated fluid is blood-tinged or bloody, cytological evaluation of the aspirate is indicated. In this instance, diagnostic tissue is required; if the cytology is not definitive, excisional biopsy of the residual mass is indicated.

Fibrocystic changes that, as in the present case, are not associated with severe symptoms generally require only reassurance once the presence of malignancy has been excluded. More severe degrees of breast pain (referred to as mastodynia or mastalgia), especially if the pain has become constant throughout the menstrual cycle ("noncyclical mastodynia"), often require treatment. Exclusion of non-breast-related causes of pain is important. Costochondritis, angina pectoris, and even cervical nerve root pain can be mistaken for breast pain. Breast pain unrelated to the menstrual cycle may be caused by infection or a large cyst. Once physical examination and history point to fibrocystic changes as the culprit, therapy should consist of appropriate reassurance to the patient that she does not have breast cancer. Over-the-counter analgesics may be suggested for mild to moderate pain. Caffeine may worsen mastodynia and patients should severely limit their caffeine consumption for 2–3 months to determine if their symptoms improve. Nicotine may also worsen symptoms and patients are well advised to stop smoking. When these conservative efforts fail, other steps can be taken. Danazol, a weak androgen, is the most effective drug for therapy of mastodynia. The side effects—including amenorrhea, body fat redistribution, hirsutism, acne, weight gain, and deepening of the voice—are so troublesome that its use is usually restricted to very severe cases with pain throughout the menstrual cycle. Oral contraceptives may either improve or worsen the discomfort of mastodynia depending upon the formulation of the birth control pills, so adjusting the patient's prescription may help. Evening primrose oil, available in many health food stores, has been shown in some studies to alleviate cyclical mastodynia, although the mechanism of action is currently unknown. Most other remedies, including vitamin E, have not been shown to work better than placebos in prospective evaluations.

Finally, it is appropriate to address the risk of developing breast cancer in patients who have fibrocystic disease. Most of these patients are not at increased risk for breast cancer. About 5% of women who undergo biopsy for what prove to be fibrocystic changes are found to have "proliferative" disease: hyperplasia of the ducts or lobules. Such patients are at increased risk of developing breast cancer; the risk increases further if the hyperplasia is associated with atypia (atypical ductal or lobular hyperplasia) especially if the atypical hyperplasia occurs in a patient with a family history of breast cancer. Patients with a strong family history of breast cancer and biopsy-proven atypical hyperplasia should be counseled about prophylactic mastectomies or participation in a clinical trial of breast cancer prevention. Outside of this small fraction of patients, the issue of surgery should rarely, if ever, arise for management of fibrocystic symptoms or for cancer prevention. Instead, women with fibrocystic changes should be counseled to perform monthly breast self-examination to detect any changes beyond those usually associated with cyclical hormonal fluctuations. When the health care provider has properly reassured and educated the patient about fibrocystic changes and actively involved the patient in her own subsequent evaluation, the patient's "disease" can be considered "treated."

BIBLIOGRAPHY

August DA, Sondak VK. Breast. In: Greenfield LJ, Mulholland MW, Oldham KT, Zelenock GB, Lillemoe KD, eds. Essentials of Surgery: Scientific Principles and Practice. Philadelphia: Lippincott-Raven, 1997:439–449.
Cancer Committee of the American College of Pathologists. Is "fibrocystic disease" of the breast precancerous? Consensus meeting. Arch Pathol Lab Med 1986; 110:171–173.
Page DL, Dupont WD. Anatomic markers of human premalignancy and risk of breast cancer. Cancer 1990; 66:1326–1335.

Case #A.1.4
Goal: To discuss the use of fine-needle aspiration

THOMAS J. KEARNEY

A 60-year-old woman presents with a 2-cm palpable breast mass. Bilateral mammograms reveal an area of increased parenchymal density corresponding to the palpable mass; the mammograms are characterized as "indeterminate." A fine-needle aspirate reveals normal mammary epithelium. What would be your next step in evaluating this patient?

It is unusual for a hard mass in a postmenopausal woman to be benign. In postmenopausal women, the replacement of glandular tissue by fat, the absence of hormone-related functional changes, and the high incidence of cancer make the evaluation of palpable breast masses relatively straightforward. Mammograms are obtained in this setting solely to screen for other occult lesions that would need to be addressed at the same time. In this particular case, the mammogram revealed a mass that was clinically suspicious. The standard treatment today for early-stage breast cancer is lumpectomy with axillary dissection followed by radiation to the breast and adjuvant therapy (when indicated). Knowledge of the nature of a lesion prior to lumpectomy allows the axillary dissection to be done at the same time, avoiding the need for a second surgery. Also, the treatment plan can be discussed in more detail with the patient if malignancy is confirmed preoperatively.

Fine-needle aspiration (FNA) permits rapid, minimally invasive diagnosis of many palpable breast masses. The incidence of false-positive findings is generally less than 0.5%. FNA is not specific enough to allow definitive surgery, particularly mastectomy, without prior confirmation of the presence of cancer with an intraoperative frozen section. The reported sensitivity of FNA ranges from 70% to 99%; 85% is a good estimate of the true sensitivity in most settings. Sensitivity is technique dependent and influenced by the experience of the clinician obtaining the specimen and the interpreting cytologist. False-negative findings are caused by inadequate sampling (missing the lesion), improper processing of the specimen, or inability of the cytologist to make a definite diagnosis. In our breast center, the cytologist is available on short notice to come to the clinic and assess the adequacy of the specimen at the bedside, allowing additional samples to be taken if needed. A diagnostic FNA reveals cells that show a specific benign entity or cells that are unequivocally malignant. A finding of normal epithelial cells or lipocytes may mean that the aspiration needle missed the intended target. These findings should be interpreted as nondiagnostic. Readings such as acellular, atypical, or suspicious are also nondiagnostic and cannot be used for decision making.

Core biopsies can be obtained in the office with hand-held instruments and may be useful when cytological expertise is not available or when definitive preoperative histology and hormone receptor analysis are important. Both spring-loaded and manual core biopsy devices are available in a variety of sizes. Larger-diameter core needles such as 16 or 14 gauge are more likely to provide diagnostic information than 20-gauge needles, although the larger needles require a local anesthetic for patient comfort.

Stereotaxic X-ray-guided core biopsy has been used for minimally invasive diagnosis of nonpalpable breast lesions detected mammographically. The technique is quite effective, especially for mass lesions, as opposed to microcalcifications. Stereotaxic mammography is used to guide an aspirating or biopsy needle into the suspicious lesion and to verify that the sampling was performed with the needle tip in proper position. Seven series comparing stereotaxic core biopsy to surgical excision have demonstrated sensitivities ranging from 71% to 100%. In all of these studies, the patients were highly selected. A report from a consortium of 20 institutions studied over 6000 women who had stereotaxic core biopsy. A total of 2237 women had no follow-up and 2456 had short-term (6 month) mammographic follow-up. A total of 1363 women had open-biopsy confirmation of their stereotaxic core biopsy. A total of 280 women had benign core biopsies with 15 cancers found on open biopsy for a false-negative rate of over 5%. This compares with a false-negative rate of under 0.5% for wire localization breast biopsy. As with FNA or core biopsy of palpable lesions, nondiagnostic samples need to be followed up by surgical biopsy. Of particular note, a stereotaxic core finding of atypical hyperplasia is associated with malignancy at excisional biopsy in about half the cases.

Most recently, use of the breast biopsy "mammotome" has become more common. This device allows mammographically guided placement of a biopsy needle within a mass or microcalcifications, and repeated "resection" of small cores of tissue. Sensitivity and specificity of this technique approach 90%.

Ultrasound-guided core biopsy of mammographically detected lesions has been offered as a cost-effective and quicker alternative to stereotaxic biopsy, particularly when performed by breast surgeons in the office. This approach allows clinicians who are comfortable with ultrasound to identify cysts and avoid biopsy altogether and to confirm the diagnosis of lesions suspected of being fibroadenomas. Drawbacks include the inability to visualize mass lesions in 20% of cases, inability to detect microcalcifications, and lack of widespread familiarity with the technique.

BIBLIOGRAPHY

Burbank F, Parker SH, Fogarty TJ. Stereotactic breast biopsy: improved tissue harvesting with the mammatome. Am Surg 1996; 62:738–744.

Kearney TJ, Morrow M. Effect of reexcision on the success of breast-conserving surgery. Ann Surg Oncol 1995; 2:303–307.

Kopans DB. Review of stereotaxic large-core needle biopsy and surgical biopsy results in nonpalpable breast lesions. Radiology 1993; 189:665–666.

Layfield LJ, Glasgow BJ, Cramer H. Fine needle aspiration in the management of breast masses. Pathol Annu 1989; 24:23.

Meyer JE, Smith DN, DiPiro PJ, Denison CM, Frenna TH, Harvey SC, Ko WD. Stereotactic breast biopsy of clustered microcalcifications with a directional, vacuum-assisted device. Radiology 1997; 204:575–576.

Parker SH, Burbank F, Jackman RL, et al. Percutaneous large core breast biopsy: a multi-institutional study. Radiology 1994; 193:359–364.

Parker SH, Jobe WE, Dennis MA. Ultrasound guided automated large core breast biopsy. Radiology 1993; 187:507–511.

Staren ED. Surgical office based ultrasound of the breast. Am Surg 1995; 61:619–627.

Case #A.1.5
Goal: To discuss the indications for use of core needle biopsies
SUSAN A. MCMANUS

A 43-year-old woman presents with a 6-cm, movable, hard breast mass, with palpable axillary lymph nodes. What are the options for approaching this problem? What would you choose?

This patient has locally advanced breast cancer until proven otherwise (clinical stage IIIA). Many of these patients are treated with neoadjuvant chemotherapy, followed by surgery, and radiation. High-dose chemotherapy is also being investigated in this setting. However, the patient has a movable 6-cm tumor, which may be operable. A diagnosis must be established before treatment can be planned.

The diagnosis should be obtained in an expeditious and cost-effective manner. This is usually possible with fine-needle aspiration (FNA). FNA provides a minimum of discomfort to the patient and has a high degree of sensitivity and specificity in the diagnosis of suspicious breast masses. Masood et al. found the accuracy of a physical examination that revealed a suspicious mass, a positive mammogram, and an FNA that showed cancer to be 99%. If two needle specimens are obtained, enough cells may be available for estrogen and progesterone receptor assays.

Core needle biopsy can also establish the diagnosis and provide additional histological information. Specifically, it can distinguish between invasive and noninvasive carcinoma; this is not possible with FNA. Disadvantages of core needle biopsy include the difficulty of targeting small lesions and patient discomfort.

Although FNA and core needle biopsy can be performed without a cytologist or pathologist present, the techniques are most reliable if the specimens are immediately assessed for adequacy. With this approach, open biopsy can almost always be avoided. Both techniques are highly sensitive and specific. The costs of the procedures are comparable.

Following examination and mammography, I would review with the patient the advantages of obtaining tissue samples as early as possible, to plan the management. I would recommend performance of an FNA with a cytotechnologist present to assure that the specimen is adequate for cytological diagnosis and for determination of the presence of hormone receptors. Core needle biopsy would be a reasonable alternative.

BIBLIOGRAPHY

Ballo MS, Sneige N. Can core needle biopsy replace fine-needle aspiration cytology in the diagnosis of palpable breast carcinoma: comparative study of 124 women. Cancer 1996; 78(42):773–777.

Ciatto S, Pacini P, Azzine V, et al. Pre-operative staging of primary breast cancer; a multicenter study. Cancer 1988; 61:1038.

Nath ME, Robinson TM, Tobon H, Clough DM, Sumkin JH. Automated large-core needle biopsy of surgically removed breast lesions: comparison of samples obtained with 14–16 and 18 gauge needles. Radiology 1995; 197:739–742.

Case #A.1.6
Goal: To discuss the multistage operative approach to breast lesions

MONICA MORROW

A 67-year-old woman presents with a 1.5-cm, palpable lesion; fine-needle aspirate is read as "suspicious for malignancy." The mammogram shows a highly suspicious spiculated lesion without other abnormalities.

When a fine-needle aspiration (FNA) is read as "suspicious," this is not sufficiently diagnostic of carcinoma to proceed directly to definitive therapy; as many as 20% of these lesions will be benign. In the case described above, there are three good options: (1) repeat the FNA in an attempt to obtain a diagnostic specimen; (2) perform a core needle biopsy (Tru-cut biopsy) in the office; (3) discuss cancer treatment options with the patient, perform a biopsy with an intraoperative frozen section to confirm the diagnosis, and proceed immediately to definitive surgery. The latter approach is appropriate only when the clinical examination and the mammogram are highly suggestive of malignancy. When considering this approach, it is important to remember that frozen section will not provide a definitive diagnosis in 100% of cases. Problems may occur in the diagnosis of papillary lesions and in identifying invasion in large areas of intraductal carcinoma.

A major problem with the use of a one-stage procedure is the difficulty patients have in selecting a local therapy when they are not sure if they have invasive cancer. I generally reserve this approach for older women who require mastectomy and are not candidates for breast reconstruction. In other patients who are potential candidates for breast preservation or those who are unsure of their preference, we perform an outpatient biopsy under local anesthesia as a lumpectomy. This has the advantage of providing a definitive histological diagnosis and allowing an evaluation of whether an axillary dissection is indicated. Some of the carcinomas that are termed "suspicious" by cytology will be well-differentiated lesions, such as tubular carcinoma, with a very low risk of axillary metastases.

The cost-effectiveness of a one-stage procedure will vary according to the number of women with suspicious cytology who turn out to have benign disease. These women will sustain increased costs with this approach as well as increased anxiety. The use of needle biopsy techniques in the office renders this approach unnecessary in the vast majority of cases.

BIBLIOGRAPHY

Foster RS. Techniques for diagnosis of palpable breast masses. In: Harris JR, Lippman ME, Morrow M, Hellman S, eds. Diseases of the Breast. Philadelphia: Lippincott-Raven, 1996:133–143.

Hamond S, Keyhani-Rofagha S, O'Toole R. Statistical analysis of fine needle aspiration cytology of the breast. A review of 678 cases plus 4,265 cases from the literature. ACTA Cytol 1987; 31:276–280.

Lannin DR, Silverman JF, Pories WJ, Walker C. Cost-effectiveness of fine needle biopsy of the breast. Ann Surg 1986; 203:474–480.

Case #A.1.7
Goal: To discuss the management of phyllodes tumors

KIRBY I. BLAND and DANIEL S. KIM

A 31-year-old woman who is 3 years post excision of a reported fibroadenoma presents with a 7-cm, recurrent breast mass. Mammogram reveals indistinct borders, but no clear indicators of malignancy.

Fibroadenoma is the most common solid breast tumor in women younger than 30 years and has a peak incidence in the years 21–25. Growth of fibroadenomas is generally self-limiting and the majority will regress or remain stable in size. Further evidence for regression is the fact that fibroadenomas are uncommon after the third decade and postmortem studies have reported rare occurrences in women older than 40 years. Although fibroadenoma is not considered a premalignant lesion, more than 100 cases of carcinoma arising in a fibroadenoma have been reported.

If this patient's breast mass was a fibroadenoma 3 years ago, is it a recurrent fibroadenoma, did it undergo malignant transformation, or did it progress to a phyllodes tumor? Alternatively, was it a phyllodes tumor 3 years ago and not a fibroadenoma?

Although fibroadenomas can recur, and do recur more commonly in black women, it is unlikely that this mass is a recurrent fibroadenoma because of its large size. Malignant transformation, if it truly occurs, is rare and is also unlikely because of the large size attained in only 3 years. The possibility of a fibroadenoma progressing to a phyllodes tumor is not well documented, although supported by some authors. This is a possibility in this patient.

Another possibility is that the initial mass was not a fibroadenoma but a phyllodes tumor. Both lesions bear a histological resemblance in that they are composed of epithelial and stromal components that are similarly arranged. The term "phyllodes tumors" is often applied to large fibroadenomas with some hypercellularity. Some authors use up to three mitoses per high-power field as a cutoff between phyllodes and fibroadenoma. Phyllodes tumors also have varying degrees of nuclear atypia and leaf-like projections of stroma. In some cases, particularly with a giant fibroadenoma or the so-called juvenile fibroadenoma, a clear distinction is impossible.

The appropriate diagnostic workup of this patient has already begun with physical examination and mammography. Next, we would proceed with a fine-needle aspiration. The combination of a mobile mass with distinct borders, mammographic findings of lobulated, benign-appearing opacities without calcifications, and cytology revealing both epithelial and stromal elements would be suggestive of a phyllodes tumor. However, as previously mentioned, distinguishing this from a fibroadenoma may be difficult. The final diagnostic test, as well as treatment, would be complete excision. Phyllodes tumor has presented clinicians with uncertainty regarding its nomenclature, diagnosis, prognostic features, and treatment. Phyllodes tumor accounts for 0.3–0.5% of breast tumors in females. The majority occur in women between the ages of 35 and 55 years. In Reinfuss et al.'s review of 170 patients, the tumor size ranged from 2 to 40 cm, with a mean of 7 cm.

Although no definite prognostic factors have been established, the histological grade may have the most long-term significance. Reinfuss et al. found that histological grading of benign, borderline, and malignant, based on tumor margin, growth of the connective tissue component, mitoses, and cellular atypia, was the only prognostic factor. Reinfuss et al. report 5-year disease-free survival for benign, borderline, and malignant tumors of 95.7%, 73.7%, and 66.1%, respectively. Others have suggested stromal overgrowth, tumor necrosis, infiltrating margins, mixed mesenchymal components, mitoses, atypia, aneuploidy, and S fraction to be prognostic. The tumor size and patient age have not been found to be prognostic.

The treatment of choice is complete surgical excision and the standard treatment should be wide local excision. Smaller tumors may be adequately treated with local excision if margins of normal breast tissue are a minimum of 1 cm. Larger tumors may require simple mastectomy if the tumor size and breast size do not allow both good margins and cosmesis. There is no indication for axillary dissection because lymph node metastases are rare, even in malignant phyllodes tumors. Local recurrences occur because of incomplete excision and do not imply malignant transformation, systemic spread, or poor prognosis. Local recurrences are treated with wide local excision or mastectomy. We would treat this patient with wide local excision if her breast size is adequate.

Metastatic disease occurs more commonly in the borderline and malignant histological types and most commonly affects the lungs, bone, and brain. Patients may receive some short-term benefit from chemotherapy and survival is poor, ranging from 2 to 11 months, with a mean survival of 4 months.

BIBLIOGRAPHY

Alle KM, Moss J, Venegas RJ, et al. Conservative management of fibroadenoma of the breast. Br J Surg 1996; 83:992–993.

Carty NJ, Carter C, Rubin C, et al. Management of fibroadenoma of the breast. Ann R Coll Surg Engl 1995; 77:127–130.

Diaz NM, Palmer JO, McDivitt RW. Carcinoma arising within fibroadenomas of the breast: a clinicopathologic study of 105 patients. Am J Clin Pathol 1991; 95: 614–622.

Iglehart JD. The breast. In: Sabiston DC, ed. Textbook of Surgery, 15th ed. Philadelphia: WB Saunders, 1997:555–593.

MacKenzie I. Breast cancer following multiple fluoroscopies. Br J Cancer 1965; 19: 1–8.

Noguchi S, Yokouchi H, Aihara T, et al. Progression of fibroadenoma to phyllodes tumor demonstrated by clonal analysis. Cancer 1995; 76:1779–1785.

Page DL, Simpson JF. Benign, high-risk, and premalignant lesions of the breast. In: Bland KI, Copeland EM, eds. The Breast: Comprehensive Management of Benign and Malignant Diseases, 2nd ed. Philadelphia: WB Saunders, 1998: 191–213.

Reinfuss M, Mitus J, Duda K, et al. The treatment and prognosis of patients with phyllodes tumor of the breast, an analysis of 170 cases. Cancer 1996; 77:910–916.

Sainsbury JR, Nicholson S, Needham GK, et al. Natural history of the benign breast lump. Br J Surg 1988; 75:1080–1082.

Stebbing JF, Nash AG. Diagnosis and management of phyllodes tumour of the breast: experience of 33 cases at a specialist centre. Ann R Coll Surg Engl 1995; 77: 181–184.

Case #A.1.8
Goal: To discuss the interpretation of fine-needle aspiration findings in a premenopausal woman over age 30

THOMAS J. KEARNEY

A 43-year-old woman presents with a new, nontender, 3-cm, mobile left breast mass. Fine-needle aspiration cytology demonstrates myoepithelial cells consistent with a fibroadenoma. The remainder of her examination is unremarkable. The family history is noncontributory.

The presence of functional glandular tissue in premenopausal women, combined with a progressively increasing incidence of cancer after the age of 30 years, makes the evaluation of palpable breast masses between age 30 and menopause problematic. The standard for the diagnosis of a palpable breast mass is excisional biopsy with pathological analysis. However, smaller tissue specimens can be diagnostic and easier to obtain. Cytology specimens obtained by fine-needle aspiration (FNA) can often distinguish between benign and malignant lesions, permitting rapid, minimally invasive diagnosis of many palpable breast masses. If FNA reveals a breast cyst containing nonbloody fluid that resolves on aspiration, no further evaluation is needed. A 4–6-week follow-up should be scheduled to ensure that the lesion has not recurred. The aspirated nonbloody fluid does not require analysis. If the mass is solid, the FNA specimen can be placed in fixative for cytological evaluation. In centers where breast ultrasound is immediately available, the distinction between a cystic mass and a solid mass can be readily made. Cystic masses require no intervention unless they are symptomatic. Solid masses require further evaluation. It would be superfluous to perform both breast ultrasound and FNA in patients with cystic masses.

The incidence of false-positive FNA is approximately 0.2%. The false-negative rate can vary greatly, between 0.5 and 35%. The most common reason for a false-negative FNA is an inadequate sample. An FNA sample that contains insufficient cells cannot be used for evaluation of a mass and must be repeated. If there are an adequate number of cells, the FNA report will result in one of three findings; malignant or atypical cells, specific benign cells such as myoepithelial cells, or nonspecific benign cells such as epithelial cells or adipose cells. The third finding raises the possibility that the lesion was missed.

The accuracy of FNA can be improved through the use of the "triple test." When an adequate FNA with a benign finding is combined with a benign physical examination and a benign appearance to the mass on mammography, observation is safe. If the mass is not seen on mammography, the triple test is invalid and excisional biopsy should be performed. The sensitivity of a concordant triple test exceeds 95%. Ultrasound can substitute for mammography to provide a modified triple test. If even one component of the triple test is discordant, a surgical biopsy must be done. If the FNA shows malignancy, definitive surgery can be planned. It would be prudent to obtain an intraoperative frozen section if mastectomy is chosen over breast conservation due to the small, but real, false-positive rate of FNA. If the triple test is concordant, repeat evaluation at 3-month intervals for 1 year is safe.

For this patient, I recommend bilateral mammography. If the results of the mammography are concordant with the physical examination and the FNA cytology, physical examination should be repeated in 3 months. If the results are discordant, excisional biopsy is indicated.

BIBLIOGRAPHY

Layfield LJ, Glasgow BJ, Cramer H. Fine needle aspiration in the management of breast masses. Pathol Annu 1989; 24:23.

Steinberg JL, Trudeau ME, Ryder DE, et al. Combined fine-needle aspiration, physical examination and mammography in the diagnosis of palpable breast masses: their relation to outcome for women with primary breast cancer. Can J Surg 1996; 39:302–311.

Vetto JT, Pomier RF, Schmidt WA, et al. Diagnosis of palpable breast lesions in younger women by the modified triple test is accurate and cost-effective. Arch Surg 1996; 131:967–974.

Case #A.1.9
Goal: To discuss the management of a recurrent simple cyst in a premenopausal woman over age 30

SUSAN A. MCMANUS

A 33-year-old woman presents with a new, tender, 4-cm, mobile right breast mass. Fine-needle aspiration obtains 12 cc of serous, nonbloody fluid and results in resolution of the palpable abnormality. No studies are performed. The patient presents 8 weeks later for reevaluation because the mass has returned.

Cyst aspiration is the best initial procedure, for it is both diagnostic and therapeutic. In today's managed care environment, it is likely that this patient had seen her gynecologist or primary care physician, who performed the aspiration. Return of the cyst would then dictate referral to a surgeon for further management. Reaspiration should be performed, for many times the cyst has not been completely aspirated, is a new cyst, or is one that was adjacent to the cyst that was aspirated. If the cyst does not resolve or if the fluid is bloody, further investigation and possible biopsy are indicated.

An ultrasound should be performed if the mass does not yield fluid on aspiration, if the mass does not resolve completely with aspiration, or if a mass is noted by the radiologist on a screening mammogram. Ultrasound of the breast can have a greater than 95% accuracy in diagnosing cysts. Typically, cysts are well circumscribed, smoothly marginated, thin-walled, and have an echo-free center with distal echogenic shadowing. Occasionally, a medullary carcinoma can resemble a cyst on ultrasound. Complex or atypical cysts require further workup with either ultrasound-guided aspiration or needle localization biopsy. While screening mammography is not routinely advised for women in their early 30s, diagnostic mammography can be very helpful. In one study of women younger than 35 years, 90% of cancers were visualized on mammography. In other studies of women younger than 40 with cancer, mammograms visualized the lesion in 65–75% of cases.

Fluid that is either grossly nonbloody or contains occult blood does not require cytological evaluation. However, if grossly bloody fluid is obtained, it is useful to send a sample for cytological evaluation. The diagnosis of intracystic carcinoma should be suspected if bloody fluid is obtained, if the cyst is not resolved with aspiration, or if a cyst occurs in a postmenopausal female who is not on estrogen replacement therapy. The patient then requires bilateral mammography followed by surgery. Leaving some fluid within the cyst will allow for easier intraoperative detection. Surgery is required even if the cytology is negative.

In all, approximately 15% of cysts recur. Biochemical analyses have been performed on cyst fluid to aid in diagnosis and prognosis. Those that contain a high K^+/Na^+ ratio are likely to have a benign apocrine epithelium and have a much higher incidence of recurrence. Some suggest that injection of air into the cyst following aspiration can decrease recurrence. Pneumocystography can often demonstrate a cyst as well as an intracystic lesion.

The absolute number of cyst aspirations is not as important as the need to determine whether the cyst resolved after aspiration and whether or not the fluid was bloody. For this patient the fluid is not bloody and merely represents the recurrence of a simple cyst. A repeat clinical examination in 4 months is recommended.

BIBLIOGRAPHY

Devitt JE. The clinical recognition of cystic carcinoma of the breast. Surg Gynecol Obstet 1984; 159:130–132.

Forrest APM, Kirkpatrick JR, Roberts MM. Needle aspiration of breast cysts. Br Med J 1995; 3:30–31.

Hughes LE, Mansel RE, Webster DJT. Cysts of the breast. In: Benign Disorders and Diseases of the Breast: Concepts and Clinical Management. London: Bailliere, Tindall, 1989:93–102.

Meyer JE, Kopans DB, Oot R. Breast cancer visualized by mammography in patients under 35. Radiology 1983; 147:93–94.

Case #A.1.10
Goal: To discuss the management of a breast cyst from the point of view of the radiologist

PHYLLIS J. KORNGUTH

A 37-year-old woman presents with a new, tender, 3-cm, mobile right breast mass. Fine-needle aspiration obtains 7 cc of blue-tinged, nonbloody fluid and results in resolution of the palpable abnormality.

From a breast-imaging standpoint, the question arises: does this woman need any breast imaging? If so, why? and what kind? If not, why not? From a clinical perspective, the simplest diagnostic (and therapeutic) step has been taken and has been effective in defining and solving this patient's immediate problem. A fine-needle aspiration has differentiated between a cystic and a solid lesion; the aspirated fluid appears typical of a benign cyst; and the palpable mass has been treated and resolved. The patient will be followed clinically and as long as the cyst does not recur, no further workup is necessary. In this particular scenario, many feel that the diagnosis of benign cyst is reliable and there is little information that will be added by mammography or ultrasound examination of this 37-year-old woman with a palpable mass.

There is another approach to this clinical problem. Many experts believe that imaging is an integral and valuable part of the workup of a palpable mass. The particular modality used may vary according to the age of the patient, with sonography being the technique of choice in very young women as it involves no ionizing radiation. The use of preaspiration and/or postaspiration imaging not only provides a means of evaluating the mass, but can determine management. If preaspiration sonography demonstrates the mass to be a simple cyst, the workup is terminated and the patient is spared an invasive procedure. If the mass is solid or is a complex cyst or has thick walls, then tissue sampling is performed either with fine-needle aspiration or biopsy. If a cyst contains a mural nodule, excisional biopsy of the mass rather than aspiration should be undertaken to exclude an intracystic papillary carcinoma. If the mass is shown to be a septated cyst or a cluster of cysts, then needle aspiration may not result in complete resolution of the mass and the mass may recur after incomplete aspiration. Since recurrence of a cyst can be a sign of underlying malignancy, it is important that the cyst be aspirated completely. Postaspiration sonography may be used to assure that the cyst has been aspirated to dryness, thus decreasing the chances that it will recur.

Table 1 Estimated New Breast Cancer Cases in Women by Age, 1996

Age	Estimate[a]	Percent of total
20–29	510	0.3%
30–39	8,700	4.7%
40–49	33,400	18.1%
50–59	30,900	16.8%
60–69	40,000	21.7%
70–79	44,700	24.3%
80+	26,000	14.1%
Total	184,300	100.0%

[a]Estimates may not add to total due to rounding.
Source: American Cancer Society, Surveillance Research, 1995. Data from SEER, 1995.

Pre-aspiration mammography is helpful not only in evaluating the mass itself, but in screening the remainder of that breast as well as the contralateral breast for nonpalpable disease. This is especially true for older women since the risk of carcinoma rises steadily with increasing age. (see Table 1.) While carcinoma is not common in women under the age of 40 (accounting for only 5% of new cases in 1996), the incidence begins to rise as a woman approaches 40, and thus, a mammogram should be performed in any woman over 35 who presents with a palpable mass, if she has not had a recent screening exam.

BIBLIOGRAPHY

Breast Cancer Facts and Figures 1996. American Cancer Society, Atlanta, GA, 1996.
Cady B. How to perform breast biopsies. Surg Oncol Clin North Am 1995; 4:47.

A.2.   NONPALPABLE BREAST LESIONS

Case #A.2.1
Goal: To discuss the management of a stable, nonpalpable, mammographic abnormality

PHYLLIS J. KORNGUTH

A 63-year-old woman undergoes routine screening mammography for the first time in 2 years. She is found to have a 1.5-cm cluster of indeterminate microcalcifications in the upper inner quadrant of the left breast. Old mammograms are obtained, and these calcifications appear unchanged from 4 years ago.

The management of any mammographic abnormality involves a number of steps beginning with a full assessment of the lesion and ending with appropriate recommendations to the woman and her referring physician. A thorough evaluation of lesion characteristics involves not only the mammographic appearance, including any special views, but also the results of adjunctive tests such as physical examination, ultrasound examination, and so forth. The sine qua non for evaluation of a cluster of microcalcifications are magnification views (Fig. 1). Calcifications are often difficult to characterize on standard mammographic views and their configuration may be more accurately determined on magnified images. It is sometimes possible to make a recommendation for management on the basis of mammographic appearance alone; for example, if the calcifications look very suspicious on the magnification views, biopsy will be recommended. If they are typically benign, no additional follow-up will be suggested. However, if the abnormality is neither typically malignant nor typically benign in its mammo-

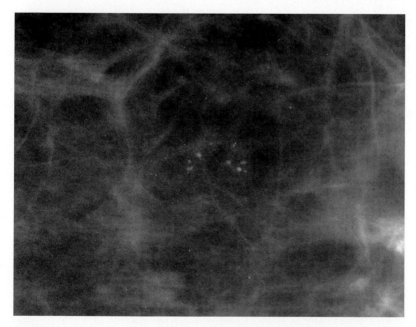

Figure 1   Microcalcifications seen on magnification view.

graphic appearance, then additional information from two more sources is necessary before a final assessment is made.

Comparison with prior studies, if they are available, speaks to the stability of the abnormality. If a lesion appears relatively benign and one can demonstrate stability on mammograms for 2–3 years, it is much more likely that one is dealing with a benign entity and tissue sampling is not necessary. If, on the other hand, there has been a change in the lesion (the mass has enlarged or the cluster of microcalcifications has increased in number), biopsy will be the recommendation for management. The final data comes from *patient* demographics and her clinical and family history. For example, an abnormality that appears fairly benign and would ordinarily be followed mammographically might be more suspicious in a woman who has had a previous contralateral breast cancer and tissue sampling will be recommended.

Once all of this information has been gathered, the radiologist will make a final assessment and recommendation for management. If a lesion is considered benign, only routine screening will be suggested. If a lesion is felt to be probably benign, it should be followed mammographically. This is considered safe since fewer than 2% of these abnormalities will turn out to be carcinoma, and more importantly, when they are biopsied because of a change in their mammographic appearance, they have the same good prognosis as if biopsied initially. A probably benign abnormality should be followed with a unilateral examination in 6 months and bilateral studies at 12 and 24 months. In the case of a cluster of microcalcifications, magnification views must be done at all of the follow-up examinations to assess possible change. An indeterminate lesion is one that is not convincingly benign in mammographic appearance. This category of lesion is most appropriately diagnosed with the least invasive and most accurate tissue-sampling technique since the majority (approximately 80%) will be benign on biopsy and the patient should be spared open surgical biopsy. Fine-needle aspiration may be the technique of choice in certain hands, but it is a very operator-dependent technique. Its reliability and accuracy depend on very experienced individuals, both the person doing the aspirating and the pathologist interpreting the breast cytology. In inexperienced hands, the rate of insufficient samples can be as high as 38% and sensitivity can vary from 68 to 93%. Image-guided needle core biopsy has been shown to be as accurate as open surgical biopsy and is ideally suited for tissue sampling of an indeterminate lesion. For lesions that are considered to have a high probability of malignancy, biopsy (either needle core or excisional) is recommended.

In the above scenario, the cluster of microcalcifications first seen on a screening examination are then examined on magnification views. The radiologist feels that they are neither typically benign nor typically malignant and must either establish their stability or tissue-sample them. Attempts to obtain old films are successful and the cluster is shown to have been stable for 4 years. Thus, they are now considered to be benign and no further immediate workup is necessary. If old films were not available, these indeterminate calcifications should be sampled by means of vacuum-assisted stereotactic needle core biopsy.

BIBLIOGRAPHY

Sickles EA. Periodic mammographic follow-up of probably benign lesions: results in 3,184 consecutive cases. Radiology 1991; 179:463–468.
Sickles EA, Parker SH. Appropriate role of core breast biopsy in the management of probably benign lesions. Radiology 1993; 188:315.

Case #A.2.2
Goal: To discuss the management of a simple cyst detected radiologically

PHYLLIS J. KORNGUTH

A 71-year-old woman undergoes annual screening mammography. She is found to have a new, 1.5-cm, well-marginated density in the outer portion of the right breast. Breast ultrasound is performed and reveals a simple cyst corresponding in location to the mammographic abnormality (Fig. 1A–D).

This case illustrates the appropriate imaging workup of a new, well-defined mass on mammogram. A mass lesion that is well circumscribed and smoothly marginated is most likely a benign mass, since the two most common entities that present with this mammographic appearance are a cyst or a fibroadenoma. If this appearance were pathognomonic of a benign abnormality, no further workup would be necessary. Unfortunately, some malignant processes (both primary malignancies and metastatic lesions) can share this mammographic presentation and it is necessary to further evaluate the mass. This is particularly true in an elderly woman, since benign cysts and fibroadenomas most commonly occur in the 35–50-year age group and are uncommon in postmenopausal women unless they are on hormonal replacement therapy. Carcinoma is much more common in older women and any new mass (whether palpable or nonpalpable) must be further evaluated in this age group.

The simplest and least invasive method of evaluation is sonographic interrogation. Ultrasound is used strictly as an adjunctive study with one purpose (and only one purpose) in mind, namely, to define a mass as cystic

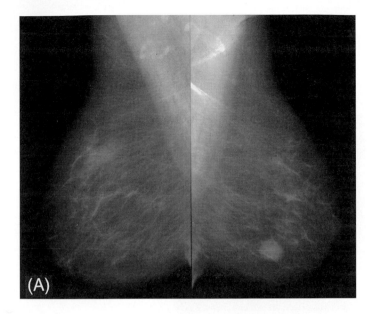

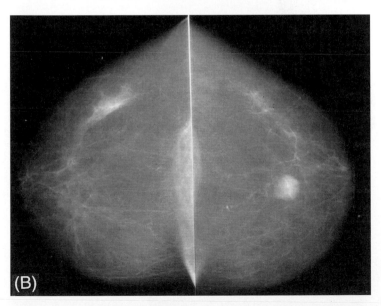

Figure 1 Mediolateral oblique (A), craniocaudal (B), and coned-down (C) views from a screening mammogram show a 1.5-cm, well-defined mass at 6:00 in the left breast. Ultrasound (D) shows the mass to be a simple cyst.

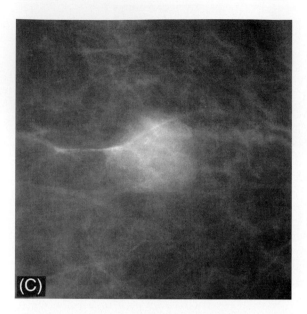

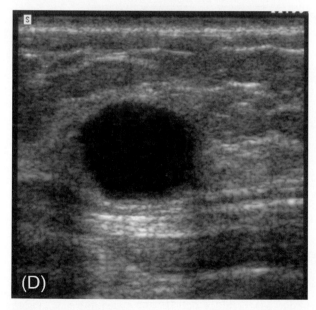

Figure 1 Continued

or solid. Ultrasound is not yet capable of accurately differentiating benign from malignant solid masses, but it is capable of defining a simple cyst. If the mass is shown to be a simple cyst, that is the end of the diagnostic workup. Neither aspiration nor imaging follow-up is required. If the size or location of the cyst is causing the patient discomfort, then aspiration should be done for symptom relief, but simple cysts are considered benign and need not be further considered.

Case #A.2.3
Goal: To discuss the management of a new, "benign-appearing" mammographic density in a postmenopausal woman

CAROL H. LEE

A 61-year-old woman undergoes her first screening mammogram; no old mammograms are available. She is found to have a smooth, well-marginated, 1.3-cm right breast mass. Breast ultrasound demonstrates the lesion as solid, homogeneous, and with distinct margins. The nodule is not palpable.

Nonpalpable, smooth, well-circumscribed masses discovered by mammography are usually benign. The likelihood of malignancy for such a finding, based on several series, is on the order of $1-2\%$. Other mammographic abnormalities that have been shown to have a low likelihood of malignancy include single or multiple clusters of smooth, round or oval calcifications, diffusely scattered tiny calcifications, focal asymmetrical densities with concave margins and interspersed fat, and asymptomatic solitary dilated ducts. In one study of over 3000 cases deemed to be "probably benign" by mammography, 0.5% ultimately proved to be malignant and all of these were small tumors with favorable prognoses. Because of the low rate of malignancy of these lesions, follow-up with short-interval mammography rather than biopsy is felt to be an appropriate management strategy.

It is generally agreed that nonpalpable, noncalcified masses with well-circumscribed, smooth margins should be included in the probably benign category (Fig. 1). There is some disagreement, however, on whether the size of the mass or the age of the patient should be taken into consideration before deciding whether a mass is probably benign. Some advocate biopsy of all well-circumscribed masses over 1 cm in diameter. Similarly, some recommend biopsy of well-circumscribed masses in younger women with the rationale that cancers in younger women tend to have a faster rate of growth and therefore should not be watched. Others recommend biopsy of these masses in older women, citing the increased incidence of breast cancer

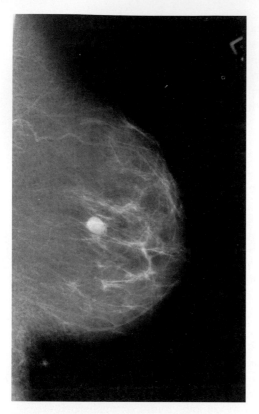

Figure 1   Mammographic appearance of a benign mass.

with increasing age and the higher positive predictive value of a mammographic abnormality among older women. In one series of 1400 well-circumscribed masses, 1.4% ultimately proved to be malignant. Although there was a slightly increased likelihood of malignancy among larger masses and among masses in older women, the differences were not statistically significant and it was concluded that neither size nor patient age should preclude an otherwise benign-appearing mass from being managed with mammographic surveillance.

In the patient presented here, ultrasound would be the next step in evaluation of the mammographically detected mass to determine whether it is cystic or solid. If the mass meets all the criteria for a simple cyst by ultrasound and is asymptomatic, no further evaluation or follow-up is needed. For solid masses, recent studies using high-resolution ultrasound equipment suggest that sonographic features can help differentiate benign from malignant masses. By ultrasound, benign masses are oriented parallel to the skin surface and have an elliptical shape, well-defined margins, and homogeneous internal echoes (Fig. 2). However, the accuracy of using ultrasound criteria alone to determine whether a mass is benign or malignant has yet to be definitively determined. In this patient, once the mass was shown to be solid by ultrasound, the next step in its evaluation would be magnification views to better assess its margins. Magnification images can reveal subtle spiculation or microlobulation of masses not readily apparent on standard views. If the mass is indeed spiculated or microlobulated, it would not fall into the probably benign category and would need to be biopsied.

In this 61-year-old woman with a smooth, 1.3-cm mass with benign mammographic and ultrasound features and a likelihood of malignancy of 2% or less, mammographic surveillance would be a reasonable management recommendation. A typical surveillance protocol would require a unilateral mammogram in 6 months. If the mass is unchanged, a bilateral mammogram 6 months after that and then yearly thereafter would be recommended. Although there have been reported cases of malignant masses that have remained unchanged for many years, this is an unusual occurrence and documented stability over 2–3 years is generally regarded as evidence that a mass is benign. Patients with mammographic abnormalities that can be classified by their appearance as probably benign should be informed of the low probability of malignancy and the importance of compliance with the short-interval surveillance recommendation.

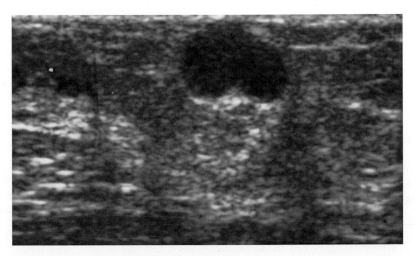

Figure 2 Ultrasound of a benign cystic lesion.

The "ideal" positive biopsy rate is a matter of debate. Some advocate that a 10% positive biopsy rate maximizes the chance of decreasing mortality through aggressive evaluation of mammographically detected abnormalities. Others, citing morbidity and cost associated with biopsy, consider a 40% yield of malignant biopsies to be more appropriate. Most would agree, however, that routinely recommending biopsy for lesions with a positive predictive value of 2% or less is not warranted. If, however, despite reassurance of the likely benign nature of the mass and the extremely low likelihood of malignancy the patient desires biopsy, this could be achieved in this case with ultrasound or stereotaxically guided core needle biopsy rather than open surgical biopsy. In this particular case, the patient elected mammographic surveillance and the mass was unchanged over 3 years of follow-up. The patient was put back into the routine screening pool and the mass has remained stable.

BIBLIOGRAPHY

Brenner RJ, Sickles EA. Acceptability of periodic follow-up as an alternative to biopsy for mammographically detected lesions interpreted as probably benign. Radiology 1989; 171:645–646.

Helvie MA, Pennes DR, Rebner M, et al. Mammographic follow-up of low-suspicion lesions: compliance rate and diagnostic yield. Radiology 1991;178:155–158.

Sickles EA. Periodic mammographic follow-up of probably benign lesions: results in 3,184 consecutive cases. Radiology 1991; 179:463–468.

Sickles EA. Nonpalpable, circumscribed, noncalcified solid breast masses: likelihood of malignancy based on lesion size and age of patient. Radiology 1994; 192: 439–442.

Stavros AT, Thickman D, Rapp CL, et al. Solid breast nodules: use of sonography to distinguish benign and malignant lesions. Radiology 1995; 196:123–134.

Varas X, Leborgne F, Leborgne JH. Nonpalpable, probably benign lesions: role of follow-up mammography. Radiology 1992; 184:409–414.

Case #A.2.4
Goal: To discuss the use of stereotaxic biopsy

CAROL H. LEE

A 47-year-old woman, who on screening mammography was found to have an 8-mm, well-defined nodule associated with indeterminate-appearing microcalcifications, presents for evaluation. Her family history is unremarkable. She is nulliparous.

A well-circumscribed mass smaller than 1 cm has a very high likelihood of being benign, and most feel such a lesion can be appropriately managed by short-interval follow-up mammography rather than biopsy. If calcifications are present within the mass, however, these must be evaluated independently, and if by their appearance they are considered indeterminate or suspicious for malignancy, the mass no longer belongs in the "probably benign" category and the lesion should be biopsied.

The traditional method for obtaining tissue diagnosis of a nonpalpable lesion is surgical excision preceded by needle localization, and this remains the "gold standard" by which other biopsy techniques are measured. More recently, however, image-guided needle biopsy has been employed with increasing frequency as an alternative to surgical biopsy in the evaluation of suspicious mammographic abnormalities. Needle biopsy can be accomplished with ultrasound or stereotaxic guidance. In stereotaxic needle biopsy, two images of the breast are obtained at 15° angles off center. The exact location of the abnormality within the breast can be calculated by measuring the relative movement of the lesion between the two images. Once the location of the lesion is determined, either by ultrasound, which is most appropriate for masses, or by stereotaxis, fine-needle aspiration (FNA) using a small-bore needle (usually 22 gauge) can be performed to obtain cells for cytology, or core needle biopsy using a large-bore needle (usually 14 gauge) can be employed to obtain actual tissue samples from the lesion. FNA has the advantages of being quick, easily performed, and minimally invasive. The disadvantages of FNA compared to core or excisional biopsy, however, include a higher rate of insufficient material, a higher chance of false-positive results, the inability to determine whether a malignancy is in situ or invasive, and the need for a skilled cytopathologist to interpret the results.

Several studies have shown good correlation between the results of stereotaxic core needle biopsy (SCNB) and subsequent surgical excision with a reported false-negative rate of 1.5% or less. Long-term follow-up studies of large numbers of patients who have undergone SCNB with benign results are not yet available; as longer follow-up is performed it is likely that the false-negative rate will be shown to be higher than is currently reported, although probably not substantially so. The potential benefits of SCNB must be weighed against the possibility of a lower sensitivity for diagnosing malignancy.

The advantages of SCNB over excisional biopsy include shorter procedure time, lower morbidity, and the absence of internal or external scarring of the breast. No special preparation is necessary by the patient prior to the procedure, only local anesthesia is used and the patient can immediately resume normal levels of activity. In addition, the cost of SCNB is substantially less than that of excisional biopsy. The use of SCNB was shown in one study to prevent the need for surgery in 77% of 182 patients with an overall decrease in cost of diagnosis of 55%. This would translate into an annual savings of $200 million nationwide. In another study of cost-effectiveness of SCNB, the procedure was found to save biopsy and save costs for all categories of nonpalpable mammographic abnormalities regardless of size, type of finding (mass or calcifications), or level of suspicion. The greatest savings occurred with lower-suspicion masses. The least savings occurred with highly suspicious calcifications, but even in this circumstance, $446 was saved per case. The cost savings associated with the use of SCNB over surgical biopsy assumes a similar positive predictive value of lesions biopsied. If lesions with a low likelihood of malignancy undergo SCNB rather than short-interval follow-up mammography, the cost of evaluating mammographic abnormalities will actually increase.

In the case presented here, the presence of indeterminate calcifications within the mass mandates that biopsy be performed (Fig. 1). After discussion

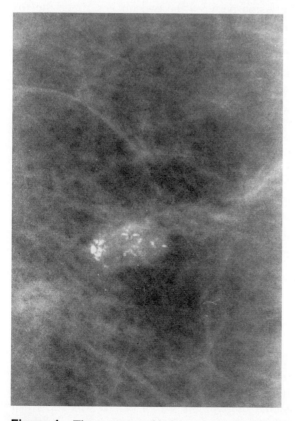

Figure 1   The presence of indeterminate calcifications within a mass mandates that biopsy be performed.

with the patient and her referring physician, SCNB was elected. Radiograph of the excised cores, similar to the specimen radiograph obtained at the time of needle localization and excisional biopsy, documented that the targeted calcifications had indeed been sampled. Histological examination of the excised cores revealed a fibroadenoma that had undergone hyaline degeneration and contained calcifications. This was considered a specific benign diagnosis, which was concordant with the mammographic finding. No further evaluation was deemed necessary and the recommendation in this case was for the patient to undergo routine yearly screening mammography in the future.

BIBLIOGRAPHY

Elvecrog EL, Lechner MC, Nelson MT. Nonpalpable breast lesions: correlation of stereotaxic large-core needle biopsy and surgical biopsy results. Radiology 1993; 188:453–455.

Hilner BE, Bear HD, Fajardo LL. Estimating the cost-effectiveness of stereotaxic biopsy for nonpalpable breast abnormalities: a decision analysis model. Acad Radiol 1996; 3:351–360.

Jackman RJ, Nowels KW, Shepard MJ, et al. Stereotaxic large-core needle biopsy of 450 nonpalpable breast lesions with surgical correlation in lesions with cancer or atypical hyperplasia. Radiology 1994; 193:91–95.

Lee CH, Egglin TK, Philpotts L, et al. Cost-effectiveness of stereotactic core needle biopsy: analysis by means of mammographic findings. Radiology 1997; 202:849–854.

Liberman L, Fahs MC, Dershaw DD, et al. Impact of stereotaxic core breast biopsy on cost of diagnosis. Radiology 1995; 195:633–637.

Parker SH, Burbank F, Jackman RJ, et al. Percutaneous large-core breast biopsy: a multi-institutional study. Radiology 1994; 193:359–364.

Case #A.2.5
Goal: To discuss the diagnostic evaluation of suspicious-appearing microcalcifications

PHYLLIS J. KORNGUTH

A 46-year-old woman undergoes her first screening mammography and is noted to have a "suspicious" (BiRads class V) cluster of microcalcifications in the left breast (Fig. 1). The radiologist recommends a stereotaxic X-ray-guided biopsy. The patient sees a surgeon, who recommends an operative excisional biopsy with wire localization. She comes to seek your opinion regarding optimal management.

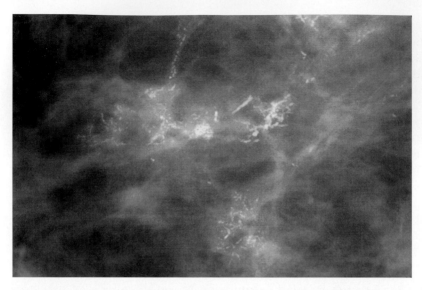

Figure 1 Mammogram, left craniocaudad view, of a 46-year-old woman revealing a suspicious cluster of microcalfications.

To date, there are two schools of thought as to the appropriate use of stereotaxic needle core biopsy (SNCB) in the diagnosis of a nonpalpable mammographic abnormality. One group of experts feels that any mammographic abnormality that has a high probability of being malignant (>20%) should be needle-localized and entirely removed at open surgical biopsy (OSB). This allows the patient and the surgeon to make therapeutic choices based on a larger volume of tissue than is taken by needle core biopsy. For example, the presence of an extensive intraductal component may not be evident on needle cores and its presence may favor mastectomy rather than lumpectomy as the treatment of choice. The use of SNCB for a suspicious mammographic lesion is felt to interpose an additional procedure and expense into the diagnostic workup and should *only* be used in those instances when it has been determined that mastectomy will be the surgical treatment, because of either (1) patient preference, (2) multiple suspicious lesions in one breast, or (3) serious comorbid conditions that preclude prolonged or multiple surgeries. SNCB is more appropriately used for more benign-appearing lesions (i.e., those having a <20% chance of being malignant), thus providing a less expensive and less invasive technique to make the diagnosis and sparing the patient an operation for benign disease.

The other point of view embraces stereotaxic needle core biopsy to make the initial diagnosis of malignancy. It is felt that if invasive carcinoma is shown to be present, then the surgeon can plan to do a lumpectomy and axillary node dissection at one operation, rather than subjecting the patient to two surgical procedures.

Both of these approaches are valid and depend on the philosophy of the breast surgeon and the informed choice of the patient. A multi-institutional, federally funded study is now underway looking at the appropriate use of stereotaxic needle core biopsy in the evaluation of nonpalpable breast lesions; the results are not yet available.

In counseling this patient, it is important to point out the advantages, disadvantages, and limitations of both SNCB and OSB. Open surgical (excisional) biopsy is considered to be the gold standard of breast biopsy diagnosis. Its accuracy is often assumed to be 100%, although false-negatives have been reported to be as high as 10% and false-positives <1%. It has the advantages of fully removing the lesion and of providing a larger volume of tissue for the pathologist to examine. However, it is expensive (~$3000), invasive, may produce cosmetic and/or mammographic deformity, and often requires a long turnaround time for operating room scheduling. SNCB has been shown to be as accurate as OSB (91–98%). It is less costly (~$700), less invasive, produces no cosmetic or mammographic deformity, and is immediately available for patient convenience. Its disadvantages are (1) not all lesions are suitable (e.g., asymmetrical densities that cannot be seen well on stereo views cannot be targeted; lesions close to the chest wall or behind the nipple; a suspected radial scar, since that diagnosis cannot easily be made on needle cores), (2) not all patients are suitable (must be able to lie prone; must weigh <300 lb; must not have breasts that are ultracompressible), and (3) certain benign diagnoses are unreliable on core biopsy (e.g., 60% of biopsies diagnosed as atypical epithelial hyperplasia may contain carcinoma on OSB and may require a subsequent operation).

In this particular case, it should be pointed out that a small cluster of microcalicifications can often be problematic for SNCB. The calcifications may be difficult to see on the stereotaxic images and may be missed without vacuum assistance. This latter technique couples a vacuum device to the needle core probe enabling a larger volume of tissue to be sampled and significantly decreasing the number of inadequate samples removed. A potential hazard with this device is the possibility of removing the entire lesion making subsequent open surgical biopsy difficult should the lesion be malignant. This drawback has now been remedied with the availability of tiny metal clips that can be inserted through the probe marking the spot for further excision or radiation therapy.

BIBLIOGRAPHY

Elvecrog EL, Lechner MC, Nelson MT. Nonpalpable breast lesions: correlation of stereotaxic large-core needle biopsy and surgical biopsy results. Radiology 1993; 188:453–455.

Gisvold JJ, Goellner JR, Grant CS, et al. Breast biopsy: comparative study of stereo-taxically guided core and excisional techniques. AJR 1994; 162:815–820.

Jackman RJ, Nowels KW, Shepard MJ, et al. Stereotaxic large-core needle biopsy of 450 nonpalpable breast lesions with surgical correlation in lesions with cancer or atypical hyperplasia. Radiology 1994; 193:91–95.

Jackman RJ, Burbank F, Parker SH, et al. Atypical ductal hyperplasia diagnosed at stereotactic breast biopsy: improved reliability with 14-gauge, directional, vacuum-assisted biopsy. Radiology 1997; 204:485–488.

Kaye MD, Vicinanza-Adami CA, Sullivan ML. Mammographic findings after stereo-taxic biopsy of the breast performed with large-core needles. Radiology 1994; 192:149.

Liberman L, Cohen MA, Dershaw DD, et al. Atypical ductal hyperplasia diagnosed at stereotaxic core biopsy of breast lesions: an indication for surgical biopsy. AJR 1995; 164:1111–1113.

Case #A.2.6
Goal: To discuss the evaluation of a suspicious mammographic mass

VERNON K. SONDAK and JULIE A. WOLFE

A 58-year-old woman undergoes screening mammography and is found to have a new, spiculated, nonpalpable, 1.1-cm mass deep within the central portion of the left breast. Ultrasonography does not definitively visualize the mass.

The lesion described, a spiculated, nonpalpable, 1.1-cm mass in the breast, is highly suspicious for malignancy and requires a thorough evaluation. Although it is not specified, we assume this 58-year-old woman is postmenopausal. Additional relevant history that would help assess this lesion includes determining the use of replacement estrogen therapy, previous history of breast lesions requiring biopsy, history of traumatic injury to the breast, and family history of breast cancer. A complete physical examination should be performed, which includes palpation of the breast and of the axillary and supraclavicular regions to detect the presence of enlarged lymph nodes.

Our current recommendation calls for annual screening mammography beginning at age 40. It is important to obtain any previous mammograms and compare the finding in question to these earlier examinations. More specific mammographic evaluation would include spot compression images and magnified views of the area in question, if not already done. Ultimately, the critical issue is to obtain diagnostic tissue utilizing one of several possible techniques.

Fine-needle aspiration or core needle biopsy, if selected as a diagnostic approach, would require some form of radiological guidance to assure adequate tissue sampling. Imaging options for a tissue sample of a nonpalpable or vague lesion include ultrasound or stereotaxic guidance. It was noted that the lesion was not visible by ultrasonography (although we would not have obtained an initial ultrasonographic evaluation under routine circumstances). Stereotaxic biopsy is therefore the preferred nonoperative diagnostic approach. For nonpalpable lesions, core needle biopsy is strongly preferred over fine-needle cytology because it allows differentiation between in situ and invasive cancer. It must be stressed that a negative or nondiagnostic finding on needle biopsy would still require an excisional biopsy. A positive finding of malignancy would, however, lead to a definitive plan for wide excision and possibly axillary lymph node dissection. The alternative to stereotaxic biopsy is wire (also called needle) localization biopsy with specimen radiograph to document excision of the mammographic lesion. If this procedure demonstrates that the lesion in question is nonmalignant (entities such as a radial scar or posttraumatic fat necrosis could present with this appearance), no further therapy is necessary.

The choice of wire localization versus stereotaxic core biopsy should be made by the patient in conjunction with her treating physician, with appropriate consultation with a radiologist skilled in the performance of stereotaxic procedures. Some patients choose to proceed directly to wire localization biopsy, desiring prompt removal of the mammographic abnormality whether or not it ultimately proves to be malignant. Other patients are eager to avoid surgery and see stereotaxic core biopsy as a less invasive alternative, particularly if the lesion proves to be benign. Recently, some investigators have suggested that using stereotaxic core biopsies to diagnose malignancy results in a more cost-effective approach to definitive surgery, as a single operation can be planned in which wide surgical margins are achieved around the primary site, and at which time an axillary dissection can be performed for appropriate patients if the lesion is invasive. New devices are being developed to do more extensive, minimally invasive stereotaxic excisions of nonpalpable mammographic abnormalities. These devices will have to be evaluated to determine whether they add materially to the evaluation of breast lesions in a cost-effective manner.

The gold standard for evaluating nonpalpable abnormalities identified on screening mammography remains wire localization biopsy with intraoperative specimen radiography. Well-informed patients may choose stereotaxic core biopsy as an attractive alternative in selected cases, provided both surgeon and radiologist agree that the lesion is amenable to such an approach.

BIBLIOGRAPHY

Balch CM. The needle biopsy should replace open excisional biopsy ... but will the surgeon's role in coordinating breast cancer treatment be diminished? Ann Surg Oncol 1995; 2:191–192.
Cross MJ, Evans WP, Peters GN, Cheek JH, Jones RC, Krakos P. Stereotactic breast biopsy as an alternative to open excisional biopsy. Ann Surg Oncol 1995; 2: 195–200.
Ferzli GS, Hurwitz JB. Initial experience with breast biopsy utilizing the advanced breast biopsy instrumentation (ABBI). Surg Endosc 1997; 11:393–396.
Lee CH, Egglin TK, Philpotts L, Mainiero MB, Tocino I. Cost-effectivenesss of stereotactic core needle biopsy: analysis by means of mammographic findings. Radiology 1997; 202:849–854.

Case #A.2.7
Goal: To discuss the pitfalls of wire localization biopsy

VERNON K. SONDAK and JULIE A. WOLFE

A 55-year-old woman presents for evaluation following a mammogram that revealed an area of architectural distortion. On physical examination there are no palpable abnormalities. A wire localization biopsy is performed. Specimen mammogram indicates that the lesion is within the surgical specimen.

Architectural distortion has been defined as a focal, asymmetrical abnormality of the breast parenchyma without a definite mass. It includes spiculations radiating from a single focal point instead of from a central mass, focal retraction, or distortion of a parenchymal edge. Architectural distortion is one of the earliest mammographic signs of breast cancer. In one report, architectural distortion or focal asymmetry was the indication for biopsy of a nonpalpable mammographic abnormality in between 4 and 26% of cases. In another report of 300 consecutive nonpalpable breast cancers detected mammographically, about 20% were identified on the basis of architectural distortion or some asymmetry compared to the contralateral breast, without any type of mass or calcifications being present.

Not all cases of architectural distortion or asymmetry are cancerous. In a prospective study of 8413 asymptomatic women undergoing mammography, when architectural distortion or an asymmetrical density was the indication for biopsy of a nonpalpable breast lesion, malignancy was found in only 33% of biopsies. This rate rose to 64% if the architectural distortion was associated with microcalcifications. Nonmalignant causes of architectural distortion include inflammation, postsurgical scarring, or radial sclerosing lesions (radial scars).

In this case, it is important to compare the area of architectural distortion to the corresponding area in the opposite breast and to the same area on previous mammograms to determine whether it is a stable finding or a recent development. Further mammographic evaluation, including magnified views or spot compression views, may help to reveal subtle microcalcifications. Physical examination in this case reveals no abnormalities. It is also important to obtain a complete history, including family history, any previous history of breast or other cancers, any history of previous breast biopsies, menopausal status, and drug history including current use of estrogen therapy.

Ultrasonography may be helpful to identify cystic lesions presenting as architectural distortion or asymmetry, but is used only if there is reason to suspect the lesion may be cystic. If the architectural distortion is not a new finding compared with previous mammograms, then follow-up mammograms at 6-month intervals with concurrent physical examination is a reasonable alternative to excisional biopsy. Generally speaking, unless the area of architectural distortion is clearly stable over time, or is demonstrated to be a simple cyst by ultrasonography, some type of biopsy is indicated to exclude the presence of cancer.

Wire localization with a hooked guidewire is the standard method of accurately guiding the excisional biopsy of nonpalpable breast lesions. A stereotaxic core needle biopsy is an alternative. The specific location of the guidewire relative to the lesion should be communicated to the surgeon by the radiologist. Confirmation of adequate excision by specimen radiograph performed prior to the completion of the biopsy procedure is an essential aspect of the wire localization biopsy. Pathological analysis should include careful evaluation of the margins at the periphery of the specimen in case malignancy is found. Postoperative mammograms may be appropriate if there are questions concerning the completeness of excision based on either the specimen radiograph or the final pathology report. In general, there is no role for frozen section in the evaluation of nonpalpable breast lesions. Subsequent treatment decisions should be based on a thorough pathological analysis of the specimen. These decisions should be made jointly with the patient after she has been made aware of and had time to understand and accept the biopsy diagnosis.

BIBLIOGRAPHY

Bassett LW, Jahan R, Fu YS. Invasive malignancies. In: Basset LW, Jackson VP, Jahan R, Fu YS, Gold RH, eds. Diagnosis of Diseases of the Breast. Philadelphia: WB Saunders, 1997:461–500.

Morrow M, Schnitt SJ, Harris JB. Ductal carcinoma in situ. In: Harris JR, Lippman ME, Morrow M, Hellman S, eds. Diseases of the Breast. Philadelphia: Lippincott-Raven, 1996:355–368.

Rosenbloom MB, Lisbona A. A prospective study of 8413 asymptomatic women undergoing mammography. Can Assoc Radiol J 1990; 41:207–209.

Sickles EA. Mammographic features of 300 consecutive nonpalpable breast cancers. Am J Roentgenol 1986; 146:661–663.

A.3.   NIPPLE DISCHARGE

Case #A.3.1
Goal: To discuss the management of a fibrocystic nipple discharge

SUSAN A. MCMANUS

A 44-year-old, premenopausal woman presents with new onset of a greenish-brown left nipple discharge. Breast examination is notable only for an expressible greenish-brown discharge emanating from two adjacent ducts at approximately 5 o'clock in the left nipple.

This patient most likely has a "physiological" nipple discharge. The discharge is greenish-brown, emanates from two ducts, and is not accompanied by a mass. The discharge should be tested for occult blood and a mammogram obtained to rule out the presence of a mass or microcalcifications. If these tests are normal, the patient can be reassured that the discharge is benign (and likely due to duct ectasia) and will likely resolve with time. Should the discharge continue to be problematic, the involved ducts can be excised.

Spontaneous discharges (bloody, serosanguineous, serous, or watery) require further evaluation, for these represent pathological discharges. They are frequently found to be associated with an intraductal papilloma (48%) (Table 1). They can also be secondary to fibrocystic changes (33%) and cancer (19%). The incidence of cancer increases with age and with the presence of a palpable mass. An entity called "bloody nipple discharge of pregnancy" does not require surgery, but almost all other pathological discharges require surgical exploration.

A patient presenting with a pathological discharge requires a careful history and physical examination. Patients with a history of breast cancer in a first-degree relative have a higher likelihood of noninvasive or invasive carcinoma causing their discharge. These patients may be in their thirties at the time of presentation. The clinical examination should include a careful search for the trigger zone, the area that when palpated produces the nipple discharge. Usually this is identified at the circumareolar margin. As noted, a concomitant mass in a postmenopausal woman increases the likelihood of malignancy.

After examination, a mammogram with magnification views of the retroareolar area should be obtained. This may visualize faint microcalcifications. Most patients should have galactograms to further aide localization of the lesion causing the discharge. In patients with discharge who were diagnosed subsequently with infiltrating and noninvasive cancer, the presence of a papilloma was frequently present in the original specimen. Therefore, all pathology must be identified when doing a nipple exploration for a pathological discharge. Several studies, including Tabar's, indicate that galactography is a highly reliable diagnostic tool. However, the results of a normal galactogram are not conclusive.

Cytological evaluation of the nipple aspirate is helpful when it is positive for malignancy, especially if a trigger zone has been identified on examination. In patients with bloody discharge who were found to have cancer, 70% had positive nipple cytology. A report that the cytology is "benign" or negative for malignancy does not obviate surgical management.

Surgical procedures for nipple discharge include major duct excision and selective duct excision (microdochectomy). Surgery may be done with local anesthesia and intravenous sedation on an ambulatory basis. Frozen section examination of the tissue is not often helpful.

Editors' comment: Not all surgeons find the use of galactograms essential in the management of nipple discharge. Complete duct excision allows thorough pathological examination of the abnormal duct.

BIBLIOGRAPHY

Chaudary MA, Millis RR, Davies GC, Hayward JL. Nipple discharge: the diagnostic value of testing for occult blood. Ann Surg 1982; 196:651–655.

McPherson VA, Mackenzie WC. Lesions of the breast associated with nipple discharge; prognosis after local excision of benign lesions. Can J Surg 1962; 5: 6–11.

Tabar L, Dean PB, Zolton P. Galactography: the diagnostic procedure of choice for nipple discharge. Radiology 1983; 149:31–38.

Winchester DP. Nipple discharge. In: Harris JR, Lippman ME, eds. Diseases of the Breast. Philadelphia: Lipincott-Raven, 1996:106–110.

Case #A.3.2
Goal: To discuss the management of bilateral galactorrhea

ROSEMARY B. DUDA

A 48-year-old woman seeks evaluation for the new onset of bilateral milky nipple discharge that is most frequent with nipple stimulation, but occasionally occurs spontaneously. She has five children, all of whom she breast-fed. Her youngest child is 8 years old. Physical examination is normal; the discharge is not expressible.

Galactorrhea is a persistent milky-white discharge from the nipples that occurs in the absence of parturition or beyond 6 months postpartum. It may be spontaneous or result from stimulation. Most patients who present with galactorrhea and have normal menses have idiopathic galactorrhea. This is a benign condition that may result from increased responsiveness of the breast tissue to normal physiological concentrations of prolactin. The prolactin level was reported to be normal in 86% of all women in one series with galactorrhea without amenorrhea.

Bilateral galactorrhea may also be associated with endocrine abnormalities. Elevated prolactin levels may indicate the presence of a pituitary adenoma with resultant bilateral galactorrhea. An analysis of 235 patients with galactorrhea revealed that 20% of all patients and 34% of women with amenorrhea had a radiologically evident pituitary tumor. These tumors are usually microadenomas of chromophobe cell origin. These patients tend to have very high serum prolactin levels.

Galactorrhea and elevated prolactin levels may be present in women who use oral contraceptives, antihypertensive medications, phenothiazines, tranquilizers, and other drugs that antagonize the physiological effects of dopamine. Galactorrhea may also occur in women who have primary hypothyroidism, or who are diagnosed with various amenorrhea syndromes, chronic renal failure, pulmonary disease, chest trauma, or following chest surgery. A variety of hypothalamic and pituitary diseases may also cause galactorrhea. These conditions all enhance prolactin secretion and stimulate milk production.

The management of this patient should include a careful history, including a review of all medications, and a thorough physical examination. The breast examination should attempt to confirm that the the nipple discharge is milky, rather than bloody. A mammogram should be obtained to identify the presence of underlying pathology. There is no role for a ductogram as the potential pathology is not in the breast tissue itself but is a response of the breast tissue to a hormonal stimulus.

If the patient does not use any suspect medications and has not been previously diagnosed with associated conditions, further evaluation is necessary. A serum prolactin level can be measured; if it is elevated, further appropriate diagnostic workup can be pursued. Thyroid function tests should be obtained to detect hypothyroidism. If the laboratory tests are normal and no underlying disease is identified, observation and reassurance is the treatment of choice. Most women with bilateral galactorrhea will not have an identifiable cause.

BIBLIOGRAPHY

Frantz AG, Wilson JD. Endocrine disorders of the breast. In: Wilson JD, Foster DW, eds. Williams Textbook of Endocrinology, 7th ed. Philadelphia: WB Saunders, 1985:402–421.

Jacobs LS, Daughaday WM. Physiologic regulation of prolactin secretion in man. In: Josimovich JB, ed. Lactogenic hormones, fetal nutrition and lactation. New York: Wiley, 1974:351–377.

Kleinberg DL, Noel GL, Frantz AG. Galactorrhea: a study of 235 cases, including 48 with pituitary tumors. N Engl J Med 1977; 296:589–600.

Case #A.3.3
Goal: To discuss the management of a bloody nipple discharge

THOMAS J. KEARNEY

A 59-year-old woman undergoes annual breast cancer screening. Bilateral mammograms are normal. Squeezing of the right nipple expresses 3 drops of blood from a single duct at 11 o'clock. No masses are palpated. The patient states that she has noted small blood stains on her nightgown on four occasions over the past 3 months.

The evaluation of women who present with nipple discharge is determined by the nature of the discharge. A milky discharge can be physiological, secondary to numerous medications that affect serum prolactin levels, or due to pathological conditions such as a pituitary tumor or ectopic prolactin production. Approximately one-third of women who have lactated can express breast secretions. Management by duct excision is indicated if the discharge is bothersome. The discharge from a fibrocystic breast is often brown, green, or black and is usually associated with duct ectasia. Fibrocystic discharge can also be treated by duct excision if bothersome.

When a bloody discharge is observed, malignancy is a concern. Clinical evaluation should be directed toward identifying palpable or mammographic abnormalities. Cytological evaluation of nipple discharge has questionable usefulness since decisions concerning surgery are made on clinical grounds. I do not use cytological evaluation of nipple discharge in my practice. Likewise, galactography is only occasionally helpful, although some feel it helps guide excision. A negative galactogram should not preclude surgery. Often, the discharge can be localized to one quadrant of the breast, or even one duct, which is useful for guiding terminal duct excision. I would recommend this procedure in this case. The bloody nature of the discharge, combined with its spontaneous expression on several occasions, raises my level of suspicion of malignancy.

The most common cause of bloody discharge is the presence of a papilloma, accounting for one-third to one-half of cases. Duct ectasia accounts for up to another third of cases of nipple discharge. Cancer is present in 5–20% of bloody nipple discharges. Terminal duct excision can be performed on an outpatient basis using local anesthesia with sedation. Patients who may wish to breast-feed should be warned that this procedure could interfere with subsequent lactation.

BIBLIOGRAPHY

Baker KS, Davey DD, Stelling CB. Ductal abnormalities detected with galactography: frequency of adequate excisional biopsy. Am J Roentgen 1994; 162:821.
Winchester DP. Nipple discharge. In: Harris JR, Lippmann ME, Morrow M, et al, eds. Diseases of the Breast. Philadelphia: Lippincott-Raven, 1996:106–110.

Case #A.3.4
Goal: To discuss the management of an intermittent bloody nipple discharge

MONICA MORROW

A 63-year-old woman presents because of intermittent bloody nipple discharge. Bilateral mammograms are negative. The nipple discharge is not expressible on physical examination.

The discharge described meets the classic criteria for a pathological discharge. Discharges caused by underlying ductal disease are spontaneous rather than induced, and are often intermittent, but persist over time. Pathological discharges may be yellow, clear, green, or bloody. The presence of a pathological discharge is an indication for surgery. Pathological discharges are the symptom of carcinoma in only 10–15% of cases, with intraductal papilloma being the most common cause of pathological discharge.

Our standard approach to pathological discharge is to first localize the quadrant of the breast from which the discharge is produced. The discharge is then tested for blood using a guaiac card, since many dark-colored discharges assumed by patients to be bloody contain no blood. A careful breast examination is then done. If a breast mass is present, it is biopsied as it would be in the absence of a discharge. A mammogram with compression views of the subareolar area is also obtained. In the most common scenario the mammogram is normal, and a terminal duct excision with the incision placed at the areolar margin in the quadrant of the breast from which the discharge is produced is done. Frequently, once the subareolar space is entered an abnormal duct is identified. This duct is then followed for a distance of 2–3 cm in the breast. Care should be taken when the duct is transected to be sure that no discharge is coming from the distal end of the duct, indicating that the pathological lesion is more distal in the breast. The other common reason that the cause of a pathological discharge is not identified is the failure to remove the most proximal end of the duct at the level of the nipple. To prevent this problem, the initial dissection of the nipple flap should occur in the plane immediately beneath the dermis.

In the case described, the history is consistent with pathological discharge, but no discharge can be expressed. Careful clinical follow-up is indicated, and I would reexamine the patient at 3-month intervals, asking her to refrain from squeezing her nipples. Once discharge is identified, I would proceed with a duct excision as described. I do not believe that there is a role for cytology in the evaluation of a discharge. Negative cytology does not reliably exclude the presence of carcinoma, and cytology cannot reliably distinguish an intraductal papilloma from a well-differentiated papillary ductal carcinoma in situ. Galactography also has a limited role. A galactogram demonstrates filling defects but does not make a histological diagnosis. A negative galactogram does not exclude carcinoma. Pathological discharges require biopsy, regardless of the findings of cytology or a galactogram. Galactography may be useful in the young woman with a discharge who wants to preserve her ability to lactate. A preoperative galactogram with needle localization of the site of pathology allows excision of a very limited ductal segment, offering the best chance for future lactation.

BIBLIOGRAPHY

Chaudary M, Millis RR, Davies GC, Hayward JC. Nipple discharge: the diagnostic value of testing for occult blood. Ann Surg 1982; 196:651–655.

Murad TM, Contesso G, Mouriesse H. Nipple discharge from the breast. Ann Surg 1982; 195:259–264.

Urban JA, Egeli RA. Non-lactational nipple discharge. Ca Cancer J Clin 1978; 28: 3–10.

B. Noninvasive Breast Cancer

B.1. LOBULAR CARCINOMA IN SITU (LCIS)

Case #B.1.1
Goal: To discuss the role of family history in the management of patients with LCIS

THOMAS J. KEARNEY

A 30-year-old woman, with a strong family history of breast cancer (mother died at age 45; sister diagnosed at age 36), felt a lump on breast self-examination. Surgical biopsy reveals a fibroadenoma with a 2-mm adjacent area of lobular carcinoma in situ (LCIS).

Lobular carcinoma in situ (LCIS) accounts for over one-third of non-invasive breast cancers. Studies of its natural history have led to a rethinking of the meaning of LCIS. Previously, it was felt that LCIS was a specific precursor of cancer and treatment, usually mastectomy, was required. The available data today suggest that LCIS, like other atypical proliferative lesions, is not so much a committed precursor of invasive lobular cancer as a marker of susceptibility of the breasts to malignant change. All the lobular and ductal elements of both breasts are marked "at risk" by the presence of LCIS anywhere in either breast. The relative risk of developing invasive breast cancer is around 8–10 compared to the average woman. As in the described case, LCIS is almost always an incidental finding. LCIS is almost never palpable. The clustered calcifications typical of ductal carcinoma in situ are usually absent in LCIS, so there are few mammographic clues to its presence. The management of LCIS is best considered as the management of the high-risk patient.

In this case, not only does the patient have a high-risk condition, she also has a strong family history. A family history of breast cancer further increases the risk in patients with moderate- to high-risk proliferative breast disease. One author estimated the 10-year risk of developing an invasive breast cancer to be 20% for a patient as described in the scenario although the risk of actually dying from invasive breast cancer is much lower. If the patient harbors a mutation in the *BRCA1* or *BRCA2* gene, her lifetime risk of developing breast cancer may be as high as 80%. Recommendations for the evaluation and management of carriers of *BRCA1* and *BRCA2* mutations are currently evolving as further studies are being done with the general population. Initial reports were based on families with multiple affected family members and information from these families is probably not accurate for the population as a whole.

169

Once a patient has been identified as being at high risk of developing invasive breast cancer, there are three management options. None of the options has been proven in large prospective studies to be superior. The options include prophylactic surgery (mastectomy), increased surveillance, and prevention.

Normal surveillance for a woman without increased risk would include annual screening mammography and clinical breast examination along with monthly breast self-examination. The age of onset of screening is controversial with both 40 and 50 years being supported by various studies. Recommendations for screening high-risk women are not based on prospective studies. One suggested regimen is to perform twice-yearly professional breast examination and annual mammography once the diagnosis of LCIS is made.

Tamoxifen has recently been studied as a preventive agent for women at high risk for breast cancer in a prospective study of over 13,000 women. The patient in our scenario would meet the risk level to be enrolled in this trial, which compared daily tamoxifen with placebo. The study was halted prematurely in April 1998 by the National Cancer Institute (NCI) when an interim analysis showed a roughly 50% reduction in the incidence of breast cancer in the tamoxifen arm. Results have not yet been published in peer-reviewed journals and an NCI consensus statement has not yet been formulated. It is possible that tamoxifen may become the preferred alternative for the patient in the scenario.

With regard to preventive surgery, it is recommended that prophylactic mastectomy be discussed as one option for managing breast cancer risk for women with known inherited cancer susceptibility or women deemed to be at high risk by virtue of histological markers such as LCIS. Women should be counseled that there are currently no prospective clinical trials with which to estimate efficacy of the procedure although a recent retrospective study demonstrated a significant reduction in breast cancer incidence compared to the expected rate. Owing to the inability to surgically remove breast tissue completely at the time of mastectomy, some level of risk remains following surgery. Residual breast tissue has been noted in the chest wall, axilla, and abdomen following mastectomy. Any residual breast cell is still at risk for mutagenesis and transformation to a breast cancer. Simple mastectomy is preferable for prophylactic procedures, with or without reconstruction. If a prophylactic simple mastectomy revealed invasive cancer, it would seem prudent to perform an axillary dissection.

The choice of management is very individualized and must consider multiple factors. There are no clear-cut answers and definitive recommendations will require further well-conducted clinical trials.

BIBLIOGRAPHY

Cady B. Duct carcinoma in situ. Surg Oncol Clin North Am 1993; 2:75–91.

Dupont WD, Page DL. Risk factors for breast carcinoma in women with proliferative breast disease. In: Bland KI, Copeland EM, eds. The Breast: Comprehensive Management of Benign and Malignant Disease. Philadelphia: WB Saunders, 1991:293.

Easton DF, Ford D, Bishop DT. Breast and ovarian cancer incidence in *BRCA-1* mutation carriers. Am J Hum Genet 1995; 56:265–271.

Garber JE, Smith BL. Management of the high-risk and the concerned patient. In: Harris JR, Lippman ME, Morrow M, et al, eds. Diseases of the Breast. Philadelphia: Lippincott-Raven, 1996:323–334.

Hartmann L, Jenkins R, Schaid D, et al. Prophylactic mastectomy (PM): preliminary retrospective cohort study, American Association for Cancer Research. San Diego, CA, 1997, pp 168 (abstract).

Rosen PP. Lobular carcinoma in situ and atypical lobular hyperplasia. In Rosen PP, ed. Breast Pathology. Philadelphia: Lippincott-Raven, 1997:507.

Case #B.1.2
Goal: To discuss the management of LCIS

VERNON K. SONDAK and JULIE A. WOLFE

A 43-year-old postmenopausal woman is found to have multiple foci of LCIS in a biopsy specimen. The pathology otherwise reveals only fibrocystic changes. The biopsy was performed for a palpable area of thickened breast tissue. The family history is negative for breast or ovarian cancer.

Lobular carcinoma in situ (LCIS) differs significantly in its clinical presentation and biological implications from ductal carcinoma in situ. LCIS is less common than ductal carcinoma in situ (DCIS), and occurs at an earlier age. Page and colleagues noted a 0.5% incidence in 1542 breast biopsies and Haagensen et al. found a 3.6% incidence of LCIS in 5000 benign breast biopsies. The mean age at diagnosis is about 45 years of age; over 75% of women diagnosed with LCIS are premenopausal. Unlike DCIS, LCIS is rarely associated with specific mammographic findings. Calcifications may be the indication for biopsy, but on pathological analysis they almost always turn out to be unrelated to the LCIS. As is true in this case, LCIS is almost always an incidental finding when diagnosed. Furthermore, while DCIS is generally unilateral, LCIS is frequently bilateral. Newman noted a 23% incidence of bilateral LCIS in 26 women undergoing "mirror image" biopsy; Urban found a 35% incidence of bilateral LCIS in 26 women. These findings, however intriguing, are not of direct relevance, and mirror image or other biopsy of the normal-appearing contralateral breast is not indicated in LCIS.

Many studies have looked at the incidence, location, and histology of subsequent invasive carcinoma following the diagnosis of LCIS. Here again, the results are strikingly different from the case of DCIS. Representative studies show the incidence of invasive cancer ranges from 6.3% at 5-year follow-up in a study by Salvadori et al. to 34.5% after 24 years of follow-up as reported by Rosen et al. More recently, Fisher et al. followed 182 patients with LCIS for a mean of 5 years and found four ipsilateral and two contralateral invasive breast cancers (3%). A meta-analysis of 389 women diagnosed with LCIS and followed for a median of 11 years revealed a 16.4% incidence rate of invasive carcinoma and a 2.8% mortality rate. Overall, it appears that the annualized risk for invasive cancer development is about 1% per year for the 30 years after diagnosis of LCIS. Patients with LCIS and a family history of breast cancer or breast and ovarian cancers may be at even greater annual risk.

The risk of invasive cancer development appears to be equal for either breast, regardless of which breast the LCIS was found in and whether or not it was found bilaterally. The subsequent invasive cancers are evenly split between invasive ductal and invasive lobular histology (ordinarily lobular histology accounts for less than 10% of invasive cancers). In contrast, patients with DCIS are at increased risk of invasive cancer development only in the treated breast, and virtually all subsequent cancers are of the invasive ductal type.

Management of LCIS is based on the recognition of the increased risk of cancer development in either breast. Management options include careful observation or prophylactic mastectomies. If surgery is considered, *bilateral* mastectomies are required, because the risk of carcinoma with LCIS is bilateral; unilateral treatment of LCIS makes no biological sense. Attempts at local excision are not warranted, as LCIS is multifocal and the risk of invasive cancer development appears to be independent of the presence or absence of residual LCIS at the biopsy site. For the same reasons, radiation therapy has never been shown to have a role in the management of LCIS.

We would carefully counsel this patient concerning her risk for invasive cancer development and discuss the options of observation and bilateral mastectomies. If, as is the case with most LCIS patients, she chooses observation, we would examine the patient every 6 months and obtain bilateral screening mammograms annually. A low threshold is maintained for biopsy of any changes detected on physical examination or mammography, to ensure early detection in the event of invasive cancer development.

Finally, there is great interest in developing strategies to prevent the development of invasive cancer in patients with LCIS. The well-characterized high-risk status of these patients makes them ideal candidates for chemoprevention trials or other interventions aimed at decreasing breast cancer development. The NSABP has recently completed a large, randomized trial evaluating the use of tamoxifen in patients with LCIS or with other risk factors for breast cancer. Over 13,000 women at increased risk of breast cancer were enrolled in this nationwide trial. Among them, 829 (6.2%) had LCIS. Overall, there was a highy significant reduction in the risk of breast cancer development for women randomized to the tamoxifen arm. Specifically for LCIS patients, there were 18 invasive breast cancers among 411 patients randomized to placebo but only 8 among 415 randomized to tamoxifen. This 56% reduction in risk of developing invasive breast cancer certainly suggests the promise that chemoprevention may have a role for women with LICS. An efficacious middle ground to the markedly disparate alternatives of observation versus bilateral mastectomies would be welcomed by patients and physicians alike.

BIBLIOGRAPHY

Fisher B, Costantino JP, Wickerham DL, Redmond CK, Kavanah M, Cronin WM, Vogel V, Robidoux A, Dimitrov N, Atkins J, Daly M, Wieand S, Tan-Chiu, Ford L, Wolmark N. Tamoxifen for prevention of breast cancer: report of the National Surgical Adjuvant Breast and Bowel Project P-1 study. J Natl Cancer Inst 1998; 90:1371–1388.

Fisher ER, Costantino J, Fisher B, Palekar AS, Paik SM, Suarez CM, Wolmark N. Pathologic findings from the National Surgical Adjuvant Breast Project (NSABP) Protocol B-17. Five-year observations concerning lobular carcinoma in situ. Cancer 1996; 78:1403–1416.

Haagensen CD, Bodian C, Haagensen DE Jr. Lobular neoplasia (lobular carcinoma in situ). In: Haagensen CD, Bodian C, Haagensen DE Jr. Breast Carcinoma: Risk and Detection. Philadelphia: WB Saunders, 1981:238–291.

Newman W. In situ lobular carcinoma of the breast: report of 26 women and 32 cancers. Ann Surg 1963; 157:591–599.

Page DL, Kidd TE Jr, Dupont WD, Simpson JF, Rogers LW. Lobular neoplasia of the breast: higher risk for subsequent invasive cancer predicted by more extensive disease. Hum Pathol 1991; 22:1232–1239.

Rosen PP, Kosloff C, Lieberman PH, Adair F, Braun DW Jr. Lobular carcinoma in situ of the breast. Detailed analysis of 99 patients with average follow-up of 24 years. Am J Surg Pathol 1978; 2:225–251.

Salvadori B, Bartoli C, Zurrida S, Delledonne V, Squicciarini P, Rovini D, Barletta L. Risk of invasive cancer in women with lobular carcinoma in situ of the breast. Eur J Cancer 1991; 27:35–37.

Urban JA. Bilaterality of cancer of the breast. Biopsy of the opposite breast. Cancer 1967; 20:1867–1870.

Case #B.1.3
Goal: To discuss the influence of LCIS on the management of invasive ductal carcinoma

KIRBY I. BLAND and DANIEL S. KIM

A 40-year-old woman with a positive family history notes a mass in the right breast. Biopsy reveals a 0.8-cm, infiltrating ductal carcinoma and extensive LCIS.

Lobular carcinoma in situ (LCIS) occurs almost exclusively in women; the peak incidence is in the fifth decade. Up to 90% of cases of LCIS occur in premenopausal women, suggesting a significant hormonal influence. There is also a greater incidence of estrogen receptor expression with LCIS than with invasive ductal carcinoma. The true incidence of LCIS cannot be reliably determined. The results of 19 published series that examined 10,149 biopsies of nonpalpable breast lesions revealed LCIS in 1.1% of all biopsy specimens and 5.7% of all 1994 evaluable malignancies detected by mammography. This woman fits into this category of coincident invasive cancer.

Between 10% and 37% of women with LCIS will develop invasive breast carcinoma over follow-up periods of up to 25 years. It is generally believed that LCIS is not a precursor lesion because 50–65% of the subsequent invasive carcinomas are of the ductal histological type. However, invasive lobular carcinoma occurs 18 times its expected rate in women with LCIS. Fisher and colleagues do not believe that LCIS can be ruled out as a precursor of invasive cancer. Therefore, the relationship between this patient's LCIS and invasive cancer is uncertain. However, her young age is not suggestive of transition from LCIS to invasive cancer, because the majority of subsequent cancer occurs more than 15 years following diagnosis of LCIS.

This woman is at high risk for future breast carcinoma of either breast. Her risk is greater than that of the usual patient with LCIS because of her young age and concurrent invasive carcinoma. The presence of LCIS with invasive carcinoma in either breast poses a fourfold greater risk of subsequent carcinoma than does either entity alone. Interestingly, family history has not been shown to increase the risk of subsequent invasive cancer in patients with LCIS. Following treatment of the invasive cancer, which should not be influenced by the presence of LCIS, this patient requires diligent follow-up with yearly mammograms and clinical examinations. A recent evaluation of the National Cancer Data Base revealed that overall survival and disease-free survival were similar for infiltrating lobular carcinoma and invasive ductal carcinoma regardless of local therapy.

Editors' comment: The influence of family history on subsequent development of invasive breast cancer is controversial. Recent retrospective analyses have shown that patients with an invasive carcinoma with a component of LCIS can be treated with conservative surgery and radiation with acceptable results.

BIBLIOGRAPHY

Fisher ER, Costantino J, Fisher B, et al. Pathologic findings from the National Surgical Adjuvant Breast and Bowel Project (NSABP) Protocol B-17 five-year observations concerning lobular carcinoma in situ. Cancer 1996; 78:1403–1416.

Frykberg ER, Bland KI. Management of in situ and minimally invasive breast carcinoma. World J Surg 1994; 18:45–57.

Frykberg ER, Bland KI. Current concepts on the biology and management of in situ (Tis, stage 0) breast carcinoma. In: Bland KI, Copeland EM, eds. The Breast: Comprehensive Management of Benign and Malignant Diseases, 2nd ed. Philadelphia: WB Saunders Co, 1998:1012–1043.

Winchester DJ, Chang HR, Graves TA, Menck HR, Bland KI, Winchester DP. A comparative analysis of lobular and ductal carcinoma of the breast: presentation, treatment, and outcome. J Am Coll Surg 1998; 186:416–422.

B.2.   DUCTAL CARCINOMA IN SITU (DCIS)

Case #B.2.1
Goal: To discuss the management of localized DCIS

VERNON K. SONDAK and JULIE A. WOLFE

A 45-year-old woman presents with suspicious microcalcifications on screening mammograms. Physical examination is normal. Needle localization biopsy reveals a 1-cm focus of DCIS. Surgical margins are free of disease.

The current guidelines put forth by the American Cancer Society and other organizations endorse annual screening mammograms for women between 40 and 50 years of age. In the course of such screening, nonpalpable lesions that may or may not be malignant are often found. Only about 25% of "suspicious" lesions in women in this age group prove to be cancer, but most of these cancers are quite small and often noninvasive. It is relevant to define the term "suspicious microcalcifications." Calcifications that are irregular, jagged, linear or branching, and variable in size and shape are more frequently associated with malignancy than calcifications that are loosely grouped or scattered or of uniform size and shape.

Biopsy of nonpalpable breast abnormalities requires some type of radiological guidance. Although nonoperative stereotaxic core biopsy would have been a reasonable first step for this patient, operative excisional biopsy offers the advantage of complete excision and hence is frequently preferred by patients over core biopsy. We prefer a hooked guidewire to a straight needle for our localizations, as the straight needle is more prone to dislodgment during transport from the breast-imaging suite to the operating room. Regardless of localization method, a specimen radiograph should be obtained during the procedure to confirm that the radiographic abnormality has been adequately sampled. It is important to orient the specimen for accurate pathological analysis. Microscopic assessment of the margins of the specimen should routinely be performed, preferably using ink to verify the microscopic relationship of the lesion to the margins.

In this case, a diagnosis of ductal carcinoma in situ (DCIS) has been made. DCIS is a noninvasive cancer, confined within the ductal system without penetrating the basement membrane of the ductal epithelium. The synonym intraductal carcinoma is often used, although DCIS is preferred. Once the diagnosis of DCIS has been made, additional information from the pathologist is critical to select appropriate treatment. The pathology report should specifically address the size of the lesion, its histological grade and subtype, and the status of the margins; it should also verify the absence of foci of invasion. If invasion across the basement membrane is identified in a case otherwise composed of DCIS, the pathology report should distinguish this from pure DCIS and the patient should be treated as having invasive ductal carcinoma.

DCIS can be classified as low, intermediate, or high histopathological grade based upon the mitotic rate and the size, atypia, and pleomorphism of the cells. Low-grade DCIS is typically composed of small cells with uniform nuclei compared with high-grade tumors, which are described as having pleomorphic nuclei within large cells. Histological subtypes of DCIS include papillary, cribriform, and comedo DCIS. Comedo DCIS appears microscopically to be a more pleomorphic entity cytologically; the presence of comedonecrosis in DCIS is generally indicative of a high histological grade. All subtypes of DCIS, however, are by definition noninvasive.

Prior to the widespread use of screening mammography, diagnosis of DCIS was a rare event and treatment was mastectomy. Either total or modified radical mastectomy proved to have a very high ($\geq$98%) cure rate; lymph node metastases were rare in pure DCIS (<1%). Therefore, routine performance of an axillary dissection should not be recommended. The advent of screening mammography ushered in a new era, and surgeons and patients alike were faced with the paradox of performing mastectomies for in situ cancer at a time when breast conservation was being used for invasive cancer. Although mastectomy and breast conservation strategies have never been directly compared in a prospective randomized clinical trial, an extensive body of literature justifies the use of breast-conserving therapy in a subset of patients with DCIS. Controversies persist, however, regarding patient selection and therapy choices for the conservative management of DCIS.

We believe that any patient with DCIS, regardless of histopathological grade or subtype, is a potential candidate for breast-conserving therapy provided the lesion is unifocal and can be excised with negative margins and an acceptable cosmetic result. If pathological evaluation does not confirm clear margins, further resection (reexcision or mastectomy) is required. Neither lymph node dissection nor adjuvant systemic therapy is routinely offered to patients with DCIS, regardless of grade or subtype. Most patients, including the patient in this case, are advised to receive postoperative breast irradiation, based on the results of a large, randomized trial cited below.

Treatment of carefully selected patients with DCIS using complete excision and postoperative radiation provides excellent results for the vast majority of patients, but in-breast recurrences occur in about 10% of cases. Approximately half of these local recurrences are found to be recurrent DCIS and approximately half are invasive carcinoma. Patients who recur with invasive carcinoma are at risk for nodal and distant metastases and require appropriately aggressive therapy. Most patients with in-breast recurrences after conservative therapy of DCIS can be salvaged with total or modified radical mastectomy. Hence, the overall cure rate closely approximates the $\geq 98\%$ rate ascribed to mastectomy as initial treatment. Despite these good results and the high degree of patient satisfaction with the cosmetic result of excision plus radiation, many investigators have searched for subsets of patients who might reasonably be treated with wide excision alone (without radiotherapy). The most definitive data in this regard, and the most influential in our decision making, is the NSABP B-17 trial, which randomized patients with DCIS and negative margin resections to receive either excision alone or excision followed by radiation therapy. This study demonstrated that "event-free survival" ("event" defined as recurrent DCIS, recurrent invasive cancer or other new cancer) was significantly better in those patients receiving radiation therapy (75% vs. 62% at 8 years, $p = 0.00003$). Importantly, the NSABP trial did not suggest any subgroup—based on tumor size, grade, or histological type—that did not benefit from postoperative radiation.

Despite the NSABP results, some investigators have treated highly selected patients with DCIS using excision alone, without irradiation. Generally, these patients have DCIS of low histological grade, noncomedo subtype, and small size (<2 cm). Lagios followed 79 such women for a mean follow-up period of 124 months. Fifteen women (19%) recurred; 53% of the recurrences were invasive carcinomas. Silverstein followed 26 similar women for a mean follow-up period of 56 months during which two (8%) women recurred, one with recurrent DCIS and one with invasive carcinoma. Silverstein also reported a study involving 103 women treated with excision and radiotherapy during which time 10 women (10%) recurred (50% invasive), with a mean follow-up period of 56 months. The NSABP B-17 trial randomized 405 women to treatment with lumpectomy alone. After a mean follow-up period of 90 months, 104 women (25.7%) had in-breast recurrences. Fifty percent of these recurrences were invasive carcinoma.

To summarize, in the case presented, it would be our recommendation to radiate the breast following excision to negative margins, provided the patient is interested in a breast-conserving approach. There is no role for axillary dissection. This patient should then be followed with repeat mammograms on the treated side 4 months after completion of radiotherapy (approximately 6 months postoperatively). Subsequent follow-up should include physical examinations every 6 months for 5 years and then annually, plus annual bilateral screening mammograms.

BIBLIOGRAPHY

Fisher B, Dignam J, Wolmark N, Mamounas E, Costantino J, Poller W, Fisher ER, Wickerham DL, Deutsch M, Margolese R, Dimitrov N, Kavanah M. Lumpectomy and radiation therapy for the treatment of intraductal breast cancer: findings from National Surgical Adjuvant Breast and Bowel Project B-17. J Clin Oncol 1998; 16:441–452.

Fisher ER, Costantino J, Fisher B, Palekar AS, Redmond C, Mamounas E. Pathologic findings from the National Surgical Adjuvant Breast Project (NSABP) Protocol B-17. Intraductal carcinoma (ductal carcinoma in situ). Cancer 1995; 75:1310–1319.

Lagios MD. Lagios experience. In: Silverstein MJ, ed. Ductal Carcinoma In Situ of the Breast. Baltimore: Williams & Wilkins, 1997:361–365.

National Institutes of Health Consensus Development Panel. National Institutes of Health Consensus Development Conference statement: Breast cancer screening for women ages 40–49, January 21–23, 1997. J Natl Cancer Inst 1997; 89:1015–1026.

Silverstein MJ, ed. Ductal Carcinoma In Situ of the Breast. Baltimore: Williams & Wilkins, 1997.

Case #B.2.2
Goal: To discuss the management of diffuse DCIS

CHRISTINA WELTZ

In a 37-year-old woman, mammogram shows diffuse microcalcifications; they are nonpalpable; needle localization biopsy reveals multiple foci of intermediate-grade DCIS with DCIS present at the surgical margins.

This case elicits some of the still unresolved, paradoxical, and difficult features in the treatment of ductal carcinoma in situ (DCIS). Although a breast cancer without the capacity for metastasis, the histological extent and distribution of DCIS, discordance between mammographic and histological findings, and association with synchronous or subsequent invasive disease confound surgical planning and often mandate more radical excisions than are commonly performed for invasive cancers. Ongoing investigation into new imaging modalities and the relative roles of resection margins and radiation treatment may improve surgical planning and offer less extensive surgical options. However, based on current knowledge and study results, only two treatments can be offered to this 37-year-old patient: simple mastectomy with the option of reconstruction or reexcision to attain negative histological margins followed by radiation therapy.

Treatment of DCIS with mastectomy has decreased dramatically from the early 1980s, when it was performed in 71% of cases in this country; in the early 1990s, it has been performed in 43.8% of patients. This trend represents a more widespread understanding of the biology of DCIS and the proven efficacy of breast conservation for treatment of invasive disease. Consideration of mastectomy for this individual centers on local resectability as well as the patient's motivation to ensure against ipsilateral recurrence. Simple mastectomy should be presented to this 37-year-old patient as the only appropriate surgical treatment if the distribution of suspicious calcifications on mammogram precludes the possibility of a cosmetically acceptable local excision of all such lesions. Residual DCIS following breast-conserving treatment is considered the most likely source of recurrent disease, and any residual suspicious calcifications on postexcision mammography place the patient at extremely high risk of such an event. If the distribution of calcifications in this patient's mammogram suggests resectability, simple mastectomy should nevertheless be discussed as the surgical option that minimizes, and even comes close to eliminating, her chance of recurrence with either DCIS or an invasive cancer. If mastectomy is chosen, the patient should be informed that this operation cannot remove all breast tissue. An approximate 1% incidence of chest wall recurrence following mastectomy for DCIS has been reported. Reconstructive options, including the use of implants or autologous tissue and immediate versus delayed timing, should be discussed with the patient through consultation with a plastic surgeon. DCIS's noninvasive nature and the frequent detection of this disease as a mammographic abnormality are such that resection of excessive skin beyond the nipple/areolar complex is not mandated and reconstruction following a skin-sparing mastectomy can be offered. Retrospective review of experience with skin-sparing mastectomy has shown comparable tumor recurrence rates relative to conventional mastectomy, whereas cosmetic issues, and particularly the need to reshape the contralateral breast to attain symmetry, are improved.

As recently as 1991, 58.5% of patients being treated for DCIS underwent axillary dissection, usually as a component of modified radical mastectomy. This astonishing figure reflects a lack of understanding of a disease process that is noninvasive, and therefore is not a potential source of regional or other metastasis. It is also not in accord with the less than 2% incidence of positive nodes reported in combined series of patients undergoing axillary dissection for DCIS, presumably as a result of the presence of occult invasive cancer. Sentinel lymph node mapping has been proposed as a staging tool for patients with DCIS. This technique has the purported advantage of detecting and staging the rare patient with clinically occult invasive disease and positive nodal disease without subjecting all patients with DCIS to the risks of a full axillary dissection. Sentinel lymph node dissection may have a role in patients with larger, clinically palpable, or high-grade DCIS. However, in this patient with mammographically detected, intermediate-grade disease, I perceive sentinel node dissection as an interesting technique without a true indication. My preference in this case is to perform simple mastectomy and certainly make note of histological findings of any low/ medial nodes that may be included with the breast tail component of the specimen. The unexpected finding of occult invasive disease in the mastectomy specimen or in an incidentally removed axillary node would prompt a subsequent formal axillary dissection and consideration of systemic treatment.

It would be reasonable and appropriate for this 37-year-old patient to desire breast-conserving surgery for treatment of her DCIS. This reflects an increasing trend toward breast conservation for treatment of invasive cancer, and is summarized by Fisher's statement on the irony of DCIS: "that an operation for noninvasive breast cancer should be more radical than one for invasive disease seems paradoxical." The appropriateness of breast conservation, however, is contingent upon complete excision of DCIS. Residual DCIS following breast-conserving resection is commonly believed to be the cause of clinical recurrences with either in situ or invasive carcinoma. This is substantiated by an association between positive or questionable margins and subsequent recurrence, as well as the finding that most recurrences are at the site of the prior excision and often have the same histology as the index lesion. Attaining negative margins in DCIS, however, can be difficult both to predict and to achieve because of the anatomical distribution and radiographic manifestations of this disease. Serial whole-organ studies described by Holland et al. reconstruct the breast in three dimensions using detailed histological and radiographic mapping. These constructs have shown that DCIS is almost never a truly multicentric process, or one in which a substantial area of uninvolved breast tissue (3–4 cm in Holland's experience) separates foci of DCIS. However, DCIS involving almost an entire quadrant of the breast (35% of specimens studies), disease involving two or more quadrants (23%), and disease extending beyond 2 cm (83%) were common. The description of this 37-year-old patient's microcalcifications as multifocal conforms to these findings. Confounding this issue of disease extent and distribution is discordance between radiological and histological findings in DCIS. Holland's work detected a high frequency of mammographic findings, most commonly microcalcifications, which underestimate the histological extent of DCIS, particularly in patients with intermediate-grade disease. In his series of 32 breasts with predominantly micropapillary/cribiform type of DCIS, there was a 47% incidence of a 20-mm or greater discrepancy between mammmographic findings and the more extensive histological distribution of disease. Hence, in a significant fraction of patients, not only is DCIS ultimately not amenable to local resection, but the ability to determine this preoperatively is also poor. Dynamic magnetic resonance imaging (MRI) has shown promise in experimental work in defining the true extent, and hence resectability, of DCIS. This technology is based on tumor angiogenesis in the breast stroma surrounding foci of DCIS and gadolinium uptake and release by these vessels producing contrast enhancement on MRI scanning. Until this technique is validated, however, patients desiring breast conservation must be advised that an attempt at complete excision based on mammographic guidance may fail to achieve negative margins, as in this case. If this patient desired breast conservation, I would offer a further attempt at reexcision to obtain negative histological margins. Such an attempt should be guided by wire localization, perhaps bracketing the remaining calcifications seen on subsequent mammogram. Excision should be performed with an awareness on the part of the patient and the surgeon of radiographic/histological discordance and thus the possibility of not being able to achieve negative margins with a cosmetically acceptable excision.

The NSABP B-17 trial has helped define the role of radiation therapy in the treatment of DCIS. After 5 years of follow-up, this study of 818 women with DCIS showed a significantly reduced incidence of second ipsilateral, noninvasive breast cancer in patients undergoing lumpectomy with negative margins (10.4%) relative to patients undergoing lumpectomy plus breast irradiation (7.5%), and an even greater reduction in invasive cancers from 10.5% to 2.9%. While radiation therapy has since become the accepted standard of care, and one I would certainly prescribe in this case if local excision with negative margins could be achieved, Silverstein has presented compelling evidence that radiation can be avoided in many cases with acceptable outcome. Silverstein's rationale partly reflects the NSABP's finding that there was no difference in breast-cancer-related deaths between the study groups, as well as a recognition of the morbidity of radiation therapy. His treatment rationale also depends heavily on margin status. Subgroup analysis of local recurrence-free survival in patients undergoing excision only of DCIS versus combined-modality treatment shows significant differences in patients with resection margins of less than 1 mm, but no difference is detected if the resection margin is greater than 10 mm. These findings are supported by data from the National Cancer Institute in Milan, Italy, a participant in the EORTC 10853 trial also evaluating DCIS treated by excision alone versus combined excision and radiation. With an emphasis on obtaining wide margins on all specimens (at least 10 mm grossly and reexcision mandated for histological margins less than 1 mm) this group has seen no difference in second ipsilateral tumors between study arms in 151 patients followed for an average of 32 months.

Silverstein and the Milan group's data suggest an interrelationship between margin status and radiation, raising the possibility that attaining widely negative margins in excising DCIS obviates the need for radiation. To date, this concept has not been prospectively studied and should not change the recommendation of radiation therapy to this 37-year-old patient, particularly given the multifocal nature of her disease. The issue of margins relative to radiation treatment should, however, be further elucidated by the ongoing NSABP B-24 trial, which randomizes patients with DCIS treated with excision and radiation to receive either tamoxifen or placebo. This protocol does not require negative resection margins. Hence, analysis of subgroups may elucidate the relationship between radiation and margins from another perspective, specifically whether radiation can compensate for the recurrence risk of residual DCIS. Until the results of this study are available, obtaining negative margins should be considered standard of care in this 37-year-old and all patients with DCIS; and whether this patient undergoes simple mastectomy or further local excision with radiation, negative margin status is the fundamental principle of her surgical care.

BIBLIOGRAPHY

Carlson GW, Bostwick J, Styblo TM, et al. Skin-sparing mastectomy: oncologic and
    reconstructive considerations. Ann Surg 1997; 225:570–578.
Fisher B, Constantino J, Redmond C, et al. Lumpectomy compared with lumpectomy
    and radiation therapy for the treatment of intraductal breast cancer. N Engl J
    Med 1993; 328:1581–1586.
Gilles R, Zafrani B, Guinebretiere JM, et al. Ductal carcinoma in situ: MR imaging–
    histopathologic correlation. Radiology 1995; 196:415–419.
Holland R, Hendriks JHCL, Verbeek ALM, et al. Extent, distribution, and mam-
    mographic/histological correlations of breast ductal carcinoma in situ. Lancet
    1990; 335:519–522.
Salvadori B, Delledonne V, Rovini D. National Cancer Institute—Milan Experience.
    In: Silverstein MJ, ed. Ductal Carcinoma In Situ of the Breast. Baltimore:
    Williams & Wilkins, 1997.
Silverstein MJ. Van Nuys experience by treatment. In: Silverstien MJ, ed. Ductal
    Carcinoma In Situ of the Breast. Baltimore: Williams & Wilkins, 1997.
Sneige N, McNeese MD, Atkinson EN, et al. Ductal carcinoma in situ treated with
    lumpectomy and irradiation: histopathological analysis of 49 specimens with
    emphasis on risk factors and long term results. Hum Pathol 1995; 26:642–
    649.
Surveillance, Epidemiology, and End Results (SEER) Program public use CD-ROM
    (1973–1992). Bethesda, MD: National Cancer Institute, DCPC, Surveillance
    Program, Cancer Statistics Branch, 1995.

Case #B.2.3
Goal: To discuss the influence of the presence of LCIS on the management of DCIS

MONICA MORROW

*A 44-year-old woman presents with suspicious microcalcifications on
mammogram; wire localization biopsy reveals extensive LCIS and a 2-mm
focus of DCIS. Margins are free of tumor.*

Although lobular carcinoma in situ (LCIS) and ductal carcinoma in
situ (DCIS) are grouped together under the heading of in situ carcinoma,
they are separate entities with different therapeutic implications. DCIS is a
proliferation of abnormal, presumably malignant cells, confined within the
basement membrane of the breast duct. DCIS is thought to be the anatomical
precursor of invasive carcinoma, although the time to the development of
invasive carcinoma may be quite prolonged. In women with untreated DCIS,
subsequent invasive carcinomas occur in the ipsilateral breast, usually in the
same quadrant, as the DCIS. In contrast, LCIS is felt to be a risk factor for

breast cancer development rather than an anatomical precursor of the disease. In women with a diagnosis of LCIS, the risk of developing invasive carcinoma is approximately 1% per year, and subsequent carcinomas are equally distributed in both breasts. The majority of carcinomas occurring after a diagnosis of LCIS are infiltrating ductal carcinomas, further evidence that LCIS is a risk factor rather than the precursor of invasive carcinoma. DCIS and LCIS differ in a number of other important ways, as summarized in Table 1.

Treatment options that are available for the patient with DCIS include total (simple) mastectomy, excision and irradiation, or excision alone. The most appropriate treatment will depend on the extent of the DCIS and the patient's attitude toward risk. Mastectomy for DCIS is curative in 98% of cases and is a treatment for which all patients are eligible. However, mastectomy is not necessary for many DCIS patients, including the one described here, who have a minimal amount of DCIS. Patients treated with a breast-conserving approach to DCIS consisting of lumpectomy and irradiation have local recurrence rates of 10–15% at 10 years, and half of these local recurrences are invasive carcinoma. The 15-year cause-specific mortality is approximately 3%. At one time, high-grade (comedo) DCIS was thought to have a higher breast recurrence rate than low-grade DCIS; studies with longer follow-up have shown that recurrence rates do not differ by grade of DCIS, although high-grade DCIS tends to recur earlier than low-grade DCIS.

The long natural history of some DCIS, and the lack of certainty that all DCIS will progress to invasive carcinoma in a patient's lifetime, have led some authors to suggest that the lesion can be treated by excision alone. The only prospective randomized trial that has compared the treatment of DCIS with and without irradiation has demonstrated a statistically significant reduction in the incidence of both invasive and noninvasive recurrences in irradiated patients, with the largest effect observed on the incidence of in-

Table 1   Comparison of DCIS and LCIS

	DCIS	LCIS
Age of onset	Pre- or postmenopausal	Premenopausal
Clinical presentation	Mass, nipple discharge, Paget's disease	None. Incidental finding
Mammographic features	Microcalcifications, occasionally mass	None
Cancer risk	Unilateral, usually same quadrant	Bilateral

vasive recurrence. However, a number of single-institution studies have reported low local recurrence rates in highly selected patients (usually those with small, low-grade lesions with widely negative margins) treated with excision alone.

The patient described here is an appropriate candidate for treatment by excision alone if complete excision of the DCIS lesion can be documented. Assessment of margins and documentation of removal of all of the suspicious calcifications with postbiopsy mammography are complementary means of ensuring complete lesion removal. DCIS is known to grow discontinuously in the ducts, particularly lesions of low and intermediate grade, so a negative margin does not obviate the need for a postbiopsy mammogram. These films can be obtained as soon as the patient can comfortably tolerate compression, and if residual calcifications are noted repeat needle localization should be undertaken.

The presence of LCIS in this biopsy specimen has no impact on patient management since DCIS is present. LCIS is known to be a multicentric lesion, and since it is a risk factor for breast carcinoma, excision to negative margins is not appropriate. The presence of LCIS has not been shown to increase the risk of local failure in the breast after breast-conserving therapy.

BIBLIOGRAPHY

Fisher B, Costantino J, Redmond C, et al. Lumpectomy compared with lumpectomy and radiation therapy for the treatment of intraductal breast cancer. N Engl J Med 1993; 328:1581–1586.

Morrow M, Schnitt SJ, Harris JR. Ductal carcinoma in situ. In: Harris JR, Lippman ME, Morrow M, Hellman S. eds. Diseases of the Breast. Philadelphia: Lippincott-Raven, 1996:355–368.

Singletary SE. Lobular carcinoma in sit of the breast. A 31 year experience at the University of Texas. MD Anderson Cancer Center. Breast Dis 1994; 7:157–163.

Case #B.2.4
Goal: To discuss the management of positive surgical margins in patients with DCIS

ALLEN S. LICHTER

A 43-year-old woman undergoes screening mammography, which shows a suspicious area of microcalcifications. There is no palpable abnormality. Needle localization biopsy reveals a 4-mm focus of low-grade DCIS with DCIS present at the surgical margins.

Breast conservation is an appropriate alternative to mastectomy for patients with ductal carcinoma in situ (DCIS). In trying to help patients make this treatment choice, a number of points need to be emphasized. Mastectomy is clearly an excellent treatment for DCIS. Virtually all patients are locally controlled, although there are occasional chest wall recurrences reported in the literature and seen in the author's personal experience. A mastectomy does not eliminate the patient's risk of subsequent breast cancer as the contralateral breast is left intact. Cosmesis can be restored with an immediate or a delayed reconstruction. Breast preservation will typically produce better cosmesis and a more intact body image compared to mastectomy with reconstruction. However, both the ipsilateral and the contralateral breast are at risk to develop subsequent carcinoma, so the chance that a patient will have another breast "event" during her lifetime is somewhat higher if the breast is preserved. There has never been a randomized, prospective trial comparing mastectomy to breast conservation in the treatment of DCIS. If one models the potential outcomes with the optimistic assumption that mastectomy has a 100% cure rate in DCIS, one sees that the survival differences between these two techniques cannot be more than a percent or two. To try to document whether there is a difference in outcome for DCIS patients treated with mastectomy versus lumpectomy plus radiation would take a trial of many thousands of patients and it is unlikely such a trial will ever be mounted. In our own practice, we believe that breast conservation for DCIS is a treatment option that can be offered with confidence in appropriately selected patients.

Our own technique involves clearing the surgical margins in all our patients with DCIS. It also involves clearing the mammogram of all suspicious microcalcifications. While specific data on the influence of positive margins on the ultimate local control of DCIS are not available, logical extension from the treatment of invasive cancer, an entity that is often associated with the presence of DCIS, makes us believe that margin clearance is a prudent course of action until data show otherwise. In some patients with DCIS that is small (less than 1 cm) and well differentiated, and in patients who have a wide margin (1 cm of normal breast tissue surrounding the lesion), radiation therapy may not be needed at all. While this case does not obviously fall within those guidelines, since there are residual microcalcifications and the ultimate size of this lesion is not known at present, if this patient had a 4-mm, well-differentiated tumor with a positive surgical margin, her treatment options could involve reexcision plus radiation or wide reexcision with no further radiation. Subsequent clinical trials will address this matter in more detail.

There is no role for axillary lymph node dissection in the treatment of DCIS. The risk of lymph node metastases is low and the author knows of no major institution that is recommending lymph node removal in such patients. There are those patients with high-grade DCIS that is located in the extreme upper outer quadrant and where there can be some question of invasion. In those cases, we may take some low axillary lymph nodes along with the surgical resection just to be on the safe side. But those cases are few and far between.

Radiotherapy is clearly an important part of breast-conserving therapy in patients with DCIS. In NSABP B-17, the rate of recurrence without radiation was more than double the rate of recurrence with radiation. Silverstein, who advocates excision alone in many situations, suggests irradiation in patients whose tumors are less well differentiated, larger, or have narrower surgical margins.

Breast cancer researchers have been interested for some time in whether an antiestrogen such as tamoxifen could both decrease the rate of reappearance of tumors in the ipsilateral breast and decrease the appearance of new tumors in the contralateral breast. Tamoxifen has clearly proven its worth in patients with invasive breast cancer. A clinical trial testing the use of tamoxifen in noninvasive breast cancer has been completed; the results are yet to be released. Similarly, tamoxifen has been evaluated in a prevention trial where women at high risk for breast cancer, but who have not had invasive or noninvasive ductal cancer, were treated. Within the next few years we should have a clear understanding of the effect of tamoxifen on patients in these populations. At present, the author's institution considers tamoxifen an unproven agent in the management of DCIS and our patients do not routinely receive it.

BIBLIOGRAPHY

Fisher B, Costantino J, Redmond C, Fisher E, Margolese R, Dimitrov N, Wolmark N, Wickerham DL, Deutsch M, Ore L, et al. Lumpectomy compared with lumpectomy and radiation therapy for the treatment of intraductal breast cancer. N Engl J Med 1993; 328:1581–1586.

Fisher ER, Costantino J, Fisher B, Palekar AS, Redmond C, Mamounas E. Pathologic findings from the National Surgical Adjuvant Breast Project (NSABP) Protocol B-17. Intraductal carcinoma (ductal carcinoma in situ). Cancer 1995; 75:1310–1319.

Morrow M, Schnitt SJ, Harris JB. Ductal carcinoma in situ. In: Harris JR, Lippman ME, Morrow M, Hellman S, eds. Diseases of the Breast. Philadelphia: Lippincott-Raven, 1996:355–368.

Silverstein MJ, ed. Ductal Carcinoma In Situ of the Breast. Baltimore: Williams & Wilkins, 1997.

Case #B.2.5
Goal: To discuss the implications of high-grade DCIS

DAVID A. AUGUST

A 53-year-old woman presents with an abnormal mammogram and a 2-cm, palpable lesion; excisional biopsy reveals a 1.4-cm DCIS with comedonecrosis. It has a high nuclear grade. The resection margins are negative.

The key point in this case is the presence of ductal carcinoma in situ (DCIS) with *comedonecrosis*. It is generally accepted that DCIS may be treated either with simple mastectomy or with negative margin lumpectomy (with or without radiation therapy). Generally, on the basis of the results of NSABP trial B-17, which required negative margin excision followed by randomization to either observation or whole-breast irradiation followed by observation, I recommend to most women presenting with focal DCIS either simple mastectomy or lumpectomy with radiation therapy. The well-informed patient should make the choice in concert with her physicians. Withholding of radiation therapy should be considered only for small (less than 1 cm), well-differentiated tumors with adequate margins of excision (greater than 1 cm).

How should the presence of comedonecrosis affect the decision-making process in the case presented? Comedo DCIS is characterized by prominent necrosis in the involved ductal lumina. DCIS tumors with comedonecrosis are generally high grade, characterized by the presence of mitotic figures in large cells with nuclear pleomorphism evident. Such tumors appear more malignant cytologically than more mundane DCIS and are more often associated with the presence of microinvasion.

Some reports suggest an increased incidence of in-breast recurrence for tumors containing comedonecrosis following lumpectomy and radiation therapy. Silverstein et al. reported an 11% incidence of in-breast recurrence following breast conservation in women with comedo DCIS versus a 2% failure rate with noncomedo DCIS. However, when this study was updated to include longer follow-up (greater than 60-month median), the effect of histological subtype disappeared. Solin and colleagues reported a multivariate analysis of 172 women with DCIS and found an increased incidence of local recurrences only in those patients with tumors exhibiting both comedonecrosis and high nuclear grade; these features are not always concordant. Finally, an analysis of pathological features in women enrolled in NSABP B-17 found breast irradiation caused a greater risk reduction of local recurrence in patients with comedo features. For some reason, radiation therapy seemed to "work better" in these women. Furthermore, there were no differences in overall survival or occurrence of metastatic disease according to histological subtype.

These data suggest that although local control may be somewhat better in the absence of comedonecrosis, this feature is not a strong predictor of the success of breast-conserving therapy (lumpectomy plus radiation) in women with DCIS. For the patient presented, even with a palpable lesion, I would discuss the options of breast conservation and simple mastectomy (with or without immediate or delayed reconstruction) as being therapeutically equivalent in relation to overall survival. The presence of comedonecrosis would not alter my recommendations or the tenor of the conversation, as long as a negative margin excision is achieved and the patient is agreeable to receiving radiation therapy. Although simple mastectomy clearly offers improved event-free survival (by virtue of a reduced incidence of local failure), the likely survival equivalence of mastectomy and breast conservation in this situation affords most women the reassurance necessary to feel comfortable choosing breast conservation.

BIBLIOGRAPHY

Fisher B, Costantino J, Redmond C, et al. Lumpectomy compared with lumpectomy and radiation therapy for the treatment of intraductal breast cancer. N Engl J Med 1993; 328:1581.

Fisher ER, Costantino J, Fisher B, et al. Pathologic findings from the National Surgical Adjuvant Breast Project (NSABP) protocol B17: intraductal carcinoma (ductal carcinoma in situ). Cancer 1995; 75:1310.

Rosen PP, Oberman H. Tumors of the Mammary Gland. Washington, DC: Armed Forces Institute of Pathology, 1993.

Silverstein MJ, Waisman JR, Gamagami P, et al. Intraductal carcinoma of the breast (208 cases): clinical factors influencing treatment choice. Cancer 1990; 66:102.

Silverstein MJ, Cohlan BF, Gierson ED, et al. Duct carcinoma in-situ: 227 cases without microinvasion. Eur J Cancer 1992; 28:630.

Solin LJ, Yeh IT, Kurtz J, et al. Ductal carcinoma in-situ (intraductal carcinoma) of the breast treated with breast-conserving surgery and definitive irradiation: Correlation of pathologic parameters with outcome of treatment. Cancer 1993; 71:2532.

Case #B.2.6
Goal: To discuss the management of "recurrence" following primary treatment of DCIS

VERNON K. SONDAK and JULIE A. WOLFE

A 50-year-old woman, who 5 years ago had undergone a lumpectomy and radiation therapy for a 5-mm DCIS, presents because a routine mammo-

gram reveals new clusters of ipsilateral suspicious microcalcifications. The patient is highly motivated for breast conservation. The biopsy reveals DCIS.

Ductal carcinoma in situ (DCIS) (also referred to as noninvasive or intraductal carcinoma) accounts for 50% or more of the nonpalpable breast malignancies identified by mammography. The most common mammographic abnormality associated with DCIS is clustered microcalcifications, with or without an associated area of architectural distortion or a spiculated mass. DCIS may also present as nipple erosion (Paget's disease), and rarely (currently <1% of cases) as a palpable mass. Although no definitive randomized trials have been performed, mastectomy has been replaced in many cases by excision to negative margins and postoperative radiation. The current case, in which the patient initially presented with a 5-mm focus of DCIS, represents a situation in which breast conservation is frequently employed. As previously discussed (Case B.2.1), we routinely advocate postoperative radiation for most patients with DCIS who are conservatively treated. Even so, in a minority of these patients DCIS will recur in the breast despite adequate therapy. We are not provided details about the initial DCIS other than its small size (5 mm), a favorable finding for breast conservation. High-grade lesions, including those with comedonecrosis, have been associated with higher rates of in-breast failure. The presence of tumor at the margin of the initial resection would also be expected to increase the risk of in-breast recurrence. Patients with conservatively treated DCIS are routinely followed with physical examination and mammography. Although the recurrence may not manifest an identical radiological appearance to the initial lesion, most in-breast recurrences are discovered on follow-up mammography of the treated breast. The site of recurrence is nearly always at or near the previous excision. Forty to fifty percent of in-breast recurrences in patients with initial DCIS prove to be invasive carcinoma.

In-breast recurrences, whether invasive or noninvasive, merit aggressive treatment. Because this patient received radiation to the breast 5 years ago, repeat radiotherapy is not a viable option. The presence of residual calcifications suggests other foci of recurrence, possibly with invasive carcinoma. Simply reexcising the site of recurrence, therefore, without addressing these other foci, would be inadequate therapy. Despite this woman's desire to preserve her breast, our recommendation for this woman is mastectomy. Although axillary lymph node dissection is not required in cases of pure DCIS—primary or recurrent—the possibility that this patient harbors additional areas of invasive cancer must be discussed with the patient. In the past, this risk of occult invasive carcinoma elsewhere in the breast prompted some surgeons to perform limited or complete axillary dissections at the time of total mastectomy (modified radical mastectomy). We no longer consider axillary dissection for DCIS patients in the absence of histologically proven invasive cancer or nodal metastases. Instead, we have been evaluating sentinel node biopsy using lymphazurin blue dye at the time of total mastectomy. Patients who have a positive sentinel node undergo completion axillary dissection, while patients whose sentinel node(s) are negative do not—regardless of the presence or absence of invasive cancer in the resected breast. It must be stressed, however, that this approach remains investigational and has not yet been accepted as standard of care. As with any patient undergoing mastectomy, the possibility of immediate reconstruction should be thoroughly discussed and consultation with a plastic surgeon encouraged. We wish to emphasize that the mastectomy performed in a case of extensive or recurrent DCIS should be just as thorough and complete (save for the axillary dissection) as that done for invasive breast cancer—subcutaneous mastectomies are not appropriate.

BIBLIOGRAPHY

Fisher B, Dignam J, Wolmark N, Mamounas E, Costantino J, Poller W, Fisher ER, Wickerham DL, Deutsch M, Margolese R, Dimitrov N, Kavanah M. Lumpectomy and radiation therapy for the treatment of intraductal breast cancer: findings from National Surgical Adjuvant Breast and Bowel Project B-17. J Clin Oncol 1998; 16:441–452.

McMasters KM, Giuliano AE, Ross MI, Reintgen DS, Hunt KK, Byrd DR, Klimberg VS, Whitworth PW, Tafra LC, Edwards MJ. Sentinel-lymph-node biopsy for breast cancer—not yet the standard of care. N Engl J Med 1998; 339:990–995.

Morrow M, Schnitt SJ, Harris JB. Ductal carcinoma in situ. In: Harris JR, Lippman ME, Morrow M, Hellman S, eds. Diseases of the Breast. Philadelphia: Lippincott-Raven, 1996:355–368.

Case #B.2.7
Goal: To discuss the significance of an incidental finding of DCIS

ROSEMARY B. DUDA

A 30-year-old woman presents with a palpable breast lesion. Excisional biopsy reveals a fibroadenoma with an incidental finding of a 2-mm focus of DCIS. The excision margins are clear.

Intraductal carcinoma, also known as ductal carcinoma in situ (DCIS), consists of cytologically malignant cells that have not penetrated through the basement membrane into the stroma surrounding the ducts. Although once an uncommon entity, it now comprises approximately 35% of new diagnoses of breast cancer. This is largely secondary to effective screening mammography where DCIS is generally identified on the basis of clustered microcalcifications. DCIS may also be detected clinically or appear as a mammographic mass in a small number of cases. True multicentricity or multifocal disease is rare. Rather, DCIS often extends along the ductal system in which it arises. An incidental finding of DCIS in the resection specimen of a fibroadenoma is uncommon.

Our understanding of the natural history of intraductal carcinoma is incomplete. In early studies, mammography was not used as a screening tool; DCIS was diagnosed as a palpable mass and represented less than 1% of new breast cancers. Most patients were treated with radical or modified radical mastectomy. Subsequent studies with long-term data are available from several small series of women treated with an excision alone, without knowledge of status of resection margins. The frequency of development of invasive cancer ranges from 11% to 28% over 3–16 years. Most of the cases of DCIS in these series were low-grade, noncomedo carcinomas and the recurrences were generally in the vicinity of the biopsy site. In a series of 80 women diagnosed with DCIS followed for 17.5 years, only two of which were high-grade lesions, 14% recurred as an invasive cancer and 6% as DCIS.

The treatment options for DCIS include wide resection alone, wide resection with radiation therapy, and total mastectomy. The goal of surgery is to remove the entire DCIS lesion and a margin of normal tissue surrounding the lesion. This particular case presentation raises the issue of the proper management of a minute focus of noncomedo DCIS. A margin of only 1–2 mm is insufficient. For small (less than 5 mm in diameter), low-grade lesions of DCIS, a margin of resection of 5 mm may be sufficient for local control while an ideal resection margin is 10 mm.

The overall management of this patient should include: (1) a mammogram with magnification views of the biopsy site to determine whether clustered microcalcifications can be identified adjacent to the biopsy site; and (2) a review of the pathology slides to determine the closest margin of resection to the focus of DCIS. If there are no abnormal findings on the mammogram and the closest margin of resection to the focus of DCIS is at least 5 mm, then the patient may be observed. If an abnormality is found on the mammogram or the margins of resection are less than 5 mm, then a wide local resection to achieve a clean margin of 10 mm is recommended. There is a high likelihood that this lesion will be controlled with an adequate surgical resection alone. The patient should then be observed closely for the possibility of an occurrence of an invasive breast carcinoma.

Editors' comment: Although most would agree with the opinion that there is a high probability of controlling a 2-mm, well-differentiated DCIS with adequate excision alone, the appropriate use of radiation therapy in DCIS is still under investigation.

BIBLIOGRAPHY

Eusebi V, Foschini M, Cook M, et al. Long term follow up of in-situ carcinoma of the breast with special emphasis on clinging carcinoma. Semin Diagn Pathol 1989; 6:165–173.

Eusebi V, Feudal E, Foschini M, et al. Long term follow up of in situ carcinoma of the breast. Semin Diagn Pathol 1994; 11:223–235.

Holland R, Peterse JL, Millis RR, et al. Ductal carcinoma in situ: a proposal for a new classification. Semin Diagn Pathol 1994; 11:167–180.

Page DL, Dupont WD, Rogers LW, et al. Intraductal carcinoma of the breast: follow up after biopsy only. Cancer 1982; 49:751–758.

Rosen PP, Braun D, Kinne D. The clinical significance of pre-invasive breast carcinoma. Cancer 1980; 46:919–925.

Wilhelm MC, Edge SB, Cole DD, et al. Nonpalpable invasive breast cancer. Ann Surg 1991; 213:600–603.

Wood WC. Management of lobular carcinoma in situ and ductal carcinoma in situ of the breast. Semin in Oncol 1996; 23:446–452.

Case #B.2.8
Goal: To discuss the meaning of microinvasion with DCIS

JAY K. HARNESS

A 70-year-old woman presents for evaluation of an abnormal mammogram. A wire localization biopsy reveals a 5-mm DCIS with comedonecrosis and "microinvasion." The hormone receptor assay is negative.

The diagnosis of ductal carcinoma in situ (DCIS) has become more common with the increased use of mammographic screening of asymptomatic women. DCIS now represents 20–30% of breast cancers detected by clinical screening. There are five histological subtypes: comedo, solid, cribriform, micropapillary/papillary, and clinging. In general, the comedo form of DCIS has a higher incidence of multicentricity, microinvasion, and local recurrence. More than 50% of DCIS lesions are estrogen receptor (ER) negative and therefore hormone independent.

There is no consensus as to the amount or extent of invasive carcinoma described by the term "microinvasive." True microinvasion involves penetration of the basement membrane. A variety of definitions have been proposed that include subjective criteria, estimated measurements, or a combination of both. As an example, one definition states that nests of malignant cells do not extend more than 0.1 mm beyond the ductal basement membrane. I believe that it is preferable to use the term "microinvasion" for lesions with no single focus of invasive carcinoma that is 1.0 mm or larger in diameter. Foci larger than 1 mm are diagnosed as invasive ductal carcinoma. If multiple foci of microinvasion are present, there is no accurate method for estimating their aggregated diameter. These cases still qualify as ductal carcinoma with microinvasion (DCISM). As the size of the DCIS increases (e.g., 0–5 mm, 6–10 mm, 11–20 mm, etc.), the incidence of microinvasion also increases from 0% to 28%.

The incidence of axillary lymph node metastasis in the face of microinvasion has had limited study. Table 1 lists the results of such studies by 11 investigators. The range of nodal involvement is 0–20%. The largest series has only 42 patients, and the total number of patients from the 11 reports is just 287. The aggregate average of nodal involvement is 5.6%. One factor that contributes to the wide range of nodal involvement with DCISM is the lack of uniformity of the definition of "microinvasion." In those reports that had a more restrictive definition, the rate of nodal involvement was 0–5.2%. In those reports that had either a more liberal definition (e.g., invasive component generally 1 or 2 mm in size) or gave no definition of DCISM, the rate of nodal involvement increased up to 20%. In the case presented for discussion, no definition has been given of the "area of mi-

Table 1 Axillary Nodal Involvement with Microinvasive DCIS

Investigator	Number of patients with microinvasion	Nodal involvement	%
Dowlatshahi et al.	21	0	0
Kinne et al.	42	4	9.5
Kopald et al.	15	0	0
Pandelidis et al.	21	0	0
Rosner et al.	36	1	2.7
Schuh et al.	30	6	20
Schwartz et al.	13	1	7.7
Silverstein et al.	24	1	4.2
Simpson et al.	5	1	20
Solin et al.	39	2	5.1
Wong et al.	41	0	0
Total	287	16	5.6

croinvasion.'' It would appear that patients who have a small (e.g., 1 mm or less) microscopic focus of invasion are unlikely to have positive nodes.

Axillary dissection potentially benefits patients with carcinoma of the breast for several reasons. First, lymph node status remains the strongest prognostic indicator. Second, the presence of involved axillary lymph nodes usually leads to recommendations for adjuvant chemotherapy or hormonal therapy. Third, resection of axillary nodes improves local control and may or may not increase survival. However, there is no question that axillary dissection carries a risk for significant morbidity. The sentinel node technique for lymphatic mapping and lymphadenectomy, with its high positive predictive value, may be a legitimate compromise between the risks and benefits of performing or not performing an axillary dissection.

The treatment options for DCIS and DCISM include: total mastectomy (which often includes level I axillary nodes around or near the tail of the breast); or lumpectomy (with negative margins) with or without adjuvant radiotherapy and with or without axillary dissection. The appropriate use of tamoxifen in this setting is under investigation. If this patient is motivated for breast conservation, I would support her decision and strongly urge her to have whole-breast adjuvant radiotherapy and not have an axillary lymph node dissection.

While not stated, I am assuming her DCIS is primarily the comedo type because of the small focus of microinvasion. Comedo DCIS has a higher incidence of in-breast recurrence, which can be reduced with adjuvant radiotherapy. Radiotherapy treatment fields include most of the level I axillary lymph nodes. If metastases were present in these nodes, they would also be treated by the radiotherapy. If this patient does not want breast conservation, I would perform a total mastectomy using the sentinel node technique to guide my removal of the level I axillary nodes.

This patient's age, tumor size, and histology (even with microinvasion) suggest an excellent prognosis. Her 10-year survival from her cancer should be at least 98%.

BIBLIOGRAPHY

Dowlatshahi K, Snider HC Jr, Kim R. Axillary node status in nonpalpable breast cancer. Ann Surg Oncol 1995; 2(5):424–428.

Kinne DW, Petrek JA, Osborne MP, et al. Breast carcinoma in situ. Arch Surg 1989; 124(1):33–36.

Kopald KH, Hiatt JR, Irving C, Giuliano AE. The pathology of nonpalpable breast cancer. Am Surg 1990; 56(12):782–787.

Pandelidis SM, Peters KL, Walusimbi MS, et al. The role of axillary dissection in mammographically detected carcinoma. J Am Coll Surg 1997; 184(4):341–345.

Rosner D, Lane WW, Penetrante R. Ductal carcinoma in situ with microinvasion. A curable entity using surgery alone without need for adjuvant therapy. Cancer 1991; 67:1498–1503.

Schuh ME, Nemoto T, Penetrante RB, et al. Intraductal carcinoma. Analysis of presentation, pathologic findings, and outcomes of disease. Arch Surg 1986; 121:1303–1307.

Schwartz GF, Patchefsky AS, Finkelestein SD, et al. Nonpalpable in situ ductal carcinoma of the breast. Predictors of multicentricity and microinvasion and implications for treatment. Arch Surg 1989; 124:29–32.

Silverstein MJ, Gierson ED, Colburn WJ, et al. Axillary lymphadenectomy for intraductal carcinoma of the breast. Surg Gynecol Obstet 1991; 172:211–214.

Simpson T, Thirlby RC, Dail DH. Surgical treatment of ductal carcinoma in situ of the breast. 10- to 20- year follow-up. Arch Surg 1992; 127:468–472.

Solin LJ, Fowble BL, Kowalyshyn MJ, et al. Microinvasive ductal carcinoma of the breast treated with breast-conserving surgery and definitive irradiation. Int J Radiat Oncol Biol Phys 1992; 23(5):961–968.

Wong JH, Kopald KH, Morton DL. The impact of microinvasion on axillary node metastases and survival in patients with intraductal breast cancer. Arch Surg 1990; 125:1298–1302.

C. Invasive Breast Cancer

C.1. OPERABLE BREAST CANCER

Introduction

We have defined operable breast cancer as T1–2N0–1M0 for purposes of constructing this decision tree. We have therefore excluded neoadjuvant therapy as an option outside of an approved clinical trial based on an analysis of the current data, which does not conclusively show a benefit for this approach.

Case #C.1.1
Goal: To clarify the distinction between operable and inoperable breast cancer

THOMAS J. KEARNEY

A 67-year-old woman presents for evaluation of a large breast mass. Physical examination reveals an 8-cm, freely movable breast mass and small, hard, mobile axillary lymph nodes.

The concept of operable versus inoperable breast cancer was originally codified in a classic paper five decades ago by Haagensen and Stout. Patients with extensive breast edema, inflammatory cancer, skin satellite lesions, arm edema, and parasternal or supraclavicular nodes had high local recurrence rates and there were no five-year survivors. Additional criteria, called "grave signs," also predicted a poor outcome, although there were some survivors. These included tumor fixation to the chest wall, fixed nodes, large nodes, skin ulceration, or limited breast edema. These observations foreshadowed the modern staging systems. Currently, patients with stage IIIA and IIIB breast cancer are considered to have locally advanced breast cancer (LABC). The term "inoperable breast cancer" refers to stage IIIB patients. Therefore, the woman described above has clinical stage IIIA (T3N1) operable LABC. Her tumor is large but not fixed and it does not involve the skin. She has clinically positive nodes but they are not large or fixed. A modified radical mastectomy could be performed.

A number of reports have demonstrated that neoadjuvant or induction therapy in stage III disease can produce response rates of 75% or greater. This has become the standard approach for patients with stage IIIB breast cancer. Following successful induction therapy, mastectomy and radiation are used to produce survival rates that appear to be the same as with a more conventional approach and local control rates are between 70 and 80%. For patients with stage IIIA breast cancer, a modified radical mastectomy followed by postoperative adjuvant therapy is a standard approach although clinical trials evaluating induction therapy for operable breast cancer, including stage II and stage I, are ongoing.

In addition, reports have appeared concerning breast-conserving surgery following induction chemotherapy. Because these studies represent experiences with highly selected patients and long-term results with the general population are not known, this approach must be considered investigational and should be restricted to clinical trials.

BIBLIOGRAPHY

Haagensen CD, Stout AP. Carcinoma of the breast: criteria of inoperability. Am Surg 1943; 118:859.

Schwartz GF. Breast conservation following induction chemotherapy for locally advanced breast cancer: a personal experience. Breast J 1996; 2:78–82.

Touboul E, Buffat L, Lefranc JP, et al. Possibility of conservative local treatment after combined chemotherapy and preoperative irradiation for locally advanced noninflammatory breast cancer. Int J Radiat Oncol Biol Phys 1996; 34: 1019–1028.

Case #C.1.2
Goal: To review the "grave prognostic" signs that help determine operability

JAY K. HARNESS

A 53-year-old woman presents with a 4-cm, hard, subareolar mass with breast erythema, edema, and warmth.

Haagensen and Stout were responsible in 1943 for identifying poor prognostic features of breast cancer. They reviewed the experience at Columbia Presbyterian Hospital in New York City during the period 1915–1942. They identified clinical features of breast cancer that were associated with a 0% 5-year cure and a greater than 50% chance of local recurrence. The "grave signs" of breast cancer defined by Haagensen and Stout include skin ulceration, fixation of the tumor to the chest wall, axillary lymph nodes greater than 2.5 cm in diameter, edema of less than one-third of the skin of the breast, and fixed axillary lymph nodes (Fig. 1). They felt that one grave sign did not make the patient inoperable. However, only one patient who had two grave signs was disease free at 5 years.

The American Joint Committee on Cancer staging manual for breast cancer defines a T4 tumor cancer as a tumor of any size with direct extension to chest wall or skin, edema of skin (*peau d' orange*), ulceration, or satellite skin nodules. Fixed axillary lymph nodes (also a "grave sign") are classified

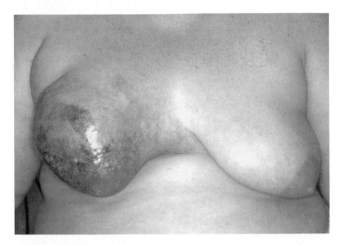

Figure 1   Example of stage IIIB breast carcinoma.

as N2. A T3 tumor is one that is more than 5 cm in greatest dimension. Most of the patients with this size tumor are also classified as stage IIIA except those who are node negative, who are classified as stage IIB. Stage IIIA and IIIB breast cancer is now generally referred to as "locally advanced breast cancer" (LABC).

Diagnosis of LABC is relatively straightforward. All patients should have mammograms, although they are technically difficult to do because of the size of the tumor and/or fixation of the tumor to the chest wall. Percutaneous core biopsies of the tumor mass can be performed quickly and easily with local anesthesia in the outpatient setting. Four to six samples should be taken. From these biopsies morphology and ER/PR status can be determined.

Punch biopsies of the edematous and erythematous skin can also be easily performed with local anesthesia in the outpatient setting. These biopsies should include some subcutaneous fat. The presence of cancer cells in dermal and/or subdermal lymphatic channels establishes the diagnosis of inflammatory breast carcinoma. There is no consistent histological type of breast carcinoma associated with inflammatory breast disease.

The clinical description of the case presented for discussion is that of a stage IIIB inflammatory breast carcinoma. A majority of inflammatory breast carcinoma patients have occult or clinically apparent axillary node involvement. The number of patients with inflammatory cancer who also have distant metastatic disease evident at diagnosis is higher than the number with the more common breast carcinomas. Appropriate initial staging of this patient should include a chest X-ray, bone scan, and liver function studies. An argument could be made for a bone marrow biopsy and cerebral magnetic resonance scanning. Once distant metastases have been ruled out, induction chemotherapy should be started.

The treatment of LABC generally includes chemotherapy, surgery, and radiotherapy. Clinical stage IIIB inflammatory carcinoma is initially considered "inoperable." Inflammatory breast carcinoma should be considered a systemic disease at the time of diagnosis. It is therefore appropriate to start induction chemotherapy not only to provide local/regional control, but to also treat probable systemic disease. Most induction chemotherapy regimens are doxorubicin based and should be given for an initial three cycles or to best response. Approximately 60–85% of patients respond to induction chemotherapy to the point where they are operable. As indicated in the clinical pathways, the next step would be modified radical mastectomy. However, some patients have both a complete clinical response (CR) and a complete pathological response (PR). I prefer to treat these patients with reexcision lumpectomy (to prove negative margins) and radiotherapy. Radiotherapy is started after completion of the postoperative chemotherapy.

Multimodality treatment of inflammatory breast cancer has greatly improved both local/regional control and long-term survival. Before the advent of systemic chemotherapy, inflammatory breast carcinoma was uniformly fatal. Currently, 3-year survival rates in the 40–70% range have been reported, and at 5 years, 30–50% of patients remain alive, most of them free of metastatic disease.

Editors' comment: The appropriate staging for inflammatory carcinoma of the breast is controversial. We recommend obtaining a chest X-ray, complete blood count, liver and renal function tests, electrolytes, bone scan, and computed-tomography scan of the chest, abdomen, and pelvis. We do not routinely examine the bone marrow or image the central nervous system.

BIBLIOGRAPHY

Beahrs OH, Henson DE, Hutter RVP, Kennedy BJ, eds. American Joint Committee on Cancer. Handbook for Staging of Cancer. Philadelphia: JB Lippincott, 1993:160–167.

Haagensen CD, Stout AP. Carcinoma of the breast. II. Criteria of operability. Ann Surg 1943; 118:859–870, 1032–1051.

Hortobagyi GN. Multidisciplinary management of advanced and metastatic breast cancer. Cancer 1994; 74(1):416–423.

Merajuer SD, Weber BL, Cody R, et al. Breast conservation and prolonged chemotherapy for locally advanced breast cancer: the University of Michigan experience. J Clin Oncol 1997; 15(8):2873–2881.

Schwartz GF, Lange AK, Topham AK. Breast conservation following induction che-
    motherapy for locally advanced carcinoma of the breast (stages IIIA and IIIB).
    A surgical perspective. Surg Oncol Clin North Am 1995; 4(4):657–669.

Case #C.1.3
Goal: To review clinical findings that define inoperability

MONICA MORROW

*A 43-year-old woman presents with a 3-cm breast mass and fixed axillary
lymph nodes.*

In the patient with a clinical diagnosis of locally advanced breast cancer, the goal of the initial evaluation should be to rapidly establish a histological diagnosis and ascertain whether metastases are present. These patients are ideal candidates for needle biopsy diagnosis either by fine-needle
aspiration cytology or by core needle (Tru-cut). Hormone receptors can be
determined with material obtained by either of these techniques. Excisional
or incisional biopsies should be avoided in this setting since they are more
expensive than the needle techniques and may delay the administration of
systemic therapy. In addition, preservation of the intact primary tumor facilitates the clinical assessment of response to chemotherapy.

The metastatic workup in this patient should include a chest X-ray,
liver function tests, serum calcium, and a bone scan. In contrast to the
asymptomatic patient with stage I or II disease where bone scans identify
metastases in fewer than 5% of patients, approximately 20% of patients with
clinical stage III disease will have bone metastases at presentation. Bilateral
mammography should be performed to document the extent of the primary
tumor and to exclude the presence of contralateral disease. In the absence
of symptoms of weight loss, abdominal pain, or abnormalities of the liver
function tests, abdominal imaging is a low-yield procedure and is not routinely indicated.

The clinical finding of fixation of the axillary mass to the chest wall
indicates that this patient has stage IIIB disease, which is inoperable and
should be treated with induction chemotherapy. Other clinical findings that
indicate inoperability include edema of the ipsilateral arm, edema of the
breast (*peau d'orange*), skin satellitosis, tumor ulceration, and inflammatory
skin changes. Large tumors (>5 cm) that lack these findings may be approached initially with surgery or chemotherapy. The use of induction chemotherapy in operable stage IIIA patients offers the potential for breast-
conserving surgery if a response is obtained, but has not been demonstrated
to have a survival advantage compared to postoperative chemotherapy.

BIBLIOGRAPHY

Hortobagyi GN, Singletary SE, McNeese MD. Treatment of locally advanced and inflammatory breast cancer. In: Harris JR, Lippman ME, Morrow M, Hellman S, eds. Diseases of the Breast. Philadelphia: Lippincott-Raven, 1996:585–599.

Case #C.1.4
Goal: To discuss the proper staging of patients with operable breast cancer

ROBERT S. DIPAOLA

A 35-year-old asymptomatic patient is found to have a 2.5-cm, infiltrating ductal carcinoma; 0/15 positive lymph nodes. Physical examination is unremarkable. Routine liver function tests, complete blood count, and serum chemistries are normal. What other tests should be ordered?

Given the need to contain cost while maintaining quality of care, the most appropriate staging workup will be of high yield and obtain data important to subsequent therapy. Radioisotope bone scanning (RBS) is highly sensitive but is not specific for metastasis. The discovery of unsuspected metastases by RBS is infrequent in early stages of breast cancer. In one study, only two of 189 patients with a T2 tumor had asymptomatic bone metastases on RBS. Therefore, RBS in patients with T2 tumors (<5 cm) is unlikely to be helpful and should be excluded from the initial workup. Similarly, a computed-tomography scan of the liver is also unlikely to be helpful, without hepatomegaly or abnormal liver function studies. Currently, tumor markers lack the sensitivity and specificity to be useful for screening or follow-up. A reasonable rule that supports not ordering any marker studies is that no clinical decision should be made on the basis of a tumor marker result until further studies develop more accurate tests.

BIBLIOGRAPHY

Ciatto S, Pacini P, Axxini V, et al. Preoperative staging of primary breast cancer: a multicenter study. Cancer 1988; 61:1038.

Case #C.1.5
Goal: To discuss breast conservation versus mastectomy

SUSAN A. MCMANUS

A 37-year-old woman in excellent health presents with a palpable, 1.2-cm right breast lesion. The axillary lymph nodes are clinically negative. If cancer is diagnosed, the patient expresses a strong initial preference for modified radical mastectomy.

This patient's initial preference for modified radical mastectomy as treatment for her breast cancer is not uncommon. Many young women view their best chance for survival as being associated with a more "aggressive" operation, i.e., a mastectomy. Although ultimately this 37-year-old may choose mastectomy with or without reconstruction for loco/regional control of her breast cancer, it is the oncologist's responsibility to present alternatives and discuss the data in a supportive and unbiased manner.

Patients who understand their options and who make their own decisions are the most likely to be satisfied with the course of treatment. Rowland and Holland, in their evaluation of the psychological reactions to breast cancer treatment, describe four types of responses: type 1, "You decide for me doctor"; type 2, "I demand you do the procedure"; type 3, "I can't decide"; and type 4, "Given the options, your recommendation, and my preferences, I chose. . . ." This particular patient best fits the type 2 description. She will likely benefit from data-based discussions of other approaches. Ideally the physician will be able to match the patient's needs with information that results in a "mutual participation or shared responsibility" for the decision making.

Six prospective, randomized trials have established that breast conservation with lumpectomy followed by radiation yields survival results equal to mastectomy. Furthermore, the risk of local recurrence after breast preservation is 5–10%, equivalent to the risk of chest wall recurrence after modified radical mastectomy. This information must be clearly explained to address this patient's impression that modified radical mastectomy offers improved survival. Next it will be necessary to explain that she has a small mass, clinically and mammographically, that is not accompanied by calcifications on the mammogram and should be amenable to breast-conserving therapy. Discussion should not be limited to merely the surgical options, for women need to understand that lumpectomy and axillary dissection should be followed by radiation for adequate local control.

Finally this patient may benefit from a two-staged procedure, i.e., lumpectomy followed by more extended surgery. This would enable her to have the pathology reviewed more completely and to meet with the radiation oncologist, a plastic surgeon, and perhaps a social worker prior to making her final decision. If the patient has presented alone for the initial visit, I would encourage including her spouse or a confidant in the discussion.

BIBLIOGRAPHY

Abrams, JS, Phillips PH, Friedman MA. Meeting highlights a reappraisal of research
results for the local treatment of early stage breast cancer. J Natl Cancer Inst
1995; 87(24):1837–1845.

Eberlien T. Current management of carcinoma of the breast. Ann Surg 1994; 220:
121–136.

Ganz PA. Advocating for the woman with breast cancer. Ca Cancer J Clini 1995;
45(2):114–126.

Rowland JH, Holland JC. Psychological reactions to breast cancer and its treatment.
In: Harris JR, Hellman S, Henderson IC, Kinne DW, eds. Breast Diseases
Philadelphia: JB Lippincott, 1991:849–866.

Winchester DJ, Menck HF, Winchester DP. The National Cancer Data Base report
on the results of a large non-randomized comparison of breast preservation
and modified radical mastectomy. Cancer 1997; 80(1):162–167.

Case #C.1.6
Goal: To discuss the role of radiation therapy in breast conservation

LAWRENCE J. SOLIN

*A 63-year-old woman who had lateral right chest wall irradiation 17
years ago for a 4-cm, malignant, fibrous histiocytoma arising in the
anterior axillary line just below the level of the breast undergoes breast
biopsy. She is found to have a 1.3-cm, invasive ductal carcinoma. The
excision margins are negative. Review of the old radiation fields suggests
that the lower outer quadrant of the breast, in the area of the newly
diagnosed breast cancer, received in excess of 3000 cGy. The patient is
strongly motivated to pursue breast conservation and asks what is the
importance of radiation therapy if her breast cancer has already been
widely excised.*

This patient presents with a favorable tumor for breast conservation
treatment. However, her clinical situation is complicated by her prior course
of radiation treatment, which appears to have included the location of the
current breast cancer. Because she has already received a course of radiation
treatment, a second course of radiation poses the potential for such complications as soft tissue fibrosis, soft tissue necrosis, rib fracture, pain, or an
unsatisfactory cosmetic outcome. These complications could seriously affect
the patient's quality of life and could even require major surgery (e.g., toilet
mastectomy with plastic surgical repair). A history of prior therapeutic radiation is commonly considered an absolute contraindication to breast con-

servation treatment with radiation, and mastectomy is recommended for the patient with such a history.

More information is needed about the prior course of radiation treatment to determine whether or not this patient is a candidate for breast conservation. The old radiation treatment records need to be reviewed in detail by a radiation oncologist. The prior radiation fields need to be reproduced on the patient as closely as possible. However, accurately reproducing the prior radiation fields may be difficult for a number of reasons. First, older treatment records are often not sufficiently detailed to reproduce accurately a prior treatment program and, in some cases, may be incomplete, lost, or destroyed. Second, tattoos may not have been used to mark the radiation fields. Third, the patient may have lost or gained weight, which would change the relationship of the skin and any tattoos to underlying structures.

The patient should be placed on a simulator table to attempt to reproduce the prior radiation fields as closely as possible and to determine the location of these fields relative to the breast and to the location of the current breast cancer. As sarcomas are generally treated to doses substantially greater than 3000 cGy, this patient likely received additional radiation treatment, via either external-beam radiation or brachytherapy. If brachytherapy was used, the dose contribution from brachytherapy to the breast should be estimated. Thus, additional information from the prior radiation treatment program is necessary before treatment recommendations can be made for the current breast cancer.

Assuming that a careful review of the prior radiation treatment records confirms that the dose to the area of the breast cancer is 3000 cGy as presented, there are three options for the local management of the breast for this patient: (1) modified radical mastectomy; (2) lumpectomy, axillary lymph node dissection, and radiation treatment; or (3) lumpectomy and axillary lymph node dissection without radiation treatment. Regardless of the local treatment of the breast, an axillary lymph node dissection should be included because this patient is a candidate for adjuvant systemic chemotherapy if her lymph nodes are pathologically positive. For patients treated with breast radiation, adjuvant systemic chemotherapy improves the local control rate after lumpectomy compared to patients treated without adjuvant chemotherapy. However, when radiation is not given, there is no difference in local control for patients treated with lumpectomy plus adjuvant chemotherapy compared to patients treated with lumpectomy alone without adjuvant chemotherapy. The relative merits of the three local treatment options are as follows:

Modified radical mastectomy (with or without reconstruction) is a standard, effective local treatment for this patient with early-stage breast cancer. Mastectomy for this patient would avoid the potential complications from a second course of radiation. In addition, the relatively low dose of radiation given 17 years ago should not increase the risk of complications from a mastectomy as initial management of this patient's current breast cancer. With the T1 lesion, the patient should be offered the option of breast reconstruction. As noted above, mastectomy, not breast conservation treatment, is recommended for a patient with a history of prior therapeutic radiation.

Breast conservation surgery (i.e., lumpectomy and axillary lymph node dissection) with radiation carries the increased risk of complications from a second course of therapeutic radiation. Should a complication develop, major surgical repair could be required. Although most prospective, randomized trials and most single-institution, retrospective studies have used radiation consisting of whole-breast treatment plus a boost to a total dose of 6000 cGy or more, a boost may not be necessary if the margins of resection are negative. The National Surgical Adjuvant Breast and Bowel Project B-06 study showed acceptable local control with 5000 cGy delivered to the whole breast after lumpectomy with pathologically confirmed negative margins of resection. Nonetheless, a total radiation dose of at least 8000 cGy (=5000 cGy + 3000 cGy), or more if a boost is used, exceeds accepted levels of normal tissue tolerance. While their study is not directly analogous to the present case, Karasek and Deutsch have reported six patients treated with radiation for lymphoma, followed 10–27 years later by treatment of breast cancer using lumpectomy and radiation; none of the six patients developed a serious complication from the two courses of radiation with 15–118 months of follow-up.

Breast conservation surgery without radiation is not generally recommended as treatment for early-stage breast cancer, but could be considered for the patient as presented. Omitting radiotherapy would eliminate the risk of complications from the second course of radiation, but is associated with a substantially increased risk of local recurrence. The value of radiation treatment following breast conservation surgery is to improve substantially the rate of local control in the treated breast.

On balance, mastectomy is the recommended local treatment of the breast for the patient as presented. The average life expectancy for a 63-year-old woman is approximately 19 years, and therefore, this patient should be treated with curative intent. Mastectomy is one of the two standard local treatments for early-stage breast cancer and allows the patient to undergo breast reconstruction; this approach offers a standard, relatively safe, and effective treatment program, while avoiding the potential risks associated with a second course of radiation treatment. A second, less desirable approach is breast conservation surgery without radiation treatment; however, the omission of radiation puts the patient at substantial risk for local recurrence requiring salvage mastectomy. Breast conservation treatment with radiation is not recommended because of the risk of complications from a second course of radiation.

BIBLIOGRAPHY

Emami B, Lyman J, Brown A, et al. Tolerance of normal tissue to therapeutic irradiation. Int J Radiat Oncol Biol Phys 1991; 21:109–122.

Fisher B, Anderson S, Redmond C, et al. Reanalysis and results after 12 years of follow-up in a randomized clinical trial comparing total mastectomy with lumpectomy with or without irradiation in the treatment of breast cancer. N Engl J Med 1995; 333:1456–1461.

Fowble BL, Solin LJ, Schultz DJ, Goodman RL. Ten year results of conservative surgery and irradiation for stage I and II breast cancer. Int J Radiat Oncol Biol Phys 1991; 21:269–277.

Harris JR, Morrow M. Local management of invasive breast cancer. In: Harris JR, Lippman ME, Morrow M, Hellman S, eds. Diseases of the Breast. Philadelphia: Lippincott-Raven, 1996:487–547.

Karasek K, Deutsch M. Lumpectomy and breast irradiation for breast cancer after radiotherapy for lymphoma. Am J Clin Oncol 1996; 19:451–454.

McCormick B. Invasive breast carcinoma: Patient selection for conservative management. Semin Radiat Oncol 1992; 2:74–81.

Case #C.1.7
Goal: To discuss the role of radiation treatment for small invasive breast cancers

LAWRENCE J. SOLIN

A 68-year-old woman presents with a 4-mm, estrogen-receptor-positive, moderately differentiated, invasive ductal carcinoma. Lumpectomy achieves "good," negative margins. Axillary dissection reveals 0/15 nodes. She lives 45 miles from the nearest radiation facility.

This patient presents with a favorable lesion for breast conservation treatment. The one potential problem is that she lives 45 miles from the nearest radiation therapy facility. The distance that this patient will need to travel on a daily basis for her radiation therapy treatments raises the issue of the importance of radiation treatment following lumpectomy with negative margins of resection for a small, T1 breast cancer.

The goals of breast conservation treatment are to achieve survival rates equivalent to mastectomy and to achieve the best possible cosmetic outcome while minimizing the risk of local recurrence and complications. The value of radiation treatment following breast conservation surgery is to improve substantially the rate of local control in the treated breast, but not survival.

These findings have been demonstrated in multiple prospective, randomized trials. In the National Surgical Adjuvant Breast and Bowel Project (NSABP) protocol B-06, the local failure rate at 12 years was reduced from 35% to 10% ($p < 0.001$) with the addition of radiation after lumpectomy, and the improvement in local control was evident for both node-negative and node-positive patients. In the NSABP B-06 trial, improved local failure rates were seen with radiation for all size tumors, including tumors ≤ 1 cm, although there was a small number of patients in this subgroup.

A number of studies have attempted to identify a subgroup of patients that can be treated with wide excision or quadrantectomy alone without radiation therapy. In a prospective, single-arm trial, Schnitt et al. treated favorable patients with wide excision alone, without radiation therapy. Favorable patients were defined in that study as having an infiltrating ductal, mucinous, or tubular carcinoma ≤ 2 cm in diameter, widely clear negative margins of resection (≥ 1 cm), pathologically negative axillary lymph nodes, no extensive intraductal component or lymphatic vessel invasion present, and adequate breast size to permit breast conservation treatment should a local recurrence develop. This study reported a local recurrence rate of 3.6% per year of follow-up; the crude 3-year local recurrence rate was 10.5%. The crude 3-year local recurrence rate was 0% for a comparison group treated with radiation therapy. After treatment with quadrantectomy alone, Veronesi et al. reported a risk of local recurrence at 42 months of approximately 16% for women aged <55 years and 4% for women aged >55 years ($p = 0.0188$); the local recurrence rate was considered to be sufficiently low in women aged >55 years to warrant the omission of radiation therapy. On balance, no reproducibly identified subgroup of women has been defined to warrant omitting radiation treatment following lumpectomy.

Although no clearly defined consensus has emerged for the minimum distance for negative margins necessary to consider omitting radiation treatment after lumpectomy or wide excision, most investigators have used a minimum distance for negative margins of 1 cm. In contrast, the acceptable distance for negative margins for a lumpectomy when radiation treatment is to be delivered is generally considered to be 1 or 2 mm, although no consensus has emerged for this distance, either. If the pathological margins for a lumpectomy have been carefully assessed, tumors with focally close or focally positive margins are acceptable for breast conservation treatment.

A phase I/II, single-arm study by the Radiation Therapy Oncology Group (RTOG) is currently accruing patients for treatment with brachytherapy alone as the sole method of radiation treatment following lumpectomy. The brachytherapy radiation for this study is designed to treat the primary tumor bed with a margin in a reduced overall treatment time. The radiation treatment in this study consists of 45 Gy using conventional low-dose brachytherapy over 3.5–6 days or 34 Gy using high-dose brachytherapy given in 3.4-Gy fractions b.i.d. in 10 fractions over 5–7 days. This study is designed to evaluate a type of radiation treatment for the patient who might benefit from radiation treatment after lumpectomy, but for whom standard daily radiation treatments over 6–7 weeks are impractical. Vicini et al. have reported a pilot study of low-dose brachytherapy as the sole radiation treatment for 60 patients with early-stage breast cancer; among these patients, no local recurrences developed with a median follow-up of 20 months.

A second RTOG protocol is currently evaluating the role of radiation for women aged ≥70 years with tumors ≤2 cm, positive or indeterminate estrogen receptors, and clinically negative lymph nodes treated with lumpectomy plus tamoxifen. This study will test whether radiation decreases the risk of local recurrence in elderly women treated with tamoxifen and whether lumpectomy plus tamoxifen is adequate treatment for these patients.

On balance, conventional radiation treatment should be recommended for the patient as presented above. The one exception to this recommendation would be if the patient had significant comorbid medical problems. The average life expectancy for a 68-year-old woman is more than 15 years. The significant improvement in local control associated with radiation treatment generally warrants radiation treatment in this setting. An important factor to be considered is whether the patient drives or can be driven for her daily radiation treatment; most 68-year-old women are sufficiently healthy and active to receive daily radiation treatment. The final argument for radiation treatment in this setting is that should the patient develop a local recurrence, the local recurrence could occur at a time when the patient is less medically fit to undergo salvage mastectomy; although radiation treatment does not eliminate the risk of local recurrence, radiation treatment substantially reduces this risk.

BIBLIOGRAPHY

Fisher B, Redmond C, and others for the National Surgical Adjuvant Breast and Bowel Project. Lumpectomy for breast cancer: an update of the NSABP experience. J Natl Cancer Inst Monogr 1992; 11:7–13.

Fisher B, Anderson S, Redmond C, et al. Reanalysis and results after 12 years of follow-up in a randomized clinical trial comparing total mastectomy with lumpectomy with or without irradiation in the treatment of breast cancer. N Engl J Med 1995; 333:1456–1461.

Peterson ME, Schultz DJ, Solin LJ. Breast cancer patients with focally positive or close pathologic margins can be adequately treated with breast-conserving therapy. Radiology 1996; 201(Suppl 1):205 (abstract).

Radiation Therapy Oncology Group Protocol RTOG 97-02. Evaluation of lumpectomy, tamoxifen, and irradiation of the breast compared with lumpectomy plus tamoxifen in women 70 years of age or older who have carcinoma of the breast that is less than or equal to 2 cm and clinically negative axillary nodes: a phase III study.

Radiation Therapy Oncology Group Protocol RTOG 95-17: A phase I/II trial to evaluate brachytherapy as the sole method of radiation therapy for stage I and II breast carcinoma.

Schnitt SJ, Hayman J, Gelman R, et al. A prospective study of conservative surgery alone in the treatment of selected patients with stage I breast cancer. Cancer 1996; 77:1094–1100.

The Uppsala-Orebro Breast Cancer Study Group. Sector resection with or without postoperative radiotherapy for stage I breast cancer: a randomized trial. J Natl Cancer Inst 1990; 82:277–282.

Veronesi U, Luini A, Galimberti V, Zurrida S. Conservation approaches for the management of stage I/II carcinoma of the breast: Milan Cancer Institute trials. World J Surg 1994; 18:70–75.

Vicini FA, Chen PY, Fraile M, et al. Low-dose-rate brachytherapy as the sole radiation modality in the management of patients with early-stage breast cancer treated with breast-conserving therapy: preliminary results of a pilot trial. Int J Radiat Oncol Biol Phys 1997; 38:301–310.

Whelan T, Clark R, Roberts R, et al. Ipsilateral breast tumor recurrence postlumpectomy is predictive of subsequent mortality: results from a randomized trial. Int J Radiat Oncol Biol Phys 1994; 30:11–16.

Case #C.1.8
Goal: To discuss the role of boost radiation therapy in the treatment of breast cancer

ALLEN S. LICHTER

A 56-year-old woman undergoes lumpectomy, axillary dissection, and radiation therapy for a 1.4-cm, estrogen-receptor-negative, moderately differentiated, invasive ductal carcinoma of the right breast. She presents for treatment planning for her radiation therapy.

The technical aspects of treating the breast with radiation are well agreed upon. The breast is approached with two tangentially directed fields. The medial field enters at the midline and exits through the midaxillary line, while the lateral field represents a mirror image. Superiorly, the field extends past all palpable breast tissue, and inferiorly, it extends about 1 cm below the inframammary fold. Because the chest wall is curved and the radiation passes in a straight line, a small area of lung is subtended by the radiation beams. Typically, this is 2 cm or less of the ipsilateral lung, which represents 5% or less of the lung volume. If more than this amount of lung appears inside the treatment field, the patient should be resimulated to try to reduce the size of this rim of lung tissue as much as possible. Each patient has a contour taken of the shape of her breast and has her dose distribution modeled in the computer (Fig. 1). Once the proper dose distribution has been developed, one typically treats the breast to a dose of 45–50 Gy in 5–51/2 weeks. Each day's treatment takes approximately 10 min and most patients go through this therapy with few, if any, acute side effects.

At the completion of the whole-breast treatment, the majority of radiation oncologists in the United States apply a boost to the tumor bed. The absolute necessity of this boost remains controversial. In the oft-sited NSABP B-06 trial, which went a long way to establish the value of lumpectomy and radiation as an alternative to mastectomy, no boost treatment was given, and the in-breast failure rate at 12 years of follow-up was 11%. This is not strikingly different from the recurrence rates reported by

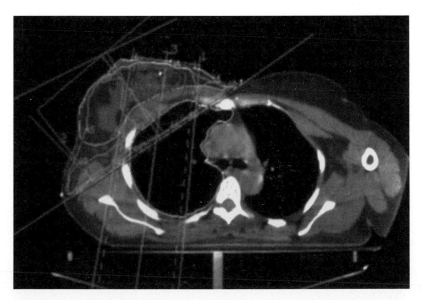

Figure 1 Each patient has a contour taken of the shape of her breast and has her dose distribution modeled in the computer.

institutions that do use a boost. Recently, a group from Lyon, France published a randomized, prospective trial comparing boost to no boost. The recurrence rate in the boost population was 3.2% and in the nonboost population it was 4.5%. However, with over 500 patients in each arm of the trial, this difference in recurrence was statistically significant. This type of study gives comfort to both sides in the boost debate. Those who do not favor the use of a boost can cite the very small difference that this treatment makes in a randomized study. Those who favor a boost can cite that a statistically significant advantage was obtained for patients who received a boost.

At the authors' institution, virtually all patients still receive a boost. This can be done in two ways. At our institution we apply an electron beam directly to the boost site to bring the total dose to the boosted area to 60 Gy. Most of our patients have clips left in the surgical bed by the surgeon at the time of the excision, which greatly facilitates the design and dose prescription for the boost field. For those patients who do not have clips left behind, a limited number of computed-tomography slices through the boost volume can usually ascertain the location of the tumor bed and its depth below the skin surface.

Complications of radiation administered in this fashion are relatively rare. Approximately 5% of patients will have an asymptomatic rib fracture secondary to the irradiation delivered to the ribs of the chest wall. The author has never seen a long-term complication resulting from these asymptomatic rib fractures; they are largely picked up incidentally when looking at a chest X-ray or a bone scan obtained for another reason. Approximately 1% of the patients or less will develop radiation pneumonitis. This typically presents as a cough, not associated with fever or shortness of breath. The chest X-ray is often clear in this setting, and a short course of oral prednisone will resolve the symptoms. Almost all patients will experience some breast discomfort following radiation and almost all patients will gradually clear this discomfort. The occasional patient has persistent pain in the breast and chest wall requiring the use of anti-inflammatory agents. For left-sided breast cancers, a small portion of the anterior heart is included inside the radiation field. In patients who have received postmastectomy chest wall irradiation, there is a small, but measurable increase in late cardiac events such as myocardial infarction. Patients treated with modern breast conservation techniques have not been followed long enough to know whether they will also share in this risk, but it is prudent to try to minimize the cardiac volume included within the radiation ports as much as possible. Finally, the most serious of all complications is the appearance of a second malignancy in the treated volume. These are typically angiosarcomas and can be quite difficult to treat. Fortunately, the incidence of this is rare, probably one in several hundreds to several thousand cases.

Case #C.1.9
Goal: To discuss the risks and benefits of radiation therapy

ALLEN S. LICHTER

A 65-year-old woman, with severe chronic obstructive pulmonary disease, presents with a 1.7-cm lesion of left breast. Core needle biopsy reveals an invasive ductal carcinoma. There are palpable axillary lymph nodes.

This is a difficult case. Clearly the breast itself needs to be treated with radiation. In studies where lumpectomy alone was used to treat invasive breast cancer, recurrence rates in the 30–40% range have been seen. A local recurrence in this case setting would be a major problem since the typical treatment for recurrence is mastectomy, and that would be a challenge in this patient. Therefore, I would certainly recommend that radiotherapy be delivered to the breast.

The next question is what to do about the palpable axillary adenopathy. Ideally, one would perform an axillary lymph node dissection in such a patient, and this would take care of the axilla as far as local therapy is concerned. If this patient cannot have an axillary lymph node dissection, there are some additional choices. One could, of course, treat with radiotherapy alone, including the enlarged axillary lymph nodes. The dose required to reliably control these nodes, however, would be relatively high, and I believe the risk of long-term complications would be high if high-dose radiation were used alone. With estrogen-receptor-positive disease, one could conceive of giving several months of tamoxifen to see if the lymph nodes would shrink and then give radiotherapy, but this would probably delay the entire treatment process for too long a period. I would prefer that the palpable adenopathy be excised. This could be done under local anesthesia. I would then direct radiotherapy to the breast, axilla, and supraclavicular fossa comprehensively in an effort to provide permanent local control.

Treating this patient with radiation is also a challenge from a pulmonary standpoint. One would have to be extremely careful to exclude as much lung as possible from all the treatment fields, but it should be possible to treat this patient without any major reduction in her limited pulmonary capacity.

Case #C.1.10
Goal: To discuss the influence of positive surgical margins on the conservative management of breast lesions

KIRBY I. BLAND and DANIEL S. KIM

A 37-year-old woman presents with a 1-cm region of clustered micro-calcifications on mammogram. Wire localization biopsy reveals infiltrating ductal carcinoma with positive margins. The patient is strongly motivated to pursue breast-conserving therapy.

Breast conservation therapy has emerged as the standard of care for many women with breast cancer. Six randomized trials have compared mastectomy to breast conservation therapy and have demonstrated no significant difference in overall survival and distant disease-free survival. However, there were highly significant differences in local recurrence, and local recurrences are usually treated with mastectomy. Since salvage mastectomy for recurrence is considered failure of conservation therapy, with psychosocial and economic consequences, local recurrence has fostered much discussion.

Positive margins have been shown to increase the risk of local recurrence. Schnitt and colleagues looked at negative, close, focally positive, and more than focally positive margins and found local recurrence rates of 0%, 4%, 6%, and 21%, respectively. Anscher et al. examined positive, close, and indeterminate margins and found local recurrence rates of 9%, 1.5%, and 6%, respectively. Some authors suggest that with an extensive intraductal component (EIC)-negative tumor and only focally positive margins, reexcision is not mandatory if radiotherapy is included.

Schnitt et al. have demonstrated a significantly higher local recurrence rate with margins that are more than focally positive, compared to focally positive margins. Any time a positive margin is evident within permanent pathological specimens, we perform wide local excision of the previous biopsy site, and would do so in this patient. If the primary lesion has diffusely positive margins, or if the reexcision has "close" or positive margins, we would perform a modified radical mastectomy, if the lesion is an infiltrating neoplasm.

The presence of EIC has been shown to correlate with positive margins and to increase the risk of local recurrence. Schnitt et al. found a true recurrence and "marginal miss" rate (TR/MM) of 20% with EIC-positive tumors and only 7% for EIC-negative tumors at 5 years. We would offer this woman breast conservation therapy if her EIC status is amenable to this approach. However, if she was EIC positive and her margins could not be cleared, the best treatment would be a modified radical mastectomy.

Contraindications for reexcision following lumpectomy would include any contraindications for breast conservation and radiation therapy. Winchester and Cox proposed the following absolute and relative contraindications: Absolute contraindications include pregnancy in the first or second trimester, two or more gross lesions in different quadrants, or diffuse microcalcifications on mammography, and a history of prior radiotherapy to the area, especially in patients with a prior history of Hodgkin's disease. The relative contraindications are a history of collagen vascular disease, a large tumor in relation to the breast size, large pendulous breasts, and centrally located tumors. A particular contraindication for reexcision when breast conservation is otherwise feasible would be an inability to maintain adequate cosmesis in achieving negative margins.

BIBLIOGRAPHY

Anscher MS, Jones P, Prosnitz LR, et al. Local failure and margin status in early-stage breast carcinoma treated with conservation surgery and radiation therapy. Ann Surg 1993; 218:22–28.

Cady B. Choice of operations for early breast cancer: an expanding role for breast conservation instead of mastectomy. In: Bland KI, Copeland EM, eds. The Breast: Comprehensive Management of Benign and Malignant Diseases, 2nd ed. Philadelphia: WB Saunders, 1998:1130–1152.

Macmillan RD, Purushotham AD, George WD. Local recurrence after breast-conserving surgery for breast cancer. Br J Surg 1996; 83:149–155.

Schnitt SJ, Abner A, Gelman R, et al. The relationship between microscopic margins of resection and the risk of local recurrence in patients with breast cancer treated with breast-conserving surgery and radiation therapy. Cancer 1994; 74: 1746–1751.

Winchester DP, Cox JD. Standard for breast-conservation treatment. CA Cancer J Clin 1992; 42:134–162.

Case #C.1.11
Goal: To discuss the management of multifocal microcalcifications

MICHAEL H. TOROSIAN

A 52-year-old woman presents with a biopsy-proven, 3.5-cm, infiltrating ductal carcinoma and a mammogram showing multifocal, indeterminate microcalcifications. She has clinically negative axillary lymph nodes.

This patient presents with a 3.5-cm infiltrating ductal carcinoma proven by surgical biopsy. Her mammogram reveals multifocal, indeterminate microcalcifications. A postbiopsy mammogram should be performed in this instance to determine the number and pattern of residual microcalcifications following lumpectomy.

The presence of residual, multifocal, indeterminate microcalcifications poses a difficulty for follow-up of breast cancer patients if breast conservation therapy is desired. A clinical judgment needs to be made whether the patient is a candidate for breast conservation therapy or would be best served by undergoing modified radical mastectomy. If there are innumerable foci of indeterminate microcalcifications, the safest approach is modified radical mastectomy. In the presence of diffuse, indeterminate microcalcifications, follow-up after breast conservation therapy would be essentially impossible and detection of recurrent cancer could be significantly delayed. Alternatively, if few areas of indeterminate microcalcifications are present and the patient strongly desires breast conservation therapy, needle localization/excision of these areas of microcalcification could be performed as an intermediate step in determining whether or not breast conservation could be pursued. If no other areas of carcinoma are demonstrated, breast conservation consisting of lumpectomy with clear surgical margins, a level I and II axillary lymph node dissection, and radiation therapy to the breast could be undertaken.

Magnetic resonance imaging is currently investigational and available only at select medical centers. To provide clinically relevant information regarding breast treatment, detailed images of the ipsilateral breast with and without gadolinium enhancement might be obtained with a specially designed breast coil. Magnetic resonance imaging has enabled the detection and localization (via guidewire insertion) of multifocal carcinoma and, thus, identified the need for mastectomy as opposed to breast conservation therapy in some patients. Accurate staging of patients with known breast cancer is likely to become an important clinical role for magnetic resonance imaging in the future.

In summary, this clinical situation requires careful clinical judgment and thorough discussion with the patient. The mammogram must be carefully examined and the patient clearly informed of the difficulties and limitations of follow-up evaluation should breast conservation therapy be pursued. The safest treatment option in this setting is to perform modified radical mastectomy—nevertheless, the patient plays an integral role in the decision-making process *if* the residual microcalcifications are *limited* and she is fully informed of the treatment and diagnostic limitations that exist.

BIBLIOGRAPHY

McKenna RJ Sr. The abnormal mammogram: radiographic findings, diagnostic options, pathology, and stage of cancer diagnosis. Cancer 1994; 74(Suppl):244.

Moskowitz M. The predictive value of certain mammographic signs in screening for breast cancer. Cancer 1983; 51:1007.

Orel SG, Schnall MD, Newman R, Powell CM, Torosian MH, Rosato EF. Initial experience with MR imaging-guided breast biopsy. Radiology 1994; 193:97.

Sickles E. Breast calcifications: mammographic evaluation. Radiology 1986; 160: 289.

Winchester D, Cox J. Standards for breast conservation treatment. CA Cancer J Clin 1992; 42:134.

Case #C.1.12
Goal: To discuss the importance of an "extensive intraductal component"

LAWRENCE J. SOLIN

A 40-year-old woman, following biopsy of a palpable lesion, presents for evaluation of a 1.5-cm, infiltrating ductal carcinoma with associated extensive intraductal component (EIC) and positive margins. The first opinion she received was to undergo a modified radical mastectomy.

This patient presents with a T1 lesion, and presumptively is interested in breast conservation treatment. A potential problem for breast conservation treatment is the presence of an extensive intraductal component (EIC)-positive tumor with positive margins of resection.

Evaluation of EIC is made on pathological examination of the primary breast cancer. An EIC-positive tumor is defined as either: (1) intraductal carcinoma prominently present ($\geq 25\%$) within the main infiltrating tumor mass and any intraductal carcinoma seen outside of the main infiltrating tumor mass; or (2) intraductal carcinoma with microinvasion. EIC-positive tumors have been associated with an increased risk of local recurrence following breast conservation treatment compared to EIC-negative tumors. However, EIC status does not impact on the rates of survival or distant metastases.

The presence of an EIC-positive tumor indicates the potential for extensive spread of intraductal carcinoma in the breast, such that radiation treatment in conventional doses may not be sufficient to control residual microscopic disease, which, in turn, may lead to local recurrence. Holland et al. reported the results from pathological evaluation of 214 mastectomy specimens. At a distance of >2 cm from the edge of the primary tumor, EIC-positive tumors had more intraductal carcinoma in the breast compared to EIC-negative tumors (58% vs. 19%, respectively; $p < 0.00001$) and more "prominent" intraductal carcinoma (33% vs. 2%, respectively; $p = 1 \times 10^{-8}$). "Prominent" intraductal carcinoma was defined in this study as the presence of intraductal carcinoma in six or more microscopic low-power fields. In the study by Schnitt et al. (1987), residual carcinoma was found in 88% of reexcisional biopsy specimens for EIC-positive tumors compared to 48% for EIC-negative tumors ($p = 0.002$).

Careful pathological evaluation of the margins of resection is necessary to obtain adequate local control for EIC-positive tumors. When the margins of resection are negative for EIC-positive tumors, no difference in local control is found compared to EIC-negative tumors. Gage et al. reported a 6% risk of local recurrence for EIC-positive tumors with negative margins of resection, but a 26% risk of local recurrence for EIC-positive tumors with positive margins of resection. To obtain negative margins of resection and adequate local control, a wider excision of the primary tumor may be necessary for EIC-positive tumors than for EIC-negative tumors.

Mammography is important in the preoperative evaluation of a primary breast tumor. The presence of mammographic microcalcifications is correlated with the presence of an EIC-positive tumor. Healey et al. found that mammographic microcalcifications (with or without an associated breast mass) were more commonly associated with an EIC-positive tumor than an EIC-negative tumor (83% vs. 27%, respectively; $p < 0.0001$), and microcalcifications alone without an associated breast mass were also more commonly associated with an EIC-positive tumor (34% vs. 5%, respectively; $p = 0.0002$).

The presence of an EIC-positive tumor does not contraindicate breast conservation treatment for the patient as presented. However, the patient's management should be altered somewhat to achieve an optimal outcome. The patient requires a reexcision before a final decision can be made regarding breast conservation treatment. If the reexcision shows substantial residual disease with positive margins, then mastectomy is indicated. However, if the reexcision shows minimal or no disease with negative margins, then breast conservation is appropriate treatment. In a 40-year-old patient, axillary lymph node dissection is indicated for pathological staging.

BIBLIOGRAPHY

Gage I, Schnitt SJ, Nixon AJ, et al. Pathologic margin involvement and the risk of recurrence in patients treated with breast-conserving therapy. Cancer 1996; 78: 1921–1928.

Harris JR, Morrow M. Local management of invasive breast cancer. In: Harris JR, Lippman ME, Morrow M, Hellman S, eds. Diseases of the Breast. Philadelphia: Lippincott-Raven, 1996:487–547.

Healey EA, Osteen RT, Schnitt SJ, et al. Can the clinical and mammographic findings at presentation predict the presence of an extensive intraductal component in early stage breast cancer? Int J Radiat Oncol Biol Phys 1989; 17:1217–1221.

Holland R, Connolly JL, Gelman R, et al. The presence of an extensive intraductal component following a limited excision correlates with prominent residual disease in the remainder of the breast. J Clin Oncol 1990; 8:113–118.

Schnitt SJ, Connolly JL, Khettry U, et al. Pathologic findings on re-excision of the primary site in breast cancer patients considered for treatment by primary radiation therapy. Cancer 1987; 59:675–681.

Schnitt SJ, Abner A, Gelman R, et al. The relationship between microscopic margins of resection and the risk of local recurrence in patients with breast cancer treated with breast-conserving surgery and radiation therapy. Cancer 1994; 74: 1746–1751.

Veronesi U, Luini A, Galimberti V, Zurrida S. Conservation approaches for the management of stage I/II carcinoma of the breast: Milan Cancer Institute trials. World J Surg 1994; 18:70–75.

Vicini FA, Eberlein TJ, Connolly JL, et al. The optimal extent of resection for patients with stages I or II breast cancer treated with conservative surgery and radiotherapy. Ann Surg 1991; 214:200–204.

Yeh I-T, Fowble B, Viglione MJ, et al. Pathologic assessment and pathologic prognostic factors in operable breast cancer. In: Fowble B, Goodman RL, Glick JH, Rosato EF, eds. Breast Cancer Treatment: A Comprehensive Guide to Management. St. Louis: Mosby Year Book, 1991:167–208.

Zafrani B, Vielh P, Fourquet A, et al. Conservative treatment of early breast cancer: prognostic value of the ductal in situ component and other pathological variables on local control and survival: long-term results. Eur J Cancer Clin Oncol 1989; 25:1645–1650.

Case #C.1.13
Goal: To discuss the treatment of excellent-prognosis lesions

THOMAS J. KEARNEY

A 37-year-old woman presents with an abnormal mammogram. Biopsy reveals a 4-mm, pure tubular carcinoma. The biopsy margins are negative.

Tubular carcinomas account for about 2% of all invasive breast cancers. This special type of invasive breast cancer is characterized by very-well-differentiated cells that are regular and arranged in well-defined tubules. A carcinoma is considered "pure tubular" when at least 75% of the tumor has tubular characteristics. This prevents some well-differentiated invasive cancers, which may have occasional areas of tubular appearance, from being incorrectly classified. They would be properly classified as mixed tubular cancers. Most pure tubular cancers are small if detected by palpation or by mammography. Almost all are estrogen receptor (ER) positive.

Patients with pure tubular carcinoma, such as the woman described, have an excellent prognosis. With appropriate local treatment alone, survival rates should be at least 95%. It is difficult to see how adjuvant therapy would be justified. A series of patients with small, pure tubular cancers and negative axillary nodes treated with surgery alone had no recurrences with over 15 years of follow-up. The rate of positive axillary nodes can be as low as 0% in some series, although others have shown much higher rates. Since the rate of positive nodes is already low in patients with T1a tumors and because tubular carcinomas are extremely favorable, it is appropriate to defer axillary dissection in women such as the one described with small pure tubular cancers. These women should be treated with breast-conserving surgery followed by radiation therapy.

The prognosis in breast cancer is based primarily on the size and the histology of the primary tumor along with the presence or absence of axillary metastases. Although numerous other prognostic markers have been described, their contribution to the overall ability to independently predict outcome is small. Patients with small tumors rarely have axillary metastases and have excellent outcomes. Special types of invasive breast cancer, such as pure tubular cancers along with medullary and mucinous cancers, tend to have better prognoses than unspecified invasive breast cancer. Patients with "microinvasive" breast cancer also have excellent prognoses although this term is poorly defined. Patients with excellent-prognosis invasive breast cancer should still receive radiation after breast-conserving surgery and in almost all instances should have axillary dissection as a small number will harbor unsuspected axillary metastases and will benefit from adjuvant therapy. Only selected patients such as those with small pure tubular cancers, less then 1 cm in size, or with clear "microinvasive" breast cancer can safely avoid axillary dissection.

BIBLIOGRAPHY

Berger AC, Miller SM, Harris MN, et al. Axillary dissection for tubular carcinoma of the breast. Breast J 1996; 2:204–208.

Masood S, Barwick KW. Estrogen receptor expression of the less common breast carcinomas. Am J Clin Pathol 1990; 93:437.

Peters GN, Wolff M, Haagensen CD. Tubular carcinoma of the breast. Clinical pathologic correlations based on 100 cases. Ann Surg 1981; 193:138–149.

Rosen PP. Breast Pathology. Philadelphia: Lippincott-Raven, 1997.

Rosen PP, Groshen S, Saigo PE, et al. A long-term follow-up study of survival in stage 1 (T1N0M0) and stage II (T1N1M0) breast carcinoma. J Clin Oncol 1989; 7:355–366.

Winchester DJ, Sahin AA, Tucker SL, et al. Tubular carcinoma of the breast: predicting axillary nodal metastases and recurrence. Ann Surg 1996; 223:342–347.

Wong JH, Kopald KH, Morton DL. The impact of microinvasion on axillary node dissection for T1a breast carcinoma: is it indicated? Arch Surg 1990; 125: 1298–1302.

Case #C.1.14
Goal: To discuss the choice of lumpectomy versus modified radical mastectomy

ROSEMARY B. DUDA

A 78-year-old woman underwent a fine-needle aspirate of a 2-cm mass, which revealed invasive ductal carcinoma. Physical examination reveals two small, hard, mobile axillary lymph nodes. Mammograms are otherwise normal.

Breast cancer in the elderly is common and presents special challenges. Before surgery, bilateral mammograms should be obtained to determine if other suspicious lesions exist in the ipsilateral or contralateral breast. They can also provide information regarding the extent of the cancer, which assists in the decision between lumpectomy and mastectomy. Lumpectomy is an option available to the elderly, as it is to a woman of any age, as long as histologically negative margins and an acceptable cosmetic result are achievable.

Treatment of breast cancer should be based on physiological status rather than chronological age. Comorbid disease should be taken into consideration when discussing options with the patient. While age is an important risk factor for surgery, coexisting disease is more important than age alone. Many elderly patients do well and benefit from surgical procedures.

Breast conservation is the standard of care for the treatment of stage I and II breast cancer according to the National Cancer Institute Consensus Conference because it results in survival equivalent to mastectomy. It can and should be offered to the elderly. In fact, a lumpectomy without axillary lymph node dissection can be performed as an outpatient procedure under local anesthesia, eliminating the risks of a general anesthesia. The decision to include an axillary dissection in a patient without palpable nodes is subject to debate. The decision should include an overall assessment of how the results of the dissection will affect treatment recommendations and the quality of the patient's life. Whether or not surgery should be followed by either radiation therapy, systemic therapy, or both should also be based on the general health of the patient.

Randomized trials have been performed to determine whether tamoxifen can be effectively used as a primary treatment for breast cancer in the elderly. Although the response rate to tamoxifen alone has been reported to be as high as 67%, the overall local failure rate is approximately 60%. Many of these patients required a subsequent resection. Although local control was better in the patients undergoing surgery, there was no difference in survival. Most elderly patients tolerate breast surgery. The reported mortality from a mastectomy in the elderly is approximately 1%. There also appears to be no significant increased risk from radiation in older compared to younger patients. Because most elderly patients will tolerate surgery, whether it is a lumpectomy with radiation therapy or a mastectomy, tamoxifen should not be used alone as the primary therapy. Tamoxifen alone should be reserved for those patients with significant comorbid disease that would be expected to significantly limit the person's life, regardless of a diagnosis of breast cancer.

In this particular patient, who apparently has no significant comorbid disease, a 2-cm breast cancer, and suspicious palpable axillary nodes, I would recommend lumpectomy with axillary dissection (provided the mammogram reveals no complicating findings).

Fine-needle aspiration (FNA) is a highly accurate diagnostic procedure. The false-positive rate is approximately 0–0.4% with an experienced cytopathologist. Hence, a positive FNA is a highly accurate diagnostic test upon which further planning and treatment recommendations can be made. Because of this high level of accuracy, some surgeons may perform a mastectomy without a frozen section or further biopsy of the cancer in the presence of a suspicious mammogram, clinical examination, and a positive FNA. Alternatively, the definitive operative procedure can be planned on the basis of the above tests, a core biopsy, or an incisional or excisional biopsy. When the patient is taken to the operating room, a frozen section can be performed and the surgeon can proceed with a mastectomy and/or axillary dissection if the result of the frozen section confirms the diagnosis of cancer. The false-positive rate of a frozen section is as low as 0.06%. This is perhaps the safest approach to a patient anticipating a mastectomy. When the patient is undergoing breast conservation surgery, the partial mastectomy can be performed and a frozen section obtained prior to proceeding with the axillary dissection. A positive FNA avoids a second operative procedure and anesthetic and assures a high level of accuracy in confirming a diagnosis of breast cancer.

The presence of palpable axillary nodes indicates that an axillary dissection should be performed. An axillary dissection can be performed as a component of either breast conservation surgery or a mastectomy and does not by itself dictate the primary breast surgical procedure.

Editors' comment: We do not rely on FNA results to proceed with a mastectomy or axillary dissection. All positive FNA results should be confirmed histologically (with a frozen section) in the operating room.

BIBLIOGRAPHY

Bates T, Riley D, Houghton J, et al. Breast cancer in elderly women: a Cancer Research Campaign trial comparing treatment with tamoxifen and optimal surgery with tamoxifen alone. Br J Surg 1991; 78:591–594.

Feldman PS, Covell JL. Breast and lung. In: Fine Needle Aspiration Cytology and Its Clinical Application. Chicago: American Society of Clinical Pathologists Press, 1985:27–43.

Gazet J, Ford H, Coombes R, et al. Prospective randomized trial of tamoxifen versus surgery in elderly patients with breast cancer. Eur J Surg Oncol 1994; 20: 207–214.

Innes DJ, Feldman PS. Comparison of diagnostic results obtained by fine needle aspiration cytology and Tru-cut or open biopsies. Acta Cytol 1983; 27:350–354.

Kantorowitz D, Poulter C, Sischy B, et al. Treatment of breast cancer among elderly women with segmental mastectomy or segmental mastectomy plus postoperative radiotherapy. Int J Radiat Oncol Biol Phys 1988; 15:263–270.

Lubin MF. Is age a risk factor for surgery? Med Clin North Am 1993; 77:327–333.

National Institutes of Health Consensus Development Panel Consensus Statement. Treatment of early-stage breast cancer. J Natl Cancer Inst Monogr 1992; 11: 11.

Robertson J, Ellis I, Elston C, et al. Mastectomy or tamoxifen as initial therapy for operable breast cancer in elderly patients: 5-year follow-up. Eur J Cancer Clin Oncol 1992; 28:908–910.

Schneiderman M, Axtell L. Deaths among female patients with carcinoma of the breast treated by a surgical procedure alone. Surg Gynecol Obstet 1979; 148: 193–195.

Thomas DR, Ritchie CS. Preoperative assessment of older adults. J Am Geriatr Soc 1995; 43:811–821.

Toonkel L, Fix I, Jacobson L, et al. Management of elderly patients with primary breast cancer. Int J Radiat Oncol Biol Phys 1988; 14:677–681.

Wanebo HL, Feldman PS, Wilhelm MC, et al. Fine needle aspiration cytology in lieu of open biopsy in management of primary breast cancer. Ann Surg 1984; 199:569–579.

Watson DP, McGuire M, Nicholson F, Given HF. Aspiration cytology and its relevance to the diagnosis of solid tumors of the breast. Surg Gynecol Obstet 1987; 165:435–441.

Case #C.1.15
Goal: To discuss indications for wide-volume brachytherapy as an alternative to 6 weeks of external-beam radiation therapy (EBRT)

ROBERT R. KUSKE

A 53-year-old woman executive discovers a lump in the lower central aspect of her right breast and presents immediately to her physician, who palpates a firm, 2-cm mass at the 6 o'clock position of the right breast, with no evidence of adenopathy. Mammography confirms a suspicious 2-cm, spiculated mass without associated microcalcifications. Fine-needle aspiration reveals carcinoma. The patient clearly prefers breast conservation. At excisional biopsy and staging right axillary lymph node dissection, the surgeon removes a specimen measuring 6 × 4 × 2.5 cm, containing a firm white tumor measuring 1.8 cm, grossly excised. Microscopically, the tumor is an infiltrating ductal carcinoma, histologic grade 3, nuclear grade 2, mitotic index 1, with a minor (<10%) comedo intraductal component. The closest inked microscopic surgical margin is 5 mm and clear. All 15 dissected axillary lymph nodes are negative. The tumor is estrogen and progesterone-receptor negative and aneuploid, with an S-phase fraction of 15%. Because she is self-employed with a 12-hr workday, 6 or 7 days per week, and the travel back and forth to the radiation oncology center would almost certainly be disruptive to her work, she considers forgoing radiation therapy and proceeding to mastectomy, rather than compromising her professional responsibilities. She is interested in alternatives to 6 weeks of external-beam radiation. After her case is presented at the weekly multidisciplinary breast tumor board for mammographic and pathology slide review, the patient is considered for enrollment in RTOG Protocol 95-17, a phase I/II study of brachytherapy as the only radiation therapy for selected T1, T2, N0, N1 breast cancers.

The Ochsner Clinic pilot trial, the predecessor of the national study, opened in January 1992 and closed in October 1994, after the accrual of 26 low-dose-rate (LDR) and 26 high-dose-rate (HDR) patients in alternating blocks of 10 patients. Since no patients have been lost to follow-up, the median follow-up reached 5 years in January 1998, with a minimum follow-up of over 3 years. There have been no breast recurrences and one infraclavicular recurrence. Toxicity primarily consisted of infection and fat necrosis. One LDR patient required an incision and drainage along with IV antibiotics for a *Staphylococcus aureus* breast abscess that developed after her 4th cycle of AC chemotherapy, 3 months after catheter removal. Two

HDR patients required surgery for symptomatic fat necrosis, manifested by a painful, inflamed quadrant of the breast. One of these patients had active (ESR = 62) collagen vascular disease, and another had a 60% gradient from the mean central dose to the peripheral dose. The total grade 3 toxicity rate is 5.8%. The RTOG protocol excludes patients with collagen vascular disease, limits the allowable dose gradient, and the HDR fractionation is extended over 5 days, measures that will hopefully minimize the potential for grade 3 toxicity in the cooperative group trial.

Cosmetic outcome is another important endpoint. A photographic review matching Ochsner brachytherapy patients to patients treated to the breast with external beam, by stage, breast size, and length of follow-up, found no significant difference in cosmetic outcome (see Table 1). In particular, women with very large breasts had better cosmesis and less acute toxicity with brachytherapy. Favorable results of the pilot trial led to the RTOG protocol, which will test the reproducibility, quality control, toxicity, cosmesis, and breast tumor control rates in a multi-institutional setting. The RTOG trial was activated in May 1997.

The issue of the clinical significance of multicentricity in breast cancer is seminal to this study. Since brachytherapy is a subtotal breast treatment, unlike modified radical mastectomy and standard breast conservation therapy with external-beam irradiation that treat the entire breast, there could be a theoretical risk for a future recurrence in a different quadrant of the breast.

Indeed, remote recurrences might be predicted based upon pathology studies demonstrating foci of carcinoma in a different quadrant of the breast in 26% of tumors 2 cm or less in size and 36% of tumors between 2 and 4 cm. Another pathologist found carcinoma 4 cm or more beyond the index tumor in 12% of patients without an extensive intraductal component (EIC) and in 32% with EIC. However, the *biological significance* of these remote foci is cast into doubt by many published series, with and without breast irradiation, which demonstrate that the vast majority of clinical recurrences occur in and around the site of the original excision (Tables 2 and 3). Only 0–3.5% of patients treated with breast conservation surgery recur in areas

Table 1 Cosmetic Outcome: Brachytherapy versus External-Beam Matched Controls

Treatment Group	Brachytherapy	Controls	Composite Brachytherapy		Composite Controls	
Excellent	37%	39%	Excellent/Good	76%	Excellent/Good	76%
Good	39%	37%				
Fair	21%	18%	Fair/Poor	24%	Fair/Poor	24%
Poor	3%	6%				

Table 2   Site of Breast Recurrence Following Breast Conservation Therapy

| | Relative % of local recurrences | | Absolute % of |
Investigator	Local	Remote	all treated patients
Fisher, 1986	100	0	0
Clark, 1992	83	17	1.0
Recht, 1988	80	20	2.0
Fowble, 1990	65	35	2.2
Kurtz, 1983	79	21	2.3
Veronesi, 1990	55	45	2.5
Haffty, 1989	67	33	3.6

of the breast remote from the original tumor site and this appears to be unaffected by whole-breast irradiation. The Harvard Joint Center for Radiation Therapy found that subsequent *contralateral* breast primaries were more frequent than remote ipsilateral breast recurrences or new primaries. Since wide-volume brachytherapy dose-intensifies radiation therapy to the tissues at greatest risk for recurrence, the hypothesis being tested in the RTOG study is that overall breast recurrence will be reduced.

This patient, with a tumor size less than 3 cm, negative inked microscopic surgical margins, less than four metastatic axillary nodes, no lobular histology, and no extensive intraductal component by the Harvard definition, qualifies for enrollment on the protocol. Systemic therapy has been recommended, and since all local-regional therapy is completed in the first week, there is essentially no delay in the initiation of systemic therapy. Chemotherapy can be started 2–4 weeks after the last brachytherapy dose, which should potentially optimize local control and the systemic treatment of po-

Table 3   Site of Breast Recurrence After Wide Local Excision Alone

| | Relative % of local recurrences | | Absolute % of |
Investigator	Local	Remote	all treated patients
Fisher, 1986	100	0	0
Crile, 1990	84	16	1.7
Liljegren, 1994	85	15	3.0
Clark, 1992	86	14	3.5

tential hematogenous micrometastatic disease better than current sequential regimens.

The patient was given two choices of treatment. If she preferred an outpatient approach, two daily, 20-min fractions of 340 cGy would be given over 5 days using our HDR iridium-192 remote afterloader. If hospitalization for 4 days was preferred, she would have LDR iridium-192 seeds placed within the catheters for continuous 24 hr/day brachytherapy. Two independent radiation biologists/physicists have used the linear quadratic model to show that each of these schemes should have similar probabilities of tumor control and late effects or complications.

The patient preferred to be hospitalized for the duration of the treatment. The strands of iridium-192 seeds and the catheters were removed after 100 hr. She was thoroughly instructed in aftercare of the catheter sites and returned home immediately. She resumed her heavy work schedule the following day.

It is estimated that breast conservation therapy is received by only 25–50% of eligible patients. One major factor, which was not an issue for the woman described above, is the distance a patient must travel to and from a radiation facility each day for 6 weeks of fractionated external-beam teletherapy. If wide-volume brachytherapy is proven to be an acceptable, effective, and tolerable alternative for breast irradiation, more women may be spared mastectomy. An important additional goal of the study is to document that quality brachytherapy is reproducible outside a single institution.

BIBLIOGRAPHY

Clark RM, McCulloch PB, Levine MV, et al. Randomized clinical trial to assess the effectiveness of breast irradiation following lumpectomy and axillary dissection for node-negative breast cancer. J Natl Cancer Inst 1992; 84:683–689.

Crile G, Esselstyn CB. Factors influencing local recurrence of cancer after partial mastectomy. Cleveland Clin J Med 1990; 57:143–146.

Fisher ER, Sass R, Fisher B, et al. Pathologic findings from the National Surgical Adjuvant Breast Project (Protocol 6). II. Relation of local breast recurrence to multicentricity. Cancer 1986; 57:1717–1727.

Fowble B, Solin LJ, Schultz DJ, et al. Breast recurrence following conservative surgery and irradiation: patterns of failure, prognosis, and pathologic findings from mastectomy specimens with implications for treatment. Int J Radiat Oncol Biol Phys 1990; 19:833–842.

Fowler J, Orton C. Personal communications, 1991, 1995.

Haffty BG, Goldberg NB, Fischer D, et al. Conservative surgery and radiation therapy in breast carcinoma: local recurrence and prognostic implications. Int J Radiat Oncol Biol Phys 1989; 17:727.

Holland R, Connolly JL, Gelman R, et al. The presence of an extensive intraductal component (EIC) following a limited excision predicts for prominent residual disease in the remainder of the breast. J Clin Oncol 1990; 8:113–118.

Kurtz JM, Spitalier J, Amalvic R. Late recurrence after lumpectomy and irradiation. Int J Radiat Oncol Biol Phys 1983; 9:1191.

Kuske RR, Bolton JS, McKinnon WM, et al. Breast conservation therapy: comparison of cosmesis with brachytherapy alone and after external beam irradiation. Radiology 1996; 201(P):205.

Liljegren G, Holmberg L, Adami HO, et al. Sector resection with or without postoperative radiotherapy for stage I breast cancer: five-year results of a randomized trial. J Natl Cancer Inst 1994; 86:717–722.

Recht A, Silver B, Schnitt S, et al. Breast relapse following primary radiation therapy for early breast cancer. I. Classification, frequency and salvage. Int J Radiat Oncol Biol Phys 1985; 11:1271–1276.

Recht A, Silen W, Schnitt SJ, et al. Time course of local recurrence following conservative surgery and radiotherapy for early stage breast cancer. Int J Radiat Oncol Biol Phys 1988; 15:255–261.

Rosen PP, Fracchia AA, Urban JA, et al. Residual mammary carcinoma following simulated partial mastectomy. Cancer 1975; 35:739–747.

Veronesi U, Salvadori B, Luini A, et al. Conservative treatment of early breast cancer: long-term results of 1232 cases treated with quadrantectomy, axillary dissection, and radiotherapy. Ann Surg 1990; 211:250–259.

Case #C.1.16
Goal: To discuss breast conservation in women with large breasts and repeatedly positive surgical margins

JAY K. HARNESS

A 42-year-old woman, strongly motivated for breast conservation, undergoes excisional biopsy, which revealed a 1.8-cm, invasive lobular carcinoma with positive surgical margins. Reexcision and axillary lymph node dissection reveal negative lymph nodes but positive surgical margins for invasive breast cancer. Physical examination reveals large breasts with ample remaining tissue on the operated side.

Invasive lobular carcinoma (ILC) is the second most common form of invasive breast cancer, with invasive ductal carcinoma (IDC) being the most common. Even as the second most common type, ILC constitutes only 10–14% of all invasive carcinomas. Patients with ILC are prone to bilateral disease. Prior and concurrent carcinoma of the opposite breast has been reported in 6–28% of patients and subsequent contralateral carcinoma in 9–14% of patients initially diagnosed with ILC.

Most patients with ILC present with a palpable mass that tends to have ill-defined margins. The mammographic appearance of ILC can vary considerably. The most common mammographic finding is a spiculated opacity, followed by architectural distortion, a poorly defined opacity, and a negative mammogram. The false-negative rate for mammography in ILC varies from 7% to 14%. Both the physical examination and mammographic findings in ILC can be explained by the morphology of this tumor. Classic ILC consists of a homogeneous population of small, bland-appearing cells, which may distribute diffusely in the stroma in a linear fashion (Indian-file) (Fig. 1), or concentrically around mammary ducts and terminal lobules (bull's-eye, targetoid) (Fig. 2). Despite the diffuse presence of tumor cells in ILC, the normal glandular anatomy of the breast is often preserved with little or no desmoplastic reaction. As a result little or no change in stromal density is seen mammographically.

In this case, no information is given about the patient's mammograms. Because she has large breasts, it is probably safe to assume that a large percentage of her breasts is fat. White et al. correlated the preoperative mammograms of patients with ILC with the chance of having positive margins at the time of reexcision. They found residual carcinoma in 100% of the reexcision specimens when the preoperative mammogram findings were architectural distortion, poorly defined opacity, or negative. In com-

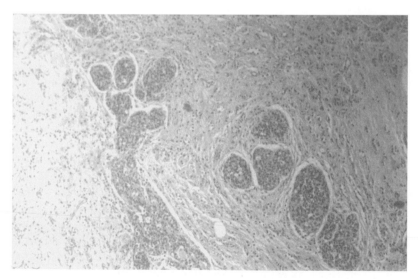

Figure 1   "Indian-file" or "single-file" pattern of uniform malignant cells in ILC.

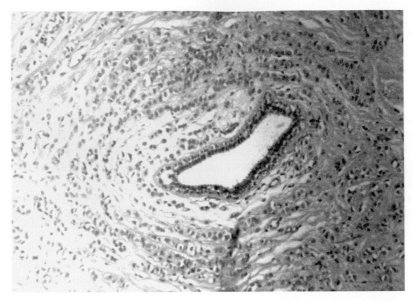

Figure 2   Single-file tumor cells surround an involved duct, producing a bull's-eye or target-like pattern.

parison, residual carcinoma was found in 18% of the reexcision specimens when a spiculated opacity was the primary preoperative mammographic finding.

ILC is associated with a higher incidence of multicentricity than IDC. Multicentricity (tumor in more than one quadrant of the breast) has been associated with an increased local recurrence rate in patients treated by lumpectomy and radiotherapy. Multifocality (multiple foci of tumor within the same quadrant of the breast), however, has not been associated with an increased risk of local recurrence. While the number of ILC patients treated by lumpectomy and radiotherapy is far less than those treated for IDC, the limited number of series that have made side-by-side comparisons of ILC and IDC patients show similar rates of ipsilateral breast recurrence.

This issue of ipsilateral breast tumor recurrence (IBTR) is a pivotal one in recommending mastectomy versus lumpectomy and radiotherapy. A number of follow-up studies have indicated that involvement of the final microscopic margins is an important and independent predictor of local recurrence for patients with invasive breast carcinoma or ductal carcinoma in situ (DCIS) treated with breast-conserving therapy. There are few situations in which breast conservation could reasonably be pursued with positive lumpectomy margins. One would be if lobular carcinoma in situ (which is not a cancer) was at the margins and the other would be a few scattered foci of DCIS at the margins. Other than these limited circumstances, positive lumpectomy margins invite a much higher incidence of ipsilateral breast recurrence. A recurrence in the treated breast is psychologically devastating for patients, and this provides a strong incentive to give the best reasonable advice on mastectomy versus breast conservation.

In this case, the patient has "large breasts" and is "strongly motivated for breast conservation." The initial stage of her cancer is the primary determinant of her ultimate prognosis. While there is some debate that an IBTR could worsen this patient's prognosis, most reports do not support that conclusion. Mammography would be the primary means of detecting an IBTR. Mammography in fatty breasts tends to be more sensitive; however, this patient's mammograms would have to be reviewed to determine whether that would be true in her case. It is also not known whether her ILC was originally seen mammographically.

The issue of how many reexcisions a patient can undergo to get clear margins depends on the size of the involved breast and the quadrant in which the cancer resides. The lower quadrants of the breast can be excised almost completely and still give a good cosmetic result. The upper quadrants are much less forgiving. It would be reasonable to offer this patient another reexcision. I would favor a third procedure in which I would push the limits of a good cosmetic result, yet resecting enough tissue to ensure negative margins around her invasive cancer. Once the limits of lumpectomy are reached and the margins are still positive, then I would recommend a completion mastectomy.

BIBLIOGRAPHY

Ashikari R, Huvos AG, Urban JA, Robbins GF. Infiltrating lobular carcinoma of the breast. Cancer 1973; 31:110–116.

Fisher ER. Lumpectomy margins and much more. Cancer 1997; 79(8):1453–1458.

Lee JSY, Grant CS, Donohue JH, et al. Arguments against routine contralateral mastectomy or undirected biopsy for invasive lobular breast cancer. Surgery 1995; 118:640–648.

Lesser ML, Rosen PP, Kinne DW. Multicentricity and bilaterality in invasive breast carcinoma. Surgery 1982; 1:234–240.

White JR, Gustafson GS, Wimbish K, et al. Conservative surgery and radiation therapy for infiltrating lobular carcinoma of the breast. The role of preoperative mammograms in guiding treatment. Cancer 1994; 74(2):640–647.

Case #C.1.17
Goal: To discuss the significance of breast size and shape in the operative management of breast cancer

MICHAEL H. TOROSIAN

An 83-year-old woman with size 40, D-cup, pendulous breasts undergoes negative-margin, right breast lumpectomy for a 2.5-cm, estrogen-receptor-positive, invasive ductal carcinoma. Axillary lymph node dissection is not performed; the ipsilateral axillary nodes are clinically normal. She is referred for radiation therapy evaluation.

Axillary dissection is not necessarily indicated in elderly patients and this decision should be made jointly by the surgeon and the medical oncologist. By avoiding an axillary dissection in this 83-year-old patient, the need for a second surgical procedure and, more importantly, general anesthesia have been avoided. Regardless of the nodal status in this patient, chemotherapy will not be considered and tamoxifen can be administered as adjuvant therapy. The large size and pendulous shape of the breast in this patient make radiotherapy planning and treatment difficult. An important surgical technique that greatly assists the radiotherapist is placement of radiopaque clips at the lumpectomy site for radiotherapy targeting. In this way, the tumor bed can be easily identified by plain radiographs when the radiation boost is administered to the lumpectomy site. In the absence of radiopaque clips, a computed-tomography scan would be required for subsequent radiotherapy planning.

A large, pendulous breast is a relative (*not* an absolute) contraindication to radiation therapy. The main problem with radiation therapy to a large breast is cosmesis. Meticulous planning and delivery of radiation therapy is required to achieve optimal therapy and cosmesis. Several techniques of administering radiation therapy (e.g., prone or lateral decubitus positioning during breast radiation) in this clinical situation have been reported to minimize postradiotherapy deformity of the breast.

In my opinion, radiotherapy should not be administered to the axillary and supraclavicular nodes if axillary dissection has not been performed. The same considerations that led to the decision to avoid axillary dissection exist for radiation therapy to this region. Fibrosis created by radiation therapy in these regions clearly increases the incidence of lymphedema. Thus, radiation therapy to the axillary and supraclavicular nodal basins should not be performed routinely in elderly patients in whom axillary dissection has not been performed.

In summary, axillary dissection should be performed only if the pathological findings will alter subsequent therapy. Radiation therapy should not be administered to the clinically negative axilla when axillary dissection has not been performed. Radiation therapy can be administered to patients with large, pendulous breasts but requires particular attention to details in pretreatment planning and administration.

Editors' comment: Radiation therapy to the undissected axilla is controversial, but available data suggest that this can be administered with a high regional nodal control rate and minimal morbidity.

BIBLIOGRAPHY

Fourquet A, Campana F, Rosenwald JC, Vilcog JR. Breast irradiation in the lateral decubitus position: technique of the Institut Curie. Radiother Oncol 1991; 22(4):261.

Fowble B, Solin L, Schultz D, et al. Frequency, sites of relapse, and outcome of regional node failures following surgery and radiation for early breast cancer. Int J Radiat Oncol Biol Phys 1989; 17:703.

Gray JR, McCormick B, Cox L, Yahalom J. Primary breast irridation in large-breasted or heavy women: analysis of cosmetic outcome. Int J Radiat Oncol Biol Phys 1991; 32(2):347.

Merchant TE, McCormick B. Prone position and breast irradiation. Int J Radiat Oncol Biol Phys 1994; 30(1):197.

C.2. NODE-NEGATIVE DISEASE

Introduction

Node-negative breast cancer now accounts for as many as 30–40% of all cases diagnosed in the United States. This entity includes both stage I (T1N0M0) and stage II (T2N0M0) patients who have survivals ranging from 70% to 95% at 5 years. Therefore, recommendations for treatment must be customized based on the overall health of the patient and the prognostic factors associated with the tumor. Although breast-conserving surgery followed by radiation is equivalent to mastectomy, many women are opting for modified radical mastectomies with reconstructive surgery. The coordination of reconstruction with adjuvant chemotherapy and radiation can present challenges for the patient and clinicians.

Case #C.2.1
Goal: To determine the role of observation in premenopausal women with breast cancer

I. CRAIG HENDERSON

A 44-year-old woman presents with a 0.7-cm, poorly differentiated, hormone-receptor-negative tumor, which is also aneuploid high S. Biopsy reveals clean surgical margins and no ductal carcinoma in situ. There is no family history of breast cancer. She is the single parent of three children and anxious about her diagnosis.

This patient has a small, invasive, and operable breast cancer. We do not know her nodal status. If she has positive axillary lymph nodes, I would definitely treat her with adjuvant chemotherapy. However, if she is node negative I would give her the option of having no treatment beyond lumpectomy and radiotherapy.

Recommendations for patients with relatively lower risk of recurrence are dependent, in part, on one's understanding of the nature of the benefit from adjuvant chemotherapy. It is well established that 4 months or more of combination chemotherapy will reduce the annual odds of death for a premenopausal woman by about 25% per year. At 10 years this translates into an absolute difference of 10% between treated and untreated patients. The median survival of treated premenopausal patients is about 1.7 years longer than that of those not randomized to adjuvant chemotherapy. It is possible that some patients are cured, but there is no evidence yet to support this. Among patients on adjuvant therapy trials who die, the proportion who die as a direct result of breast cancer is nearly the same among those who received adjuvant chemotherapy as among those who did not. In light of this, it is likely that most patients treated with adjuvant chemotherapy derive some transient benefit, but this is highly variable. Thus, the life of one patient may be prolonged by only a few months as a result of therapy whereas another may derive a survival benefit of several decades. An understanding of all of these facts is likely to affect a patient's decision to have adjuvant therapy, particularly if she already has a high probability of being cured and is faced with a relatively toxic treatment.

The proportional effects of adjuvant therapy are generally the same across all risk groups. The absolute benefits vary depending on the underlying risk. (Exceptions to this principle are the greater benefits from adjuvant tamoxifen among women with higher levels of estrogen receptor or the lack of benefit from adjuvant chemotherapy in high-risk patients with tumors that overexpress Her-2-*neu*.) Thus, the proportional effect of adjuvant chemotherapy will be the same in a group of women with 10 positive lymph nodes as in those with one positive node. The absolute affects will be greater in those with many positive nodes. This is illustrated in Table 1.

The reduction in the annual odds of death from adjuvant chemotherapy for a premenopausal woman will be about 25%; if her risk of death without adjuvant chemotherapy exceeds 30–40%, her survival at 10 years will be about 10% better than if she had not had adjuvant chemotherapy. If her risk is below 40%, the reduction in the annual odds of death will still be about

Table 1 The Effects of Adjuvant Combination Chemotherapy and Adjuvant Tamoxifen on the Reduction in Annual Odds of Death in Patients at Low, Moderate, and High Risk of Recurrence Based on Nodal Status, and on the Absolute Survival Differences Between Patients With and Without Axillary Lymph Node Involvement

Nodal Group	No. of pts.	Reduction in annual odds of death	Survival difference at 10 years
A. Combination chemotherapy trials			
N0/−	2,833	16% ± 8	4.0% ± 2.8
N1−3	2,244	18% ± 7	
N4+	1,424	13% ± 8	
Any N+			6.8% ± 1.6
Test for trend		$p > 0.1$	
B. Tamoxifen trials			
N0/−	12,813	17% ± 5	3.5% ± 1.4
N1−3	6,053	21% ± 5	
N4+	3,941	16% ± 5	
Any N+			8.2% ± 1.1
Test for trend		$p > 0.1$	

Patients of all ages are included in the analysis.
Reduction in annual odds of death would be somewhat larger if the analysis were limited to younger or premenopausal women, but statistical power would be lost as the size of each of the nodal subsets decreased.
Source: Based on data previously published in references cited.

25%, but her survival benefit will be smaller. Thus, if it is determined that her risk of dying from breast cancer in the first 10 years after diagnosis is 10%, her absolute increase in survival will be only 2.5% (0.25 × 10%). For some patients this benefit is too small to justify treatment. Others would consider this worthwhile, even if they fully understand that this does not represent a cure. In general, however, patients with a lower risk of recurrence appear to be more risk averse.

The real challenge in this patient is determining her risk of recurrence and death. If she has no positive lymph nodes and a tumor less than 1 cm, her risk of dying in the next 10 years is about 10%. Her chance of recurrence is likely increased by another 4−5% because she is receptor negative. The difficult question is how much her risk is further increased by the fact she has a high S-phase fraction. Although it is well established that a high S-phase fraction increases the risk of recurrence, it is not yet clear how great this increase is in this particular patient. A similar situation existed in the 1970s when we knew that patients with a receptor-negative tumor had an increased risk, and most of us thought that in node-negative patients this factor increased this risk by 20–50%. However, as the data matured it became apparent that the *additional* risk from a negative receptor was much smaller. This appears to be even more true of S-phase fraction. Based on calculations from a computer-assisted program developed from a neural network for a similar patient, I believe the likelihood of this patient dying of breast cancer in the next 10 years is about 20%. If this is correct, then 4–6 months of adjuvant chemotherapy is likely to reduce this to about 15% (20% − (0.25 × 20%)). In my experience most, but not all, patients would consider this a worthwhile benefit and would elect chemotherapy in this situation.

BIBLIOGRAPHY

Allred DC, Clark GM, Tandon AK, Molina R, Tormey DC, Osborne CK, Gilchrist KW, Mansour EG, Abeloff M, Eudey L, McGuire WL. HER-2/*neu* in node-negative breast cancer: prognostic significance of overexpression influenced by the presence of in situ carcinoma. J Clin Oncol 1992; 10:599–605.

Bonadonna G, Valagussa P, Moliterni A, Zambetti M, Brambilla C. Adjuvant cyclophosphamide, methotrexate, and fluorouracil in node-positive breast cancer: the results of 20 years of follow-up. N Eng J Med 1995; 332:901–906.

Early Breast Cancer Trialists' Collaborative Group. Systemic treatment of early breast cancer by hormonal, cytotoxic, or immune therapy: 133 randomised trials involving 31,000 recurrences and 24,000 deaths among 75,000 women. Lancet 1992; 339:1–15, 71–85.

Fisher B, Redmond C, Fisher ER, Caplan R. Relative worth of estrogen or progesterone receptor and pathologic characteristics of differentiation as indicators of prognosis in node negative breast cancer patients: findings from National Surgical Adjuvant Breast and Bowel Project Protocol B-06. J Clin Oncol 1988; 6:1076–1087.

Gusterson BA, Gelber RD, Goldhirsch A, Price KN, Save-Soderborgh J, Anbazhagan R, Styles J, Rudenstam D-M, Golouh R, Reed R, Martinez-Tello F, Tiltman A, Torhorst J, Grigolato P, Bettelheim R, et al. Prognostic importance of c-*erb*B-2 expression in breast cancer. J Clin Oncol 1992; 10:1049–1056.

Henderson IC. Adjuvant systemic therapy for early breast cancer. Cancer 1994; 74: 401–409.

Henderson IC. Paradigmatic shifts in the management of breast cancer. N Engl J Med 1995; 332:951–953.

Hilsenbeck SG, Ravdin PM, de Moor CA, Osborne CK, Clark GM. Paradoxical decreases in prognostic utility as datasets mature: time-dependent lack of proportional hazards in prognostic factors in primary breast cancer. Breast Cancer Res Treat 1996; 37:35 (meeting abstract).

Ravdin PM. A computer based program to assist in adjuvant therapy decisions for individual breast cancer patients. Bull Cancer 1995; 82:561s–564s.

Simes RJ, Margrie SJ. Patient preferences for adjuvant chemotherapy in breast can-
    cer. NHMRC Clinical Trials Centre, Sydney, 1991.

Case #C.2.2
Goal: To discuss the timing of chemotherapy and radiation therapy

I. CRAIG HENDERSON

*A 43-year-old woman is diagnosed with a 2.8-cm, infiltrating ductal
carcinoma. She is status postlumpectomy with a positive axillary lymph
node dissection; hormone receptors are negative. She is confused
regarding the timing of radiation therapy in relationship to chemotherapy
and particularly concerned about delaying radiation therapy for 6 months
so that she can complete chemotherapy.*

This is a patient with invasive, operable breast cancer, clinical stage I,
node positive (T1N1M0). She is premenopausal and her tumor is estrogen-
and progesterone-receptor negative. I would offer her adjuvant chemotherapy with either cyclophosphamide/methotrexate/fluorouracil (CMF) (4–6
months) or cyclophosphamide/doxorubicin (CA) (five cycles) followed by
radiotherapy to the breast and lower axillary lymph nodes.

There has been considerable controversy surrounding the sequence of
adjuvant chemotherapy and primary radiotherapy. On the one hand, a delay
in the initiation of radiotherapy may result in a higher failure rate in the
breast or regional lymph nodes. On the other hand, a delay in the initiation
of adjuvant systemic treatment may result in a smaller survival benefit. Not
only will metastatic tumor foci be larger and possibly less responsive to
adjuvant chemotherapy or tamoxifen, but the prior use of adjuvant radiotherapy may compromise the dose of adjuvant chemotherapy that can be
given. While theoretically this should not be a problem because radiotherapy
suppresses lymphocytes and has little impact on leukocytes, practically it is
problematic because most physicians adjust chemotherapy dose on the basis
of total white blood cell count rather than leukocyte count.

Some of these questions regarding the optimal sequence of these two
modalities may have been answered by a modest-sized, randomized trial
performed by investigators at the Dana-Farber Cancer Institute and the Joint
Center for Radiation Therapy. Following initial treatment with lumpectomy,
patients were either treated immediately with about 4 months of adjuvant
chemotherapy followed by adjuvant radiotherapy or the reverse. The results
of this study are summarized in Table 1.

These data appear to confirm all concerns. There was a greater local
failure rate among patients with a delay in the initiation of radiotherapy and

Table 1 Outcome by Treatment Arm for Patients Randomized to Receive Either Adjuvant Chemotherapy Followed by Radiotherapy or Radiotherapy Followed by Adjuvant Chemotherapy ($N = 242$)

Outcome	Actuarial rate (%) for each outcome		p value
	Radiotherapy first	Chemotherapy first	
Any failure	38	31	0.17
Distant failure	36	24	0.05
Overall survival	73	81	0.11
1st site of failure			
Local	5	14	0.07
Distant/regional	32	20	

a higher distant failure rate with a nonsignificant trend toward worse survival among those with a delay in chemotherapy. The chemotherapy used in this regimen consisted of cyclophosphamide, 500 mg/m^2, doxorubicin 45 mg/m^2, 5-fluorouracil on day 1 and 15, leucovorin 10 mg/m^2 on day 2 and 16, and prednisone 40 mg days 1–5. Adjustments in dose were based entirely on the absolute neutrophil count rather than total white cell count. When chemotherapy was administered first, 88% of the cyclophosphamide, 88% of the doxorubicin, and 75% of the methotrexate were given at full protocol doses. When radiotherapy was given first, significantly less chemotherapy was administered: 81% of the cyclophosphamide ($p = 0.01$), 81% of the doxorubicin ($p = 0.01$), and 50% of the methotrexate ($p = 0.0001$).

The International Breast Cancer Study Group has inadvertently conducted two trials in which the interval from surgery to radiotherapy was randomly varied in 718 women. In these studies patients were randomized to different durations of adjuvant CMF chemotherapy, and radiotherapy was administered following the completion of all chemotherapy. There were no significant differences in the total failure rate, rate of developing distant metastases, or overall survival.

Some physicians might choose to administer concomitant chemotherapy and radiotherapy to obviate the need to delay either modality. While theoretically attractive, the logistics of this are often difficult. Physicians who use this approach usually avoid drugs known to be synergistic with radiotherapy, such as methotrexate and doxorubicin, while the radiotherapy is being given. In addition, some investigators have observed a less than satisfactory cosmetic result more often when chemotherapy and radiation therapy are given concomitantly than when given separately.

BIBLIOGRAPHY

Beadle GF, Harris JR, Come S, Henderson IC, Silver B, Hellman S. The influence of adjuvant chemotherapy on the cosmetic result after primary radiation treatment. Am J Clin Oncol 1984; 7:117–118.

Lippman ME, Lichter AS, Edwards BK, Gorrell CR, d'Angelo T, DeMoss EV. The impact of primary irradiation treatment of localized breast cancer on the ability to administer systemic adjuvant chemotherapy. J Clin Oncol 1984; 2:21–27.

Overmoyer B, Fowble B, Solin L, Goldstein L, Glick J. The long-term results of conservative surgery and radiation with concurrent chemotherapy for early stage breast cancer. Proc Annu Meet Am Soc Clin Oncol 1992; 11:A185 (abstract).

Recht A, Come SE, Henderson IC, Gelman RS, Silver B, Hayes DF, Shulman LN, Harris JR. The sequencing of chemotherapy and radiation therapy after conservative surgery for early-stage breast cancer. N Engl J Med 1996; 334:1356–1361.

Wallgren A, Bernier J, Gelber RD, Goldhirsch A, Roncadin M, Joseph D, Castiglione-Gertsch M. Timing of radiotherapy and chemotherapy following breast-conserving surgery for patients with node-positive breast cancer. International Breast Cancer Study Group. Int J Radiat Oncol Biol Phys 1996; 35: 649–659.

Case #C.2.3
Goal: To discuss the sequence of radiation and chemotherapy from the radiation oncologist's point of view

KIRAN MEHTA and BRUCE G. HAFFTY

A 52-year-old white woman undergoes lumpectomy and axillary dissection for a 2.1-cm, estrogen-receptor-positive, node-negative, invasive ductal carcinoma. Adjuvant therapy with CMF plus tamoxifen as well as breast radiation therapy has been recommended.

It is well established that breast conservation therapy with lumpectomy, axillary lymph node dissection, and radiation therapy (RT) provides equivalent survival to mastectomy for the majority of women with early-stage breast cancer. In addition, clinical trials have demonstrated the efficacy and survival advantage to adjuvant systemic therapies. Therefore, we are commonly faced with the need to combine RT and systemic therapy in patients following conservative surgery.

Unfortunately, there is little randomized data on which treatment decisions can be based. Options of combining RT and chemotherapy (CT) include a variety of schedules such as: RT first followed by CT, CT first followed by RT, RT and CT simultaneously, or RT administered after several cycles of CT followed by additional CT (commonly referred to as "sandwich" therapy). The Joint Center for Radiation Therapy (JCRT) experience has shown no difference in local control (LC), disease-free survival (DFS), or overall survival (OS) between patients treated with concurrent or sequential CT and RT. In making decisions regarding sequencing, one must take into consideration several factors including the extent of surgical resection, margin status, lymph node status, as well as the competing risks of local failure and distant metastasis.

A number of studies examined the effect of delays in the initiation of RT on local recurrence. Some studies have found that delays were associated with an increased rate of local recurrence. Other retrospective studies have not found that delays are associated with increased local recurrence. Interestingly, in the studies that failed to show increased local recurrence, wider local excisions were performed with strict attention to margins and reexcision for positive margins. Therefore, in this patient we would review the pathology paying close attention to the size of the resection specimen as well as the status of all margins. If all margins are negative, this may suggest a lower tumor burden, and a subsequent delay may not be harmful in terms of local control. If, however, on review of the pathology, there is question regarding a close or positive margin, one must consider reexcision. With a focally positive margin, in which a reexcision is not planned, the initiation of radiation therapy without significant delay would be recommended.

It would seem logical that delays in the initiation of CT may decrease its effectiveness. However, conflicting results have been seen in many of the retrospective reviews of patients treated with either mastectomy or breast-conserving therapy. Another question regarding sequencing is whether full-dose RT precludes the ability to deliver full-dose CT. Unfortunately, these data are also controversial. Radiation has different effects on different subsets of white blood cells. Lymphocyte counts are generally more suppressed than granulocyte counts. If dose reductions are made on the basis of granulocyte count rather than total lymphocyte count, one may be able to deliver higher doses of chemotherapy.

Another question that often arises in these situations is whether RT and CT can be given concurrently. The obvious advantages would be eliminating the delay of one of the modalities as well as a possible additive synergistic interaction between RT and CT. However, one must weigh this against the possibility of increased morbidity and/or decreased cosmetic result. In some studies patients treated with both modalities simultaneously have had greater skin reactions. However, this has not been seen in all studies. In one series acute skin reactions were more severe especially in patients who received concurrent methotrexate. This group has also noted an increase in radiation pneumonitis (particularly when a supraclavicular field was matched) as well as inferior cosmetic results.

On the other hand, Glick et al. found no increase in complications or decrease in cosmetic result in patients treated with concurrent RT and CT (in which methotrexate was omitted during RT). Thus, when considering administering both therapies concurrently one must precisely plan the administration of these two modalities taking into account the possibility for enhanced toxicity.

The ultimate goal of adjuvant therapy in any breast cancer patient is to obtain the highest rate of survival. The only randomized study comparing the sequencing of CT and RT after conservative surgery was performed at JCRT. In this study, 244 patients were randomized to receive a 12-week course of CT either before or after RT. The results of this study showed a higher rate of local recurrence in the CT-first group. However, a higher rate of distant recurrence was noted in the RT-first group. The researchers concluded that a 12-week course of CT given prior to RT is preferable as distant metastases are more likely to ultimately impact on survival. Also of note, patients in the RT-first group receive significantly lower doses of CT and suffer increased hematological toxicity.

It seems reasonable in this patient to initiate adjuvant therapy with six cycles of CMF. This can be followed by RT to the intact breast with a boost to the tumor bed.

The final question arises as to when tamoxifen should be incorporated. The theoretical concern is that the concurrent use of tamoxifen with RT might result in a decreased sensitivity to radiation if the cancer cells are growth-arrested by tamoxifen. Similar issues have been raised regarding this potential interaction of tamoxifen with CT. Laboratory data have not clearly demonstrated a decrease in the sensitivity of cancer cells to radiation in the presence of tamoxifen. Unfortunately, there is little clinical data regarding the timing of tamoxifen with RT. In the study by Wazer et al. tamoxifen was shown to worsen the cosmetic result after breast-conserving treatment. However, this is not a uniformly held opinion. At present there is little information regarding the timing of the initiation of tamoxifen and its effect on ultimate survival. Therefore, we would initiate tamoxifen after the completion of RT.

BIBLIOGRAPHY

Abner A, Recht A, Vincini F, et al. Cosmetic results after surgery, chemotherapy, and radiation therapy for early breast cancer. Int J Radiat Oncol Biol Phys 1991; 21:331.

Botnick L, Come S, Rose C, et al. Primary breast irradiation and concomitant adjuvant chemotherapy. In: Harris J, Hellman S, Silen W, eds. Conservative Management of Breast Cancer. Philadelphia: JB Lippincott, 1983:321.

Bucholz T, Austin-Seymour M, Moe R, et al. Effect of delay in radiation in the combined modality treatment of breast cancer. Int J Radiat Oncol Biol Phys 1993; 26:23.

Buzdar A, Kau S, Smith T, et al. The order of administration of chemotherapy and radiation and its effect on the local control of operable breast cancer. Cancer 1993; 71:3680.

Buzzoni R, Bonnadonna G, Valagussa P, et al. Adjuvant chemotherapy with doxorubicin plus cyclophosphamide, methotrexate, and fluorouracil in the treatment of resectable breast cancer with more than three positive nodes. J Clin Oncol 1991; 9:2134.

Fowble B, Fein DA, Hanlon AL, et al. The impact of tamoxifen on breast recurrence, cosmesis, complications, and survival in estrogen receptor positive early stage breast cancer. Int J Radiat Oncol Biol Phys 1995; 32(Suppl):150.

Glick J, Fowble B, Haller D, et al. Integration of full-dose adjuvant chemotherapy with definitive radiotherapy for primary breast cancer: four-year update. NCI Monogr 1988; 6:297.

Hansen R, Erickson B , Komaki R, et al. Concomitant adjuvant chemotherapy and radiotherapy for high risk breast cancer patients. Breast Cancer Res Treat 1990; 17:171.

Hartsell W, Recine D, Griem K, et al. Does delay in the initiation of radiation therapy adversely affect local control in treatment of the intact breast? Radiother Oncol 1992; 24(Suppl):537 (abstract).

Lingos T, Recht A, Vincini F, et al. Radiation pneumonitis in breast cancer patients treated with conservative surgery and radiation therapy. Int J Radiat Oncol Biol Phys 1991; 21:355.

McCormick B, Begg C. Norton L, et al. Timing of radiotherapy in the treatment of early stage breast cancer. J Clin Oncol 1993; 11:191 (letter).

Meek A. Order S, Abeloff M, et al. Concurrent radiochemotherapy in advanced breast cancer. Cancer 1983; 51:1001.

Moliterni A, Bonadonna G, Valaguessa P, et al. Cyclophosphamide, methotrexate and fluorouracil with and without doxorubicin in the adjuvant treatment of resectable breast cancer with one to three positive axillary nodes. J Clin Oncol 1991; 9:1124.

Piccart M, DeValeriola D, Paridaens R, et al. Six-year results of a multimodality treatment strategy for locally advanced breast cancer. Cancer 1988; 62:2501.

Recht A, Coleman C, Harris J, et al. Timing of radiotherapy in the treatment of early stage breast cancer. J Clin Oncol 1993; 11:191 (letter).

Recht A, Come S, Gelman R, et al. Integration of conservative surgery, radiotherapy, and chemotherapy for the treatment of early stage node-positive breast cancer: sequencing, timing, and outcome. J Clin Oncol 1991; 9:1662.

Recht A, Come SE, Henderson IC, et al. The sequencing of chemotherapy and radiation therapy after conservative surgery for early-stage breast cancer. N Engl J Med 1996; 334:1356.

Sponzo R, Cunningham T, Caradonna R. Management of nonreversable (stage III) breast cancer. Int J Radiat Oncol Biol Phys 1979; 5:1475.

Wazer D. Joyce M, Chan W, et al. Effects of tamoxifen on the radiosensitivity of hormonally responsive and unresponsive breast carcinoma cells. Radiat Oncol Invest 1993; 1:20.

Case #C.2.4
Goal: To discuss the treatment of a high-risk, 1-cm tumor

WILLIAM N. HAIT

A 55-year-old woman presents with a suspicious mammogram. Excisional biopsy shows 1.0-cm, invasive ductal carcinoma, hormone receptor negative, aneuploid, high-S breast cancer. The past medical history is negative. Staging evaluation yields a T1N0M0 tumor. Would your management differ if this was a mucinous carcinoma?

The treatment of choice in this woman is a lumpectomy, axillary lymph node dissection, and radiation to the breast with boost to the tumor bed. Adjuvant treatment with chemotherapy or tamoxifen is not indicated owing to the small size and lack of hormone receptors.

The decision not to treat a node-negative patient is based on the estimation of her chances of relapse and the potential risks and benefits of adjuvant therapy. The prognosis of this patient is estimated to be approximately 90% disease-free at 10 years based on the size and histological type. An additional variable is the influence of aneuploidy and high S fraction, which may worsen the overall prognosis. There are no randomized trials that have included a large enough subset of these patients to know whether this patient would benefit from adjuvant chemotherapy.

The meta-analysis of Peto suggests that the overall reduction in risk of recurrence with adjuvant chemotherapy is independent of the absolute risk of recurrence; therefore, her expected reduction in risk would be approximately 30% from adjuvant chemotherapy, or approximately 3%, given a risk of relapse of approximately 10% ($10 \times 0.3 = 0.33$).

If her histology was neither invasive ductal nor lobular, e.g., mucinous, her prognosis is probably even better. Rosen et al. have estimated that a 3-cm "special histology" is approximately equivalent risk to a 1-cm lobular or infiltrating ductal carcinoma.

T1a and b (0.5–1.0 cm) lesions have excellent prognoses and should not receive adjuvant chemotherapy outside of a clinical trial. This woman is at risk of subsequently developing a second breast cancer during her lifetime (approximately 1%/year) and should be considered for prevention trials. Special lesions have an overall better prognosis than infiltrating ductal and lobular carcinoma and should be considered separately in regard to adjuvant therapy.

BIBLIOGRAPHY

Carter C, Allen C, Henson D. Relation of tumor size, lymph node status and survival in 24,740 breast cancer cases. Cancer 1989; 63:181.

Early Breast Cancer Trialists' Collaborative Group. Systemic treatment of early breast cancer by hormonal, cytotoxic, or immune therapy. Lancet 1992; 339: 1,71.

Koscielny S, Tubiana M, Le M, et al. Breast cancer: relationship between the size of the primary tumor and the probability of metastatic dissemination. Br J Cancer 1984; 49:709.

Rosen PP, Saigo PE, Braun DW Jr, et al. Predictors of recurrence in stage I (T1N0M0) breast carcinoma. Ann Surg 1981; 193:15.

Wenger CR, Beardslee S, Owens MA, et al. DNA ploidy, S-phase and steroid receptors in more than 127,000 breast cancer patients. Breast Cancer Res Treat 1993; 28:9.

Case #C.2.5
Goal: To discuss the management of medial lesions

JAMES F. HOLLAND

A 39-year-old woman presents with a 2-cm, palpable mass in the upper inner quadrant of her right breast. Excisional biopsy reveals a 1.3-cm, well-differentiated, estrogen-receptor-positive, infiltrating ductal carcinoma. Medial margin is positive for invasive tumor. Her oncologist recommends reexcision with axillary lymph node dissection. Results give clean margins and 0/12 positive lymph nodes. She comes seeking an opinion regarding additional therapy.

The anatomical location in the breast has little relationship to metastatic potential, or to location of metastases. Thus survival, size for size, is the same for lesions in the inner quadrant as for lesions in the outer quadrant. With a 1.3-cm, ER-positive, well-differentiated tumor and negative axillary nodes at age 39, this patient has about a 15% chance of micrometastatic disease and thus eventual recurrence. She should be encouraged to take tamoxifen for 5 years by which time more information will be available about other antiestrogens that might further extend effective tumor suppression. Faced with a 15% chance of losing at age 39, I believe she also should be encouraged to accept chemotherapy.

BIBLIOGRAPHY

Fisher B, Shank NH, Ausman RK, Bross IDJ. Location of breast carcinoma and prognosis. Surg Gynecol Obstet 1969; 129:705–716.

Case #C.2.6
Goal: To discuss issues of adjuvant therapy in the elderly patient

SANDRA F. SCHNALL

A 75-year-old woman presents with a 1.8-cm, infiltrating ductal carcinoma, hormone receptor negative, aneuploid, low-S-phase breast cancer. She has undergone a lumpectomy, has clean surgical margins, and negative lymph nodes. She has mild hypertension and a history of a myocardial infarction 1 year ago. She is currently on aspirin and a thiazide diuretic.

The treatment of breast cancer in women over age 65 is of increasing importance in the United States. It is estimated that by the year 2000 almost 50% of newly diagnosed breast cancer patients will be in this age group. Moreover, death rates for breast cancer have also increased in women over age 65. Unfortunately, older patients with breast cancer are more likely to have comorbid medical problems that may compromise treatment options.

The patient described has a T1N0M0 stage I tumor. Unfortunately, her estrogen receptor (ER) and progesterone receptor (PR) were negative, provoking alternative treatment discussions. At the minimum she will require adjuvant radiation therapy for local control of the remaining breast tissue. However, she has significant prognostic findings that likely require/demand some form of systemic therapy. These include the tumor size being greater than 1 cm, the negative hormone receptor status, and the aneuploid nature of the tumor.

For most patients, the ER/PR content of the tumor correlates with the benefit from hormone treatment. However, in the overview analysis the reduction of the annual odds of recurrence was up to 16%, even in hormone-receptor-negative, postmenopausal patients. Unfortunately, those odds are not high and therefore one must consider treatment with chemotherapy in these women. In postmenopausal women up to age 69, adjuvant chemotherapy regimens have decreased the odds of recurrence by 22% and decreased the odds of death by 14%, in both node-negative and node-positive patients. Performance status, not age, was the best indicator of tolerance of these treatments, which included anthracycline-based regimens or cyclophosphamide/methotrexate/5-FU (CMF). Dose intensity may ultimately prove to be a major factor in outcome. Dose reduction should not be employed routinely in elderly patients, unless toxicity develops. Women of all ages are likely to develop some degree of neutropenia. Unfortunately, it may be more severe in the age group over 70.

In node-positive elderly patients, who maintain a good performance status with minimal comorbid medical problems, I advocate adjuvant chemotherapy, possibly followed by hormonal treatment. In an elderly patient with a node-negative breast cancer, who is ER/PR positive, one could still consider chemotherapy followed by hormone therapy, again depending upon prognostic indicators of the tumor as well as performance status.

A cost-benefit analysis of adjuvant chemotherapy in postmenopausal women in the age group 60–80 showed an improved survival in older women, but still less than in younger women up until age 75. Above age 75, the oncologist should determine the cost/benefit/toxicity ratio in conjunction with the comorbid medical issues.

In this patient, I would likely offer six cycles of CMF chemotherapy. She may require the addition of colony-stimulating factors. I would not advocate the use of an anthracycline owing to her history of coronary artery disease and node-negative status. Despite the hormone receptor status, she may still obtain some benefit from tamoxifen, given at completion of chemotherapy. These benefits could include some cytostatic advantage, as well as amelioration of cardiovascular and osteoporotic conditions.

Trials in node-negative, node-positive, ER/PR-negative, and ER/PR-positive patients are ongoing. It is likely that treating the elderly with chemotherapy is reasonable in several settings as long as there is otherwise a reasonable life expectancy.

BIBLIOGRAPHY

Desch CE, Hillner BE, Smith TJ, et al. Should the elderly receive chemotherapy for node negative breast cancer? A cost effectiveness analysis examining total non-active life expectancy outcomes. J Clin Oncol 1993; 11:777–782.

Early Breast Cancer Trials Collaborative Group. Effects of adjuvant tamoxifen and of cytotoxic therapy on mortality in early breast cancer. N Engl J Med 1988; 319:1681–1692.

Muss HB. Breast cancer in older women. Semin Oncol 1996; 23(Suppl 2):82–88.

Case #C.2.7
Goal: To discuss the management of "large" lesions in postmenopausal women

TERESA GILEWSKI and LARRY NORTON

A 52-year-old, postmenopausal woman presents for evaluation of a 5.2-cm, estrogen-receptor-positive, node-negative, infiltrating ductal carcinoma. The tumor is diploid, low S phase.

Prognosis is primarily a function of axillary lymph node involvement but tumor size is also important. Since this is a T3 or stage IIB lesion, the patient is at an increased risk of recurrence compared to smaller node-negative tumors. The S-phase fraction must still be considered a research prognostic tool, as results are highly variable between laboratories and even within the same tumor. Ploidy is not a useful prognostic factor either. Yet even with negative axillary nodes, this patient's odds of recurrence are high because of the large tumor size.

Systemic adjuvant therapy reduces the annual odds of recurrence and death by a fixed degree regardless of the actual odds of recurrence or death. Hence, patients at high risk of recurrence would be helped considerably by systemic therapy (a fixed percent of a high risk is a large benefit), whereas patients at low risk of recurrence are helped less by the same treatment (the same fixed percent of a low risk is a small benefit). Because this patient's odds of recurrence are high, systemic therapy will help her substantially, and should be included in the treatment plan.

Because the tumor is ER-positive and because the patient is older than 50, tamoxifen will have a marked beneficial impact on her odds of recurrence . Even with the use of tamoxifen, however, her residual risk of recurrence is still high. Chemotherapy will have its fixed effects on that residual risk, so the impact of chemotherapy will be significant. Several randomized trials support a role for combination chemoendocrine therapy in postmenopausal, node-positive patients. It is anticipated that similar benefit will also occur in node-negative disease. For this reason we would advise treating such a patient with chemotherapy and with tamoxifen.

Several chemotherapy options are available. Which chemotherapy would we use? The chemotherapy regimen most commonly used in node-negative breast cancer has been cyclophosphamide plus methotrexate plus 5-fluorouracil (CMF). However, data from the NSABP in node-positive breast cancer demonstrate the equivalency of doxorubicin plus cyclophosphamide (AC) chemotherapy to CMF in efficacy. Compared to doxorubicin-based regimens, CMF is less leukemogenic, causes less alopecia, and is especially well tolerated if all three drugs are given intravenously every 3 weeks for eight cycles. There is no evidence that one form of CMF is superior to any other in the adjuvant setting. Although AC therapy has been preferred by some because it is shorter in duration, it is associated with a small, but real chance of clinically important cardiotoxicity. The argument that it causes fewer days with nausea is now not as major given the efficacy of modern antiemetic drug therapy. Therefore, AC has become frequently used in clinical practice.

Based on the large tumor size, a more dose-intensive regimen is also reasonable. For example, outpatient chemotherapies that promise to be better than AC or CMF include doxorubicin followed by CMF (A-CMF) and sequential doxorubicin-paclitaxel-cyclophosphamide (ATC); however, neither has been compared directly with AC or CMF. A Canadian study comparing cyclophosphamide plus epirubicin plus 5-fluorouracil with CMF is not yet reported. Since A-CMF is superior to CMF alternating with doxorubicin, and it is unlikely that CMF alternating with doxorubicin is inferior to CMF alone, A-CMF would be a reasonable treatment for this high-risk patient.

A research study in node-positive primary disease comparing AC with AC followed by paclitaxel has recently completed accrual in the American Intergroup. Should this variant on ATC prove superior in this trial, it would likely replace A-CMF in the high-risk setting.

Following the completion of chemotherapy, the patient should be treated with radiation to the remaining breast if she had breast-conserving surgery or should consider radiation to the chest wall if she had a mastectomy. Tamoxifen for 5 years is also indicated. A study comparing chemotherapy followed by tamoxifen versus simultaneous chemotherapy plus tamoxifen has completed accrual, but is not yet reported. The advantage of starting tamoxifen after the completion of chemotherapy is that if a toxicity common to both modalities occurs during simultaneous use, it may be unclear which modality to discontinue.

The above discussion breaks the decision regarding the use of chemotherapy, hormonal therapy, or both into two parts. The first step is to estimate prognosis; the second is to estimate the benefits to be expected with the use of either or both therapy types. Of course, issues of comorbidity, social concerns, and patient preference are also important, and must contribute to an informed opinion. A frail, elderly patient might experience more toxicity from chemotherapy than benefit, especially because the efficacy of CMF seems to decline with patient age. Tamoxifen's benefit is level at about a one-third reduction in recurrence rate in spite of patient age, as long as the patient is postmenopausal. Hence, a decision to use tamoxifen alone in this setting is quite rational and would be appropriate for many patients.

BIBLIOGRAPHY

Bonadonna G, Zambetti M, Valagussa P. Sequential or alternating doxorubicin and CMF regimens in breast cancer with more than three positive nodes. JAMA 1995; 273:542–547.

Carter CL, Allen C, Henson DE. Relation of tumor size, lymph node status, and survival in 24,740 breast cancer cases. Cancer 1989; 63:181–187.

Early Breast Cancer Trialists' Collaborative Group: Systemic treatment of early breast cancer by hormonal, cytotoxic, or immune therapy. Lancet 1992; 339: 1–15, 71–85.

Fisher B, Anderson S, Redmond CK, et al. Reanalysis and results after 12 years of follow-up in a randomized clinical trial comparing total mastectomy with lumpectomy with or without irradiation in the treatment of breast cancer. N Engl J Med 1995; 333:1456–1461.

Fisher B, Brown AM, Dimitrov NV, et al. Two months of doxorubicin-cyclophosphamide with and without interval reinduction therapy compared with 6 months of cyclophosphamide, methotrexate, and fluorouracil in positive-node breast cancer patients with tamoxifen-nonresponsive tumors: results from the National Surgical Adjuvant Breast and Bowel Project B-15. J Clin Oncol 1990; 8:1483.

Fisher B, Dignam J, Bryant J, et al. Five versus more than five years of tamoxifen therapy for breast cancer patients with negative lymph nodes and estrogen receptor-positive tumors. J Natl Cancer Inst 1996; 88:1529–1542.

Fisher B, Redmond C, Legault-Poisson S, et al. Postoperative chemotherapy and tamoxifen compared with tamoxifen alone in the treatment of positive-node breast cancer patients aged 50 years and older with tumors responsive to tamoxifen: results from the National Surgical Adjuvant Breast and Bowel Project B-16. J Clin Oncol 1990; 8:1005–1018.

Hedely DW, Clark GM, Cornelisse CJ, et al. Consensus review of the clinical utility of DNA cytometry in carcinoma of the breast. Br Cancer Res Treat 1994; 28: 52–60.

Hudis C, Norton L. Adjuvant drug therapy for operable breast cancer. Semin Oncol 1996; 23:475–493.

International Breast Cancer Study Group. Effectiveness of adjuvant chemotherapy in combination with tamoxifen for node-positive postmenopausal breast cancer patients. J Clin Oncol 1997; 15:1385–1394.

Overgaard M, Hansen PS, Overgaard J, et al. Postoperative radiotherapy in high-risk premenopausal women with breast cancer who receive adjuvant chemotherapy. N Engl J Med 1997; 337:949–955.

Ragaz J, Jackson SM, Le N, et al. Adjuvant radiotherapy and chemotherapy in node-positive premenopausal women with breast cancer. N Engl J Med 1997; 337: 956–962.

Riccio L, Hudis C, Seidman A, et al. Long-term distant disease-free survival (DFS) from two pilot studies of dose-dense sequential adjuvant chemotherapy (CRX) in women (pts) with resected breast cancer (BC) and >3 positive lymph nodes (positive lymph nodes) Proc Am Soc Clin Oncol 1997; 16:145a (abstract).

Tumor Marker Expert Panel. Clinical practice guidelines for the use of tumor mark-
    ers in breast and colorectal cancer. J Clin Oncol 1996; 14:2843–2877.

Case #C.2.8
Goal: To discuss the coordination of reconstruction with adjuvant therapies

DANIEL F. HAYES

*A 35-year-old woman presents with a T2N1M0 infiltrating ductal
carcinoma. She has opted for modified radical mastectomy with
reconstruction. You would like to treat her with four cycles of cyclophosphamide and doxorubicin (CA). She has a tissue expander in place.*

The issue of sequencing and coordination of breast reconstruction in
women who choose to have a mastectomy for breast cancer has been of
concern for many years. In the past, women were often counseled that they
should wait for 2 or more years after their mastectomy before they consider
reconstruction. This time was felt to be appropriate so that the individual
patient could grow accustomed to her mastectomy scar, and it would also
avoid masking a chest-wall recurrence. However, there is no medical reason
to be concerned about masking a chest-wall recurrence, as there is little, if
any, benefit to early detection of these lesions. Furthermore, most, if not all,
chest-wall recurrences will be within the dermis or subdermis of the overlying skin and rarely, if ever, are deep to the reconstruction. Importantly, the
advent of early reconstruction, even to the point of being immediate at the
time of the mastectomy, appears to have dramatically improved an individual's taking her first step toward recovery after the devastating diagnosis of
breast cancer. Therefore, in a patient for whom mastectomy appears to be a
preferable choice over breast preservation, initiating her reconstruction at
the time of modified radical mastectomy appears to be appropriate.

The theoretical disadvantage of this approach might include the very
long procedure required to perform both a modified radical mastectomy and
the first steps of reconstruction. However, in carefully selected patients with
no other complicating medical illnesses, short-term complications appear to
be no higher than in those patients for whom a two-step procedure is performed. A second potential disadvantage might be that such complications
result in a delay of initiation of chemotherapy. Of course, the concern in
this regard would be the potential loss of benefit that early (adjuvant) systemic therapy may provide. Again, however, the reported complication rate
from immediate reconstruction appears to be quite low, and immediate reconstruction rarely results in a prolonged delay in initiation of adjuvant
chemotherapy. Furthermore, although some uncontrolled reports several

years ago suggested that perhaps the delay of initiation of chemotherapy of a few weeks might result in adverse outcomes, results from several randomized trials suggest that this is not the case. However, one must be aware of the results of a single randomized trial of patients undergoing breast-conserving therapy. In this study, delay of initiation of adjuvant chemotherapy due to preceding application of radiation therapy to the breast resulted in a higher distant disease-free recurrence rate and a nonstatistically significant lower survival rate when compared to chemotherapy before radiation. However, these results need to be confirmed.

In summary, this patient should be treated with appropriate chemotherapy as was planned all along. It does not appear that she had any complications from her early reconstruction, and I would recommend that the tissue expander be treated as would normally be done. However, replacement of the tissue expander with the permanent prosthesis, which is usually performed a few months after placement of the tissue expander, should be delayed until after chemotherapy is complete. This will avoid a second major operation during the four cycles of chemotherapy, which might significantly prolong a subsequent cycle.

BIBLIOGRAPHY

Fisher B, Brown A, Mamounas E, Wieand S, Fisher E, Robidoux A, et al. Effect of preoperative therapy for primary breast cancer on local-regional disease, disease-free survival, and survival: results from NSABP B18. Proc Am Soc Clin Oncol 1997; 16:127a.

Gabriel S, Woods J, O'Fallon W, Beard CM, Kurland L, Melton LJ. Complications leading to surgery after breast implantation. N Engl J Med 1997; 336:677–682.

Ludwig Breast Cancer Study Group. Prolonged disease-free survival after one course of perioperative adjuvant chemotherapy for node-negative breast cancer. N Engl J Med 1989; 320:491–496.

Mackay G, Bostwick J. Breast reconstruction. In: Harris J, Lippman M, Morrow M, Hellman S, eds. Diseases of the Breast. Philadelphia: JB Lippincott, 1996: 601–619.

Recht A, Come S, Henderson IC, Gelman R, Silver B, Hayes DF, et al. Five-year results of a randomized trial testing the sequencing of chemotherapy and radiation therapy following conservative surgery for patients with early stage breast cancer. N Engl J Med 1996; 334:1356–1361.

Recht A, Hayes DF, Eberlein T, Sadowsky N. Local-regional recurrence after mastectomy or breast conserving therapy. In: Harris J, Lippman M, Morrow M, Hellman S, eds. Diseases of the Breast. Philadelphia: JB Lippincott, 1996: 649–667.

C.3. NODE-POSITIVE DISEASE

Introduction

Node-positive breast cancer accounts for 60–70% of newly diagnosed cancer in women in the United States. The survival of node-positive patients is inversely correlated with the number of positive nodes. We have chosen for the sake of convenience to split node-positive patients into those with 1–3, 4–9, and >10 positive nodes, recognizing the somewhat artificial nature of these groupings. An important question in women with positive lymph nodes is when to recommend high-dose chemotherapy with autologous stem cell rescue. Until large randomized trials are completed, the use of this approach must be considered experimental, and its use outside of well-controlled clinical trials must be discouraged.

Case #C.3.1
Goal: To discuss the treatment of a young, hormone-receptor-negative patient with 1–3 positive lymph nodes
MAX S. WICHA

A 33-year-old woman presents following lumpectomy with a T2N1M0, high-grade, infiltrating ductal carcinoma. Three of 20 lymph nodes are positive. The tumor is aneuploid, high S, and hormone receptor negative.

This young patient presents with a poor-prognosis, high-grade, infiltrating ductal carcinoma with three of 20 positive lymph nodes. The aneuploid status, high S phase, and ER/PR negativity add to the negative prognostic features. Although the size of the tumor is not stated, the T2 staging indicates that the tumor is between 2 and 5 cm. Given these prognostic factors, one would calculate that the patient's risk of recurrence in the absence of chemotherapy is greater than 50%. This premenopausal patient should definitely be advised to receive chemotherapy. The standard option is 6 months of CMF. A number of studies have examined the addition of doxorubicin and have found no significant advantage to CMF. The NSABP's randomized node-positive trial compared CMF for 6 months to four cycles of doxorubicin plus cyclophosphamide (doxorubicin 60 mg/m^2 and cyclophosphamide 600 mg/m^2 IV every 21 days). There was no significant difference in disease-free or overall survival for doxorubicin and cyclophosphamide. However, owing to the shorter duration of treatment, this would be a reasonable alternative. More recently, regimens utilizing sequential doxorubicin for four cycles followed by eight cycles of CMF have been utilized in high-risk breast cancer. Trials comparing doxorubicin followed by CMF against CMF alone are currently in progress. These studies, however, require patients to have four or more positive lymph nodes. Current studies utilizing high-dose chemotherapy with stem cell rescue are being employed in two groups of women; one with 10 or more positive nodes and others with four to nine positive nodes. Although single-arm studies in these groups appear superior to historical controls, until the randomized studies are completed this will not be conclusively established.

The timing of radiation therapy and chemotherapy has been addressed in several studies. There has been a recent report of comparing initial chemotherapy followed by radiation versus radiation therapy followed by chemotherapy. This study indicated that patients who receive radiation therapy first had a lower incidence of local recurrence but a higher incidence of systemic recurrence compared to those receiving chemotherapy as the initial treatment. Thus, in this patient with a high risk of recurrence, I would recommend utilizing chemotherapy first, followed by radiation therapy.

BIBLIOGRAPHY

Bonadonna G, Zambetta M, Valagussa P. Sequential or alternating doxorubicin and CMF regimens in breast cancer with more than three positive nodes. JAMA 1995; 273:542.

Fisher B, Brown A, Dimitrov N, et al. Two months of doxorubicin-cyclophosphamide with and without interval reinduction therapy compared with 6 months of cyclophosphamide, methotrexate, and fluorouracil in positive-node breast cancer patients with tamoxifen-nonresponsive tumors. J Clin Oncol 1990; 8: 1483.

Gianni A, Siena S, Bregni M, et al. Five-year results of high-dose sequential adjuvant chemotherapy in breast cancer with >10 positive nodes. Proc Am Soc Clin Oncol 1995; 14:90.

Nemoto T, Natarajan N, Bedwani R, Vana J, Murphy GP. Breast cancer in the medial half: results of the 1978 national survey of the American College of Surgeons. Cancer 1983; 51:1333.

Peters W, Ross M, Vredenburgh J, et al. High-dose chemotherapy and autologous bone marrow support as consolidation after standard-dose adjuvant therapy for high-risk primary breast cancer. J Clin Oncol 1993; 11:1132.

Recht A, Come S, Silver B, et al. Sequencing of chemotherapy and radiotherapy following conservative surgery for patients with early-stage breast cancer: results of a randomized trial. Radiat Oncol Biol Phys 1995; 32(1):148.

Somlo G, Doroshow JH, Forman SJ, Odom-Maryon T, Lee J, Chow W, Hamasaki V, Leong L, Morgan Jr R, Margolin K, Raschko J, Shibata S, Tetef M, Yen Y, Simpson J, Molina A. J Clin Oncol 1997; 15(8):2882–2893.

Case #C.3.2
Goal: To discuss postmastectomy radiation therapy

KIRAN MEHTA and BRUCE G. HAFFTY

*A 47-year-old woman undergoes a modified radical mastectomy (MRM)
for a palpable, 4.8-cm, invasive ductal carcinoma, located in the upper
inner quadrant of the right breast. The tumor is hormone-receptor-
negative and margins of resection are clear. Four of 14 axillary nodes are
involved with tumor with microscopic extracapsular extension. The patient
receives four cycles of doxorubicin/cyclophosphamide (AC) chemotherapy
and is referred for postmastectomy radiation therapy. The patient has a
T2N1M0 invasive ductal carcinoma.*

Local chest wall and/or regional nodal recurrences occur in 10–40%
of patients undergoing mastectomy for operable breast cancer. Factors predicting locoregional failure (LRF) following mastectomy include: the presence of positive axillary nodes; size of the primary; margin status; and young
age. The finding of positive axillary nodes is the major predictor of LRF.
Patients with greater than or equal to four positive lymph nodes have a
22–42% chance of LRF. Also, patients with tumors greater than or equal to
5 cm have an 18–30% incidence of local/regional recurrence following
modified radical mastectomy (MRM) without adjuvant radiation therapy
(RT). Patients with both of these features have even greater chance of LRF.

The goals of postoperative adjuvant RT are twofold: prevention of a
local/regional recurrence and improvement in disease-free and overall survival. It has been repeatedly shown that postmastectomy RT results in a
significant reduction in LRF. The significance of preventing LRF on quality
of life cannot be understated. The development of LRF can be devastating
to a woman, and the rate of control of a LRF once it develops is disap-
pointing. Even with optimal radiotherapy, about 50% of patients suffering a
LRF will die with uncontrolled disease on the chest wall. In most trials,
however, even with this substantial improvement in local/regional control,
RT has been reported to have little or no impact on overall survival. A meta-
analysis published in 1987 by Cuzick et al. further reduced the support for
chest wall radiation by suggesting that radiation may actually reduce the
survival of patients. For these reasons, the role of postmastectomy radiation
has come under great scrutiny.

Many of the trials of postmastectomy RT originated 20–30 years ago.
In reviewing some of the earlier trials of postmastectomy RT one can see
that by today's standards, patient selection was poor. Many of the earlier
trials treated patients with stage I and II disease. Also of great importance

is that the techniques and doses of radiation used in many of the earlier trials are considered inadequate by today's standards. The most common location for LR recurrence following MRM is the chest wall. The chest wall is involved in up to 70% of all LR recurrences. Failure to include the chest wall in some of the earlier trials no doubt contributed to the lack of benefit seen in these trials.

However, further follow-up of the patients treated on these earlier trials and an update of the meta-analysis by Cuzick et al. show that irradiated patients did suffer fewer deaths from breast cancer. The cardiac morbidity and mortality continued to be higher in the irradiated patients because of high fraction size as well as high radiation doses to the heart. It is suggested in the reanalysis that in addition to significantly improved local control, radiation may have a positive impact on overall survival. Interestingly, when one looks at even the older trials in which patient selection was more stringent and modern RT techniques were utilized, a reduction in mortality was seen.

Recently, two randomized trials have been reported that examine the efficacy of radiation given to patients in an era when routine chemotherapy is also administered. These studies have shown clearly that postmastectomy radiation in addition to adjuvant chemotherapy can improve overall survival in appropriately selected patients.

This patient should be treated to the chest wall and pertinent lymph-node drainage areas. It is essential to include the chest wall in any post-mastectomy patient in whom one is considering RT. The chest wall can be treated utilizing tangential fields, similar to that of an intact breast, to a total dose of approximately 50 Gy. Bolus is routinely employed on alternate days to ensure adequate skin dose. Although there is no clear data to support the use of a "boost," it is reasonable to consider an additional 10–14 Gy with *en face* electrons to the surgical scar as most failures occur in this region.

A separate anterior supraclavicular field should be employed to treat the supraclavicular lymph nodes. In an adequately dissected axilla without evidence of gross extracapsular extension (ECE) or gross residual disease, we do not routinely employ axillary radiation. The presence of microscopic ECE is not an indication to treat the axilla. The presence of microscopic ECE does not necessarily predict for increased local failure. Axillary failure in patients with adequately dissected axillae appears to be low and the potential toxicity of lymphedema warrants careful consideration before employing RT. The supraclavicular field can be treated by a single half/blocked field matched to the tangential fields. A total dose of 50 Gy should be prescribed at a depth of 3 cm.

The role of internal mammary node (IMN) radiation has been and continues to be controversial. Although many previous studies have routinely treated the IMNs, it is clear that without proper treatment planning this may be detrimental to a patient as many patients suffer cardiac morbidity and mortality. The use of techniques that minimize cardiac dose is critical in reducing the morbidity of IMN RT. Today, with sophisticated treatment planning available it may be possible to include the IMNs with little morbidity to the underlying cardiac and pulmonary structures. However, in an era in which the use of doxorubicin is routine, with this drug's inherent cardiac toxicity, we do not routinely extend the field (or add a separate field) to include the IMNs. In addition, clinical recurrences occur infrequently in the IM nodes. Although, the two randomized studies that show survival benefit to postmastectomy radiation did incorporate nodal radiation to the IM chain, neither trial included doxorubicin chemotherapy.

At present, no large randomized trials are being performed in the United States to further verify and support the role of postmastectomy radiation. The EORTC has recently mounted a trial randomizing all lymph-node-positive and lymph-node-negative patients with medial lesions to tangential radiation verses tangents and regional radiation to the supraclavicular, axillary, and internal mammary nodes. It will be years until the results of this trial are available. However, with the recent reanalysis of the meta-analysis as well as the recent randomized data, it is clear that postmastectomy radiation has a potential impact far greater than improved local control.

BIBLIOGRAPHY

Bedwinek J. Natural history and management of isolated local-regional recurrence following mastectomy. Semin Radiat Onol 1994; 4:260–269.

Cuzick J, Stewart H, Peto R, et al. Overview of randomized trials of postoperative adjuvant radiotherapy in breast cancer. Cancer Treat Rep 1987; 71:15–29.

Cuzick J, Stewart H, Rutquist L, et al. Cause-specific mortality in long-term survivors of breast cancer who participated in trials of radiotherapy. J Clin Oncol 1994; 12:447–453.

Donegan WL, Perez-Mesa CM, Watson FR. A biostatistical study of locally recurrent breast carcinoma. Surg Gynecol Obstet 1966; 122:529–540.

Fisher B, Montague E. Comparison of radical mastectomy with alternative treatments for primary breast cancer. Cancer 1977; 39:2829–2839.

Fisher B, Redmond C, Fisher ER, et al. Ten-year results of a randomized clinical trial comparing radical mastectomy and total mastectomy with or without radiation. N Engl J Med 1985; 312:674–681.

Haagensen CD, Bodian G. A personal experience with Halsted's radical mastectomy. Ann Surg 1984; 199:143–150.

Halverson KJ, Perez CA, Kusken RR, et al. Isolated local-regional recurrence of breast cancer following mastectomy: radiotherapeutic management. Int J Radiat Oncol Biol Phys 1990; 19:851–858.

Klefstrom P, Grohn P, Heinonen E, et al. Adjuvant postoperative radiotherapy, chemotherapy and immunotherapy in stage III breast cancer. Cancer 1987; 60: 936–942.

Leonard C, Corkill M, Tompkin J, et al. Are axillary recurrences and overall survival affected by axillary extranodal tumor extension in breast cancer? Implications for radiation therapy. J Clin Oncol 1995; 13:47–53.

Overgaard M, Hansen PS, Overgaard J, et al. Postoperative radiotherapy in high-risk premenopausal women with breast cancer who receive adjuvant chemotherapy. N Engl J Med 1997; 337:949–955.

Pierce LJ, Oberman HA, Strawderman MH, et al. Microscopic extracapsular extension in the axilla: is this an indication for axillary radiotherapy? Int J Radiat Oncol Biol Phys 1995; 33:253–259.

Ragaz J, Jackson SM, Le N, et al. Adjuvant radiotherapy and chemotherapy in node-positive premenopausal women with breast cancer. N Engl J Med 1997; 337: 956–962.

Rosenman J, Bernard S, Kober C, et al. Local recurrences in patients with breast cancer at the North Carolina Memorial Hospital (1970–82). Cancer 1986; 57: 1421.

Rutquist LE, Patterson D, Johansson H. Adjuvant radiation therapy versus surgery alone in operable breast cancer: long-term follow-up of a randomized clinical trial. Radiother Oncol 1993; 26:104–110.

Schwaibold F, Fowble BL, Solin LJ, et al. The results of radiation therapy for isolated local regional recurrence after mastectomy. Int J Radiat Oncol Biol Phys 1991; 21:299–310.

Toonkel L, Fix I, Jacobson L, et al. The significance of local-regional recurrence of carcinoma of the breast. Int J. Radiat Oncol Biol Phys 1983; 9:33–39.

Valagussa P, Bonnadonna G, Veronesi U. Patterns of relapse and survival following radical mastectomy. Analysis of 716 consecutive patients. Cancer 1978; 41: 1170–1178.

Case #C.3.3
Goal: To discuss the treatment of a young, healthy, premenopausal female with >10 positive lymph nodes

WILLIAM P. PETERS

A 41-year-old woman presents to your office after the diagnosis of a T2N1M0 breast cancer, with 14 positive lymph nodes, hormone receptor negative, aneuploid, low S-phase fraction. She has decided on a modified radical mastectomy and has a tissue expander in place. She is the mother of two children and has no prior medical problems. She has heard about the use of "bone marrow transplantation for women like her" and seeks an opinion on adjuvant treatment.

We would recommend that this patient participate in one of the on-going prospective, randomized trials examining the role of high-dose consolidation in patients with 10 or more positive lymph nodes. The trial being undertaken by the Cancer and Leukemia Group B/South West Oncology Group/National Cancer Institute of Canada as an Intergroup effort compares high-dose consolidation after four cycles of CAF with either high-dose cyclophosphamide, cisplatin, and BCNU with the use of autologous cellular support or in the second arm the same cyclophosphamide, cisplatin, and BCNU at the highest dose that could be administered without the use of cellular and cytokine support. Both groups receive local regional radiation therapy and tamoxifen in patients who are hormone-receptor positive.

This treatment protocol has enrolled more than 900 patients and was projected to complete accrual by the beginning of 1998. Unfortunately results of the trial will not be available until the year 2000.

For patients who are not eligible or otherwise not interested in the use of high-dose consolidation, we would recommend intensive conventional-dose regimens utilizing either doxorubicin and cyclophosphamide or doxorubicin and cyclophosphamide followed by one of the taxanes. The risk of recurrence remains very high despite the use of conventional-dose therapy. Therefore, a patient in good general health should be encouraged to participate in one of the ongoing clinical research studies in this area.

The use of a tissue expander in this treatment setting should not be seen as a major impediment to the use of high-dose consolidation. As long as the expander is in place and well healed, the ability to tolerate therapy appears to be satisfactory with no increased risk of local infections or evidence of tissue breakdown.

BIBLIOGRAPHY

Antman KH, Rowlings PA, Vaughan WP, et al. High-dose chemotherapy with autologous hematopoietic stem-cell support for breast cancer in North America. J Clin Oncol 1997; 15:1870–1879.

Klein JL, Peters WP. High-dose chemotherapy with autologous haematopoietic progenitor cell transplantation for adenocarcinoma of the breast.

Peters WP. High-dose chemotherapy with autologous bone marrow transplantation for the treatment of breast cancer: yes. In: DeVita VT, Hellman S, Rosenberg SA, eds. Important Advances in Oncology 1995. Philadelphia: JB Lippincott, 1995:215–229.

Peters WP, Dansey R, Klein J, Berry D. High-dose chemotherapy for high-risk primary breast cancer. In: Salmon S, ed. Adjuvant Therapy of Cancer VIII. Philadelphia: Lippincott-Raven, 1997:117–122.

Peters WP, Ross M, Vredenburgh J, et al. High-dose chemotherapy and autologous bone marrow support as consolidation after standard-dose adjuvant therapy for high-risk primary breast cancer. J Clin Oncol 1993; 11:1132–1143.

Case #C.3.4
Goal: To discuss the use of adjuvant hormonal therapy in premenopausal women with multiple positive lymph nodes

MAX S. WICHA

A 41-year-old woman presents 8.5 years after treatment of a 2.1-cm, infiltrating ductal carcinoma (17 positive lymph nodes, hormone receptors strongly positive) with modified radical mastectomy, radiation therapy to the chest wall, supraclavicular lymph nodes, and six cycles of CMF. Following completion of CMF she was started on tamoxifen. After 7.5 years of tamoxifen her oncologist discontinued hormonal therapy. She has concerns over recurrence of her menses, cyclical swelling of the right breast, and fear of unopposed action of estrogens.

The role of adjuvant hormonal therapy in premenopausal women has been examined in a number of studies. Unlike the case for postmenopausal women where there are clear benefits to adding tamoxifen to chemotherapy, the value of adding tamoxifen in addition to chemotherapy in younger patients has not been clearly established. For instance, in a study by Kaufmann et al. a combination of doxorubicin, cyclophosphamide, and tamoxifen was equivalent to doxorubicin and cyclophosphamide alone. The current Intergroup study 0101 is examining the treatment of premenopausal, receptor-positive, node-positive patients comparing CAF alone to CAF followed by the LHRH agonist, zoladex, versus CAF followed by zoladex and tamoxifen. However, given the strong ER/PR-receptor positivity in this case, one can certainly argue that a course of tamoxifen following CMF might be reasonable. There have been a number of trials examining the optimal duration of tamoxifen. The Scandinavian trial in node-positive patients found that 5 years of tamoxifen is superior to 2 years. However, the NSABP study showed that treatment with tamoxifen beyond 5 years was no better than 5 years of use. On the basis of this, the National Cancer Institute has recommended 5 years of treatment with tamoxifen. There are also indications in animal models that long-term tamoxifen use can lead to enhancement of tumor growth, although this has not been proven in clinical settings.

There are several reasons to advise stopping tamoxifen after 5 years. The first is the small, but definite increase in uterine cancer related to tamoxifen use. This patient apparently has had recurrence of her menses and cyclical swelling of the right breast since discontinuing the tamoxifen. Although the patient is concerned that the return of her estrogen might precipitate breast cancer recurrence, there is no conclusive evidence that this occurs. As a matter of fact, the use of estrogen replacement therapy in postmenopausal women who have previously had a diagnosis of breast cancer remains quite controversial. Many women undergo early menopause after adjuvant chemotherapy treatment. There have not been definitive randomized studies of estrogen replacement therapy in postmenopausal breast cancer patients. Retrospective studies have shown either no or very minimal elevations in breast cancer incidence in women more than 5 years after diagnosis of breast cancer who are placed on hormone replacement therapy. Women who are willing to accept the unknown risks of hormone replacement therapy, who have severe postmenopausal symptoms, should be informed that the absolute risk of this intervention is currently unknown. However, the current patient should be advised that there is no conclusive evidence that her endogenous estrogen will accelerate breast cancer growth. Although the usual follow-up for a patient 6 years after treatment is once per year, I would recommend seeing this patient twice a year because of her unfavorable presentation at the time of the diagnosis and treatment.

BIBLIOGRAPHY

Fisher B, Costantino J, Redmond C, et al. Endometrial cancer in tamoxifen treated breast cancer patients: findings from the National Surgical Adjuvant Breast and Bowel Project (NSABP) B-14. J Natl Cancer Inst 1994; 86:527–537.

Kaufmann M, Janor W, Abel U, et al. Adjuvant randomized trials of doxorubicin/cyclophosphamide versus doxorubicin/cyclophosphamide tamoxifen and CMF chemotherapy versus tamoxifen in women with node-positive breast cancer. J Clin Oncol 1993; 11:454.

Ludwig Breast Cancer Study Group. Randomized trial of chemo-endocrine therapy, endocrine therapy, and mastectomy alone in postmenopausal patients with operable breast cancer and axillary node metastasis. Lancet 1984; 1:1256.

National Cancer Institute Clinical Announcement. Adjuvant therapy of breast cancer-tamoxifen update. Washington, DC: US Department of Health and Human Services, National Institutes of Health, 1995.

Spicer D, Pike MC, Henderson BE. The question of estrogen replacement therapy in patients with a prior diagnosis of breast cancer. Oncology 1990; 4:49–54.

Theriault RL, Sellin RV. A clinical dilemma: estrogen replacement therapy in postmenopausal women with a background of primary breast cancer. Ann Oncol 1991; 2:709–717.

A Second Opinion

LARRY NORTON and TERESA GILEWSKI

Discontinuing tamoxifen after 5 years of adjuvant use is rational. At present, there is no evidence that more than 5 years of use conveys any benefit, and there is at least a theoretical risk that the drug may actually be stimulatory to some breast cancer cells after prolonged exposure. This statement is based on laboratory studies that have proven to be predictive of clinical results and on suggestive evidence from the National Surgical Adjuvant Breast and Bowel Project (NSABP) that 10 years of use might actually be slightly inferior in disease-free survival to 5 years in the node-negative adjuvant setting. Anecdotally, some patients have shown regression of disease that recurred on adjuvant tamoxifen when the drug was discontinued and no other therapy was applied. Further follow-up of the NSABP trial is in progress as are several other randomized, prospective trials evaluating tamoxifen duration, the largest of which is the ATLAS trial, centered in England. Although data in node-positive cases are lacking, the Early Breast Cancer Trialists' Collaborative Group (EBCTCG) has clearly shown that drug effects in node-positive disease qualitatively parallel those in node-negative disease, differing only in degree as a function of the relative risks of recurrence or death in the absence of systemic adjuvant therapy. Hence, 5 years of use is advised in the node-positive situation until other data are available.

The issue of adjuvant tamoxifen in premenopausal patients is less clear. The 1992 analysis of EBCTCG data does demonstrate that, while tamoxifen is most active in older patients, the drug is also active in older premenopausal patients. However, the effect is minimal below age 40. One possible mechanism is that tamoxifen competes stoichiometrically with estrogen for estrogen-receptor-binding sites, so the presence of circulating estrogen in premenopausal women reduces the tamoxifen effect. A complicating feature is that some premenopausal women respond to the use of tamoxifen with a dramatic increase in their serum estradiol levels, presumably by an interference with the pituitary-gonadal endocrine axis. Even if the usual dose of oral tamoxifen results in blood levels that can block physiological levels of estrogen, the superphysiological levels achieved in some women may nullify tamoxifen's influence on the cancer cell. It is therefore unlikely that this patient, who started adjuvant tamoxifen in her early 30s, received much or any benefit, unless the CMF had rendered her biochemically postmenopausal.

Another point to be considered is that the 1992 EBCTCG analysis has not found that tamoxifen adds appreciably to the therapy of premenopausal patients if they had already received polychemotherapy. Hence, even if she were postmenopausal at the end of CMF, which is not likely in such a young patient, real questions about the efficacy of additional tamoxifen could be raised. It is fair to say, however, that this situation is not clear, as most of the trials summarized by the EBCTCG did not use an adequate tamoxifen duration of 2 years or more. As there is no convincing evidence that adjuvant tamoxifen for 5 years harms a biochemically postmenopausal patient, therefore, its use in this high-risk patient could be justified. Monitoring of the serum estradiol levels may be helpful.

From the information provided, it appears that this patient is most likely postmenopausal because of her concern for recurrence of menses. Tamoxifen use does not cause menopause, so if she is still amenorrheic 8.5 years later, she is probably iatrogenically postmenopausal from the CMF. On the other hand, if the cyclical swelling of her contralateral breast does indicate persistent menstrual cycling, then the former situation applies. The issue could be settled by simply measuring follicle stimulating hormone (FSH), luteinizing hormone (LH), and estradiol once or twice (to gauge cyclical fluctuations). Medical or surgical castration is undoubtedly an active therapy for high-risk premenopausal breast cancer patients, but we would not advocate this here because of the prior use of CMF and the long disease-free interval that has eliminated most of the risk of recurrence.

Hence, the only breast-cancer-specific management that is indicated at this point is a physical examination and contralateral mammogram each year. Genetic counseling might be advised if the risk of familial breast cancer seems high (note the young age of onset), especially because attention might profitably be paid to a high risk of ovarian cancer should a *BRCA1* or *BRCA2* germline mutation be documented.

BIBLIOGRAPHY

ATLAS. Personal communication, Richard Peto.

Early Breast Cancer Trialists' Collaborative Group. Systemic treatment of early breast cancer by hormonal, cytotoxic, or immune therapy. Lancet 1992; 339: 1–15, 71–85.

Fisher B, Dignam J, Bryant J, et al. Five versus more than five years of tamoxifen therapy for breast cancer patients with negative lymph nodes and estrogen receptor-positive tumors. J Natl Cancer Inst 1996; 88:1529–1542.

Jordan VC, Fritz NF, Langan-Fahey S, et al. Alteration of endocrine parameters in premenopausal women with breast cancer during long-term adjuvant therapy with tamoxifen as the single agent. J Natl Cancer Inst 1991; 63:1488–1491.

Offit K, Brown K. Quantitating familial cancer risk: a resource for clinical oncologists. J Clin Oncol 1994; 12:1724–1736.

Ribeiro G, Swindell R. The Christie Hospital adjuvant tamoxifen trial-status at 10 years. Br J Cancer 1988; 57:601–603.

Rivkin SE, Green S, O'Sullivan J, et al. Adjuvant CMFVP versus adjuvant CMFVP plus ovariectomy for premenopausal, node-positive, and estrogen receptor-positive breast cancer patients: a Southwest Oncology Group study. J Clin Oncol 1996; 14:46–51.

Sunderland MC, Osborne CK. Tamoxifen in premenopausal patients with metastatic breast cancer: a review. J Clin Oncol 1991; 9:1283–1297.

Wolf DM, Langan-Fahey SM, Parker CJ, et al. Investigation of the mechanism of tamoxifen stimulated breast tumor growth with nonisomerizable analogues of tamoxifen and metabolites. J Natl Cancer Inst 1993; 85:806–812.

Case #C.3.5
Goal: To discuss the treatment of premenopausal patients with >3 positive lymph nodes

WILLIAM N. HAIT

A 45-year-old woman presents with a diagnosis of T2N1M0 hormone-receptor-negative breast cancer. Seven lymph nodes are positive for carcinoma. There is no invasion of the lymph nodes capsule. The past medical history is remarkable for rheumatoid arthritis that is well controlled on aspirin.

I would treat this patient with chemotherapy on a well-designed clinical trial followed by local regional radiation therapy. The meta-analysis included 31 randomized trials of chemotherapy versus no chemotherapy in premenopausal patients. Overall, chemotherapy produced a 30% annual reduction in the odds of recurrence and an 18% reduction in the odds of death in premenopausal, node-positive patients. Patients with four or more positive lymph nodes have a high recurrence rate, approaching 60% at 5 years. Therefore, standard chemotherapy regimens, which decrease recurrences by 20–30%, would expect to result in a recurrence rate of 42–48%, an unacceptably poor result. Therefore, the optimum treatment for this patient is unknown and all such patients should be encouraged to participate in approved clinical trials.

Recent data suggest that the use of sequential doxorubicin/CMF may form the basis of a promising approach for women with four or more positive lymph nodes. Specifically, Buzzoni et al. reported that delivering four cycles of doxorubicin at a dose of 75 mg/m^2 followed by intravenous CMF (C 600 mg/m^2; methotrexate 40 mg/m^2; 5-FU 600 mg/m^2 intravenous. day 1 every 21 days) × 8 cycles was superior to CMF × 8 followed by doxorubicin × 4 for a total of 12 cycles. Whether this regimen will be as good as or better than doxorubicin alone, other sequential regimens, doxorubicin-containing combination regimens, or paclitaxel-containing regimens are important experimental questions remaining to be answered.

The use of high-dose chemotherapy followed by stem cell rescue is also being evaluated in the 4–10 lymph nodes group. To date, no definitive results are available. The Dutch trial of Ruidenhuis et al. found no significant differences in outcome in a group of very-high-risk patients treated with high-dose chemotherapy followed by stem cell rescue compared to standard chemotherapy; this trial was too small to draw definitive conclusions. Future high-dose trials must take into consideration the potential benefit of sequential chemotherapy or full-dose doxorubicin alone before firm conclusions can be drawn.

The presence of rheumatoid arthritis and the use of aspirin are relatively minor issues in the management of this patient, as long as there was no evidence of pulmonary, hepatic, renal, or other organ dysfunction. I would switch to a reversible prostaglandin synthase inhibitor and pay careful attention to platelet counts during therapy.

BIBLIOGRAPHY

Buzzoni G, Bonadonna G, Valagussa P, et al. Adjuvant chemotherapy with doxorubicin plus cyclophosphamide, methotrexate, and fluorouracil in the treatment of resectable breast cancer with more than three positive axillary nodes. J Clin Oncol 1991; 9:2134–2140.

Carter C, Allen C, Henson D. Relation of tumor size, lymph node status and survival in 24,740 breast cancer cases. Cancer 1989; 63:181.

Early Breast Cancer Trialists' Collaborative Group. Systemic treatment of early breast cancer by hormonal, cytotoxic, or immune therapy. Lancet 1992; 339:1.

Rodenhuis S, Richel DJ, Baars JW, et al. A randomized single-institution study of high-dose chemotherapy with cyclophosphamide, thiotepa and carboplatin in high-risk breast cancer. Proc Am Assoc Cancer Res 1997; 38:438.

Case #C.3.6
Goal: To discuss the optimal time of initiation of adjuvant chemotherapy

I. CRAIG HENDERSON

A 40-year-old woman presents with a diagnosis of T1N1M0, estrogen-receptor positive (three positive lymph nodes), carcinoma of the breast, 6 months after lumpectomy and completion of radiation therapy. She did not initially accept her oncologist's recommendation of adjuvant chemotherapy but now has changed her mind.

This patient has invasive, operable breast cancer, lymph node positive. She is under age 50 and presumably premenopausal. Even though she is now 6 months post diagnosis, I would offer her adjuvant chemotherapy with either 6 months of cyclophosphamide/methotrexate/fluorouracil (CMF) or 5 cycles of doxorubicin/cyclophosphamide (CA).

I would also inform her, however, that recent overviews suggest ovarian ablation or 5 years of adjuvant tamoxifen may be as effective as chemotherapy in premenopausal women with estrogen-receptor (ER)-positive tumors (Table 1). In a Scottish trial, women randomized to receive adjuvant ovarian ablation did as well as those given adjuvant chemotherapy, and among premenopausal women with ER+ tumors, there appeared to be an advantage for ovarian ablation. However, because of the small size of the Scottish trial this subset analysis in patients with receptor-positive tumors is unreliable. In addition, the adjuvant chemotherapy used in this study, intravenous CMF, is arguably inferior to classic CMF (oral cyclophosphamide days 1–14 of a 28-day cycle) or CA, the regimens used in most adjuvant chemotherapy trials to date. In the context of the overviews and the Scottish trial, it is impossible to argue that chemotherapy, tamoxifen, or ovarian ablation has been proven superior to the other two.

It might also be reasonable to offer this patient with an ER+ tumor both chemotherapy and 5 years of adjuvant tamoxifen. Until very recently, all of the published data, including that from overviews, failed to demonstrate an advantage for adding tamoxifen to chemotherapy in premenopausal

Table 1 Indirect Comparisons of the Reduction in Annual Odds of Death from the Use of Adjuvant Chemotherapy, Tamoxifen, or Ovarian Ablation

	Reduction in annual odds of death (%)
Chemotherapy vs. no chemotherapy (combination regimens, ≥4 months)	27 ± 7
Ovarian ablation vs. no adjuvant therapy (ER+ and ER− patients)	25 ± 7
Tamoxifen for >2 years vs. no tamoxifen (ER+ and ER− patients)	27 ± 10

These comparisons are not as valid as direct comparisons, such as a randomized trial of chemotherapy vs. ovarian ablation vs. tamoxifen. However, there are no three-way comparisons available, and even two-way comparisons, such as adjuvant tamoxifen vs. adjuvant chemotherapy, are rare. In this context, these indirect comparisons represent the best available evidence.
Source: From the 1998 Overview of Adjuvant Therapy.

women. This is not surprising if you accept the possibility that a substantial part of the benefit from adjuvant chemotherapy derives from its effect on the ovaries and you recall that multiple randomized trials among women with metastatic breast cancer have shown that two or three endocrine therapies provide little or no benefit beyond that obtained with one endocrine treatment. However, a recently reported Intergroup trial in which premenopausal, node-negative women were randomized to CAF or CMF, each with or without 5 years of adjuvant tamoxifen, reported a highly significant improvement in disease-free survival and overall survival among women given both chemotherapy and tamoxifen compared to those given chemotherapy alone. In addition, the most recent overview has also shown that *5 years* (but not shorter durations) of tamoxifen added to chemotherapy imparts a survival advantage. From these observations it is plausible that the duration of adjuvant tamoxifen treatment is a more important determination of benefit in younger than in older women.

When the era of adjuvant systemic therapy for early breast cancer began, it was not uncommon for therapy to be initiated 3–6 months and, occasionally, as long as several years after diagnosis. For example, in a randomized adjuvant chemotherapy trial begun at the Dana-Farber Cancer Institute in 1973, patients were eligible up to 2 years after diagnosis but stratified by the length of the interval from biopsy to the initiation of chemotherapy. This changed when Nissen-Meyer et al. reported the results of a *retrospective* analysis of the Norwegian randomized trial comparing a short course of adjuvant cyclophosphamide with no adjuvant treatment of any type. They found that only a 2-week delay in the initiation of treatment obviated the benefit seen when chemotherapy was initiated immediately after biopsy. Overnight this report changed the way oncologists gave adjuvant chemotherapy. However, many investigators subsequently performed similar retrospective analyses of their data. Some obtained results similar to those of Nissen-Meyer et al., but others found no relationship at all between the interval from diagnosis to initiation of chemotherapy and outcome.

Nissen-Meyer's hypothesis about the detrimental effect of delaying the initiation of chemotherapy was prospectively tested in a randomized trial conducted by the Ludwig Group (now the International Breast Cancer Study Group). Patients with positive axillary lymph nodes were treated within 24 hr of surgery with adjuvant therapy followed by 6 months of CMFp (classic CMF with daily oral prednisone) or waited 1 month to begin the 6-month course of CMFp. There was no difference in the survival of these two groups. In a recent trial that randomized patients after lumpectomy to receive either radiotherapy followed by chemotherapy about 4 months later or the reverse sequence, there was a significant increase in distant recurrence and a nonsignificant increase in mortality among those with a delay in the initiation of chemotherapy. Finally, the large NSABP trial in which women with stage I and II breast cancers were randomized to preoperative (so-called neoadjuvant) chemotherapy followed 3 months later by definitive local treatment versus the reverse has thus far failed to demonstrate a survival advantage for the early initiation of chemotherapy.

Timing is important. Otherwise adjuvant systemic therapy would not impart a survival advantage compared to treating only when metastases have appeared. A delay in initiating chemotherapy after the completion of definitive local treatment likely decreases that benefit, but the reduction of benefit from each month of delay is probably not sufficiently large to measure in our clinical trials. There are no data to conclude that there is a time after which the initiation of adjuvant systemic therapy offers no benefit. Therefore, even if a delay reduces the benefit from adjuvant therapy, it is probably better than waiting until metastases have occurred.

BIBLIOGRAPHY

Early Breast Cancer Trialists Collaborative Group. The effects of adjuvant tamoxifen and of cytotoxic therapy on mortality in early breast cancer: an overview of 61 randomised trials among 28,896 women. N Engl J Med 1988; 319:1681–1692.

Early Breast Cancer Trialists' Collaborative Group. Systemic treatment of early breast cancer by hormonal, cytotoxic, or immune therapy: 133 randomised trials involving 31,000 recurrences and 24,000 deaths among 75,000 women. Lancet 1992; 339:1–15, 71–85.

Early Breast Cancer Trialists' Collaborative Group. Ovarian ablation in early breast cancer: overview of the randomised trials. Lancet 1996; 348:1189–1196.

Early Breast Cancer Trialists' Collaborative Group. Tamoxifen for early breast cancer: an overview of the randomised trials. Lancet 1998; 351:1451–1467.

Engelsman E, Klijn JGM, Rubens RD, Wildiers J, Beex MA, Rotmensz N, Sylvester R. "Classical" CMF versus a 3-weekly intravenous CMF schedule in postmenopausal patients with advanced breast cancer. Eur J Cancer 1991; 27:966–970.

Fisher B, Brown A, Mamounas E, Wieand S, Robidoux A, Margolese RG, Cruz AB Jr, Fisher ER, Wickerham DL, Wolmark N, DeCillis A, Hoehn JL, Lees AW, Dimitrov NV. Effect of preoperative chemotherapy on local-regional disease in women with operable breast cancer: findings from National Surgical Adjuvant Breast and Bowel Project B-18. J Clin Oncol 1997; 15:2483–2493.

Henderson IC. Adjuvant systemic therapy of early breast cancer. In: Harris JR, Hellman S, Henderson IC, Kinne DW, eds. Breast Diseases, 2nd ed. Philadelphia: JB Lippincott, 1991a:427–486.

Henderson IC. Endocrine therapy of metastatic breast cancer. In: Harris JR, Hellman S, Henderson IC, Kinne DW, eds. Breast Diseases, 2nd ed. Philadelphia: JB Lippincott, 1991b:559–603.

Hutchins L, Green S, Ravdin P, Lew D, Martino S, Abeloff M, Lyss A, Henderson C, Allreld C, Dakhil S, Pierce I, Goodwin J, Thompson I, Rivkin S, Chapman R, et al. CMF versus CAF with and without tamoxifen in high-risk node-negative breast cancer patients and a natural history follow-up study in low-risk node-negative patients: first results of Intergroup Trial INT 0102 (abstr). Proc Am Soc Clin Oncol 1998; 16.

Ludwig Breast Cancer Study Group. Combination adjuvant chemotherapy for node-positive breast cancer. Inadequacy of a single perioperative cycle. N Engl J Med 1988; 319:677–683.

Nissen-Meyer R, Kjellgren K, Malmio K, Mansson B, Norin T. Surgical adjuvant chemotherapy. Cancer 1978; 41:2088–2098.

Recht A, Come SE, Henderson IC, Gelman RS, Silver B, Hayes DF, Shulman LN, Harris JR. The sequencing of chemotherapy and radiation therapy after conservative surgery for early-stage breast cancer. N Engl J Med 1996; 334:1356–1361.

Scottish Cancer Trials Breast Group and ICRF Breast Unit. Adjuvant ovarian ablation versus CMF chemotherapy in premenopausal women with pathological stage II breast carcinoma: the Scottish Trial. Lancet 1993; 341:1293–1298.

Case #C.3.7
Goal: To discuss the influence of age and comorbidities on treatment of high-risk patients

JAMES F. HOLLAND

A 78-year-old woman presents with a 3-cm, infiltrating ductal carcinoma, hormone receptor negative, moderately differentiated, diploid, high-S tumor, with three positive lymph nodes. She has enjoyed excellent health with the exception of non-insulin-dependent diabetes, which she controls with glyburide.

After a mastectomy in a healthy, 78-year-old woman with T2N1 high-risk disease (hormone receptor negative, high S phase), this patient deserves the full information about her options. A healthy diabetic at age 78 has several years of anticipated survival, although there are doubtless many occult pathologies that may surface with the additional stress of treatment. After assessment demonstrating the absence of metastatic disease and historical, physical, and laboratory evidence of clinically threatening comorbidities, I would treat her with full-dose chemotherapy *for her age.*

The "elderly old" as a general rule have less resilience in marrow recovery, in mucosal recovery, less renal capacity, and less hardiness than do younger patients. A full equivalent dose for this patient might start at half or two-thirds the standard dose. In a recent CALGB study, patients with less than 50% staining for Her-2-*neu* achieved equal disease-free survival on 30 mg/m^2 of doxorubicin as on 60 mg/m^2 together with cyclophosphamide and fluorouracil. Therefore, I would obtain a Her-2-*neu* assay on her tumor. I would not hesitate to use doxorubicin, but as in all other considerations, I would follow this particularly closely for evidence of hematological, mucosal, cardiac, and other toxicities. The second dose would be calibrated based on response to the first, usually upward. Toxicity may not be taken to intolerable levels, however, because although the treatment is given for the possibility of micrometastatic disease, which is high, the possibility of lethal toxicity must always be avoided. At the dose the patient tolerates as her maximum, treatment should be adopted for four cycles, not counting the lower-dose run-in cycle.

Although I believe doxorubicin alone or in combination is better chemotherapy than methotrexate, if the patient expressed apprehension about her heart, I would use CMF. Although CMFVP (vincristine, prednisone) has been proven superior to CMF in the presence of four nodes or more and this benefit has persisted in 18 years of follow-up, the prednisone effect on carbohydrate metabolism and the vincristine effect on an aged nervous system would deter me from this choice.

Although no drug is excluded from use in the elderly old, I would avoid drugs, where possible, that inflict irreversible toxicity on the organs where their effects are manifest. Excellent health at age 78 does not imply that the slings and arrows of aging have not targeted their usual nephrons, neurons, and scattered cells in every other organ system, diminishing the resilient response to cytocidal stress.

Prophylactic antibiotics during granulocytopenia, the use of filgrastim (GCSF) if granulocytopenia is prolonged, and transfusion if necessary to keep the hemoglobin above 9 gm/dl are supportive care measures of potential applicability.

BIBLIOGRAPHY

Early Breast Cancer Trialists Collaborative Group. Systemic treatment of early breast cancer by hormonal, cytotoxic or immune therapy. Lancet 1992; 339:1–15.

Tormey DC, Weinberg VE, Holland JF, Weiss RB, Glidewell OJ, Perloff M, Falkson G, Falkson HC, Henry PH, Leone LA, Rafla S, Ginsberg SJ, Silver RT, Blom J, Carey RW, Schein PS, Lesnick GJ. A randomized trial of five- or three-drug chemotherapy and chemoimmunotherapy in women with operable node positive breast cancer. J Clin Oncol 1983; 1:138–145.

Wood WC, Budman DR, Korzun AH, Cooper MR, Younger J, Hart RD, Moore A, Ellerton JA, Norton L, Ferree CR. Dose and dose intensity of adjuvant chemotherapy for stage II, node-positive breast carcinoma. N Engl J Med 1994; 330:1253–1259. Erratum. N Engl J Med 1994; 331:139.

Case #C.3.8
Goal: To discuss the use of hormonal therapy plus chemotherapy in the adjuvant setting in postmenopausal women
WILLIAM N. HAIT

A 60-year-old woman presents with a T2(4 cm)N1(2 positive lymph nodes)M0 breast cancer. Estrogen (ER) and progesterone (PR) receptors are both strongly positive. The tumor is diploid low S. She is in excellent health. She has been treated with a modified radical mastectomy and seeks opinions regarding adjuvant therapy. Her surgeon recommends tamoxifen for 5 years.

The best treatment for this woman is unknown. The least controversial statement is that a 60-year-old patient with a tumor that is strongly ER/PR positive should receive at least 5 years of adjuvant treatment with tamoxifen. Whether this patient should also receive chemotherapy, a longer duration of treatment with tamoxifen, and/or radiation is unknown. NSABP B-16 demonstrated an increased disease-free survival when patients were treated with chemotherapy plus tamoxifen versus tamoxifen alone. However, other studies have either confirmed or failed to confirm this finding. A SWOG trial compared CMFVP to tamoxifen to concurrent CMFVP plus tamoxifen and found no benefit to the addition of chemotherapy in postmenopausal patients. The meta-analysis suggested that a benefit from adding tamoxifen to chemotherapy would only emerge after 2 years of treatment and these patients were treated with tamoxifen for only 1 year.

As a general rule, women less than age 50 should receive adjuvant chemotherapy and women over age 50 should receive adjuvant hormonal therapy as the basis of their treatment. This recommendation is based on the view that young women experience a superior result from chemotherapy whereas older women do better with hormonal treatment. The overview analysis also suggests that the outcomes from chemotherapy and hormonal therapy are magnified as one moves further away from 50 age. As a result, it becomes progressively more difficult to demonstrate an advantage to adding tamoxifen to chemotherapy in very young women and equally difficult to show an advantage for adding chemotherapy to very old women. However, the use of oophorectomy in younger patients may offer superior benefits to tamoxifen and rival the benefits seen with chemotherapy.

Recently, a SWOG/Intergroup trial (SWOG 8814) compared tamoxifen, to CAF plus tamoxifen, to CAF followed by tamoxifen in postmenopausal women with N1 and N2 disease; all patients were ER positive. A total of 1470 eligible patients were randomized. The early analysis of these data revealed a benefit in terms of disease-free survival for the CAFT group, and the benefit was more striking in women with >4 positive nodes and age <65. No data are yet available to compare the concomitant to the sequential CAF T. If the tumor overexpressed Her-2-*neu*, one might be more inclined to add chemotherapy, as these patients may not do as well with tamoxifen alone.

NSABP B-20 compared tamoxifen, to sequential methotrexate 5-FU plus tamoxifen, to concomitant CMF plus tamoxifen in ER-positive, node-negative patients. A total of 2363 patients were enrolled. In this trial, chemotherapy plus tamoxifen was superior to tamoxifen alone in terms of DFS (20–25% reduction in relapse rate). As in the previous SWOG study, the benefit was greater in the younger (<50 year old) patients, raising the possibility that had chemotherapy alone been given, the benefits in the younger patients from adding tamoxifen may not have been seen.

The optimal duration of treatment with tamoxifen in this patient is also uncertain. To date we appreciate that 5 years is superior to 2 years of treatment, and that treatment beyond 5 years may not be appropriate in node-negative patients. In node-positive patients, the benefit of treatment beyond 5 years has not been determined.

Finally, what does one recommend to a patient with a 4-cm tumor with two positive lymph nodes in regard to radiation therapy? Before the publication of two recent articles on the subject, I would not have recommended radiation therapy for a T2 lesion with two positive lymph nodes following a mastectomy. The guidelines for recommending radiation that I used were T3 lesions, positive margins, or ≥4 positive lymph nodes. The Danish Breast Cancer Cooperative Group evaluated the role of postoperative radiotherapy in high-risk (stage II or III) premenopausal women following mastectomy and adjuvant chemotherapy (CMF). Their results suggest a benefit from radiation (50 Gy) in terms of locoregional recurrences (1% vs. 68%), 10-year disease-free survival (48% vs. 34%), and overall survival (54% vs. 45%) in both node-positive and node-negative subgroups, as well as for T2 and T3 tumors. The second study reported by the British Columbia Cancer Agency included node-positive premenopausal patients treated with mastectomy and adjuvant chemotherapy (CMF). A benefit in terms of locoregional control (87% vs. 67%), disease-free (50% vs. 33%), and overall survival (54% vs. 48%) was seen at 15 years of follow-up in both the 1–3 node group and the ≥4 node subset of patients. Although these studies addressed postmastectomy radiation in *premenopausal* patients, they raise several important considerations for all women. First, are the results obtained in pre-menopausal women able to be extrapolated to postmenopausal women? Second, is a lumpectomy plus radiation and adjuvant chemotherapy equivalent to mastectomy plus radiation and adjuvant chemotherapy? The answer to the latter may never be known.

In summary, in this healthy 60-year-old woman with a relatively high risk of recurrence, I would recommend 5 years of tamoxifen plus the option of adding chemotherapy once the patient understood the risks and benefits of this approach.

BIBLIOGRAPHY

Albain K, Green S, Osborne C, et al. Tamoxifen versus cyclophosphamide, adriamycin and 5-FU plus either concurrent or sequential tamoxifen in postmenopausal, receptor (positive) breast cancer: a Southwest Oncology Group phase III Intergroup trial (SWOG-8814, INT-0100). Proc Am Soc Clin Oncol 1997; 16:128a.

Early Breast Cancer Trialists' Collaborative Group. Systemic treatment of early breast cancer by hormonal, cytotoxic, or immune therapy. Lancet 1992; 339: 1, 71.

Fisher B, Dignam J, Bryant J, et al. Five versus more than five years of tamoxifen therapy for breast cancer patients with negative lymph nodes and estrogen receptor-positive tumors. J Natl Cancer Inst 1996; 88:1529–1542.

Fisher B, Dignam J, DeCillis DL, et al. The worth of chemotherapy and tamoxifen over tamoxifen alone in node-negative patients with estrogen receptor positive invasive breast cancer: first results from NSABP B-20. Proc Am Soc Clin Oncol 1997; 16:1a.

Fisher B, Redmond C, Legault-Poiisson S, et al. Postoperative chemotherapy and tamoxifen compared with tamoxifen alone in the treatment of positive-node breast cancer patients aged 50 year and older with tumors responsive to tamoxifen: results for the National Surgical Adjuvant Breast and Bowel Project B-16. J Clin Oncol 1990; 8:1005.

Overgaard MO, Hansen PS, Overgaard J, et al. Postoperative radiotherapy in high-risk premenopausal women with breast cancer who receive adjuvant chemotherapy. N Engl J Med 1997; 337:949–955.

Ragaz J, Jackson SM, Le N, et al. Adjuvant radiotherapy and chemotherapy in node-positive premenopausal women with breast cancer. N Engl J Med 1997; 337: 956–962.

Rivkin SE, Green S, Metch B, et al. Adjuvant CMFVP versus tamoxifen versus concurrent CMFVP and tamoxifen for post-menopausal, node-positive and estrogen receptor-positive breast cancer patients: a Southwest Oncology Group study. J Clin Oncol 1994; 12:2078.

Case #C.3.9
Goal: To discuss the use of high-dose chemotherapy in postmenopausal women

WILLIAM P. PETERS

A healthy 62-year-old woman presents with a T2N1M0, hormone-receptor-negative infiltrating ductal carcinoma. Thirteen of 20 lymph nodes contain carcinoma.

A patient with a T2 lesion involving more than 10 positive axillary lymph nodes carries a very poor prognosis with conventional chemotherapy. Given the experience within cooperative groups, the vast majority of these patients will relapse within 10 years despite the use of conventional chemotherapy. It is the opinion of some investigators that contemporary regimens using taxanes may improve somewhat on this dismal prognosis, but only further follow-up will be able to validate the enthusiasm for taxane-based regimens.

The data obtained with patients who have been treated with standard-dose chemotherapy regimens, such as CAF, followed by high-dose intensification using autologous cellular support has been encouraging. A follow-up of patients treated with this strategy by our group indicates that an excess of 50% of these patients are alive and disease free at 10 years. This is substantially better than the comparison to similarly selected patients who have been treated with conventional dose regimens. Overall survival appears to be 30–40% better at 10 years compared to patients treated with conventional-dose regimens who are similarly selected from contemporary or historical control groups. Randomized studies are currently underway.

While in the past high-dose consolidation had been generally restricted to patients under the age of approximately 55, with increased experience the toxicities and morbidity associated with the use of high-dose consolidation have been largely mitigated and a therapy-related mortality in the range of approximately 2–4% is what could be expected at experienced centers. This can be seen even in patients in their early sixties, and the mere fact that the patient is over 60 should not automatically exclude consideration of high-dose consolidation. The major factors, of course, represent patient performance, organ function, and, in general, the physician's impression about the ability of the patient to tolerate the therapy.

The results of prospective randomized trials for patients in this setting are not yet available. This type of patient should be enrolled, wherever possible, in an ongoing clinical research study attempting to evaluate this area. The result of the randomized trials will likely not be available until near the year 2000.

Patients being considered for high-dose consolidation would also receive local regional radiation therapy approximately 6–12 weeks after completion of transplant, followed by the use of adjuvant tamoxifen therapy for 5 years in the hormone-receptor-positive patient.

BIBLIOGRAPHY

Antman KH, Rowlings PA, Vaughan WP, et al. High-dose chemotherapy with autologous hematopoietic stem-cell support for breast cancer in North America. J Clin Oncol 1997; 15:1870–1879.

Klein JL, Peters WP. High-dose chemotherapy with autologous haematopoietic progenitor cell transplantation for adenocarcinoma of the breast.

Peters WP. High-dose chemotherapy with autologous bone marrow transplantation for the treatment of breast cancer: yes. In: DeVita VT, Hellman S, Rosenberg SA, eds. Important Advances in Oncology 1995. Philadelphia: JB Lippincott, 1995:215–229.

Peters WP, Dansey R, Klein J, Berry D: High-dose chemotherapy for high-risk primary breast cancer. In: Salmon S, ed. Adjuvant Therapy of Cancer VIII. Philadelphia: Lippincott-Raven, 1997:117–122.

Peters WP, Ross M, Vredenburgh J, et al. High-dose chemotherapy and autologous bone marrow support as consolidation after standard-dose adjuvant therapy for high-risk primary breast cancer. J Clin Oncol 1993; 11:1132–1143.

Case #C.3.10
Goal: To discuss the treatment of a postmenopausal patient with 4–9 lymph nodes

MICHAEL REISS

A healthy, 63-year-old woman presents with a T2N1M0, infiltrating ductal carcinoma. The tumor is estrogen-receptor-positive /progesterone-receptor-negative, aneuploid, high S. Eight of 13 lymph nodes are positive.

A healthy, 63-year-old woman presents with a T2N1M0 infiltrating ductal carcinoma of the breast. The tumor is ER-positive/PR-negative, aneuploid, with a high fraction of cells in S phase. Eight of 13 axillary lymph nodes are positive for metastatic carcinoma. The prognosis of this patient is grave, because the involvement of a large number of lymph nodes with tumor strongly correlates with the presence of overt or occult metastatic disease.

The first step in her management should include staging for detectable metastatic disease. In a recent study, 28% of patients with >10 metastatic lymph nodes were found to harbor asymptomatic metastases. If metastases are discovered, the initial management should consist of endocrine therapy, most likely tamoxifen. If metastases are not detectable, based on the number of positive lymph nodes, the patient's estimated 5-year disease-free survival is 56%, and her overall survival 47%. Standard adjuvant therapy for post-menopausal women with ER-positive breast cancer and positive lymph nodes also consists of tamoxifen endocrine therapy for extended periods, probably a minimum of 5 years. At least seven randomized trials have been conducted to address the question whether the addition of systemic CCT to tamoxifen would improve the outcome in this group of women. Whereas some of these have failed to convincingly demonstrate a greater efficacy for combined modality treatment (CMT), three studies have indicated that patients who received CMT had a significantly better disease-free and overall survival. Some of the differences between these studies can be ascribed to the intensity of the cytotoxic chemotherapy (CCT), the inclusion of anthracyclines, the duration of tamoxifen therapy, and, perhaps, the fact that tamoxifen and CCT were administered concurrently. A pivotal trial that addresses some of these issues was recently completed by the North American Intergroup. In this study, women were randomly assigned treatment with tamoxifen alone, cyclophosphamide-doxorubicin-fluorouracil (CAF) plus concurrent tamoxifen, or CAF followed by tamoxifen. Tamoxifen was given for 5 years in all three groups. The results of this trial have not yet been reported.

Because of the relatively poor prognosis of women who present with extensive nodal involvement (high-risk stage II), several studies have addressed the question whether dose-intensive or dose-dense CCT might improve their outcome. Several single-arm studies of dose-intensive CCT have been conducted in women with ≥10 positive lymph nodes. In most of these, the disease-free survival appears to be superior to that of historical controls. This experience has led to the investigation of this approach in women in the intermediate risk group, i.e. with four to nine involved lymph nodes. Specifically, a number of clinical trials are ongoing in Europe and the United States in which a conventional CCT dose schedule is compared to dose intensification with peripheral blood stem cell (PBSC) rescue. One particularly interesting approach is sequential dose-dense therapy using non-cross-resistant agents or combinations. The first example of this was provided by the group in Milan in a study of alternating versus sequential doxorubicin and cyclophosphamide-methotrexate-fluorouracil (CMF) chemotherapy. The outcome of postmenopausal women with ≥4 positive nodes was significantly better when they were treated with the sequential CCT than the alternating regimen. Based on promising results in pilot studies conducted at Memorial Sloan-Kettering Cancer Center and at the Yale Cancer Center using sequential treatment with doxorubicin, taxol, and cyclophosphamide (ATC), the North American Intergroup has recently embarked on a study in which women with four to nine positive nodes are randomly assigned to ATC versus dose-intense doxorubicin-fluorouracil followed by high-dose cyclophosphamide-cisplatin-carmustine with PBSC rescue. While the outcome of these new approaches is still unknown, all women with high-risk, stage II disease should probably be treated with CCT, followed by tamoxifen in the cases in which the tumor expresses hormone receptors.

Finally, these patients should receive locoregional radiation therapy following chemotherapy, even if they have undergone a modified radical mastectomy, because the risk of local chest wall recurrence is significantly increased in patients who present with extensive nodal involvement.

BIBLIOGRAPHY

Boccardo F, Rubagotti A, Amoroso P, et al. Chemotherapy versus tamoxifen versus chemotherapy plus tamoxifen in node-positive, oestrogen-receptor positive breast cancer patients. An update at 7 years of the 1st GROCTA (Breast Cancer Adjuvant Chemohormone Therapy Co-operative Group) trial. Eur J Cancer 1992; 28:673–680.

Burtness B, DiStasio S, Orell J, Farber L, Haffty B, Reiss M. Adjuvant sequential dose intense doxorubicin, paclitaxel and cyclophosphamide for high risk breast cancer. Br Cancer Res Treat 1996; 41:233.

Castiglione-Gertsch M, Johnsen C, Goldhirsch A, Gelber RD, Rudenstam CM, Collins J, Lindtner J, Hacking A, Cortes-Funes H, Forbes J, et al. The International (Ludwig) Breast Cancer Study Group Trials I–IV: 15 years follow-up. Ann Oncol 1994; 5:717–724.

Crump M, Prince M, Goss P. Outcome of extensive evaluation of women with >10 positive axillary lymph nodes prior to adjuvant therapy for breast cancer. AntiCancer Drugs 1995; 6:71 (abstract).

Fisher B, Redmond C, Legault-Poisson S, et al. Postoperative chemotherapy and tamoxifen alone in the treatment of positive-node breast cancer patients aged 50 years and older with tumors responsive to tamoxifen. Results from the National Surgical Adjuvant Breast and Bowel Project B-16. J Clin Oncol 1990; 8:1005–1018.

Gerard JP, Hery M, Gedouin D, Monnier A, Goudier MJ, Jacquin JP, Plat F, Cabarrot E, Serin D, Namer M, et al. Postmenopausal patients with node-positive resectable breast cancer. Tamoxifen vs FEC 50 (6 cycles) vs FEC 50 (6 cycles) plus tamoxifen vs control—preliminary results of a 4-arm randomised trial. The French Adjuvant Study Group. Drugs 1993; 45:60–67.

Hudis C, Seidman A, Raptis G, Baselga J, Gilewski T, Fennelly D, Lebwohl D, Surbone A, Currie V, Moynahan M, Theodolou M, Sklarin N, Uhlenhopp M, Yao T-J, Norton L. Event-free survival after sequential dose-dense doxorubicin (A), paclitaxel (T) and cyclophosphamide (C) in women (pts) with ≥4 positive

(positive) axillary lymph nodes (lymph nodes). Br Cancer Res Treat 1996; 41: 232.

International Breast Cancer Study Group. Effectiveness of adjuvant chemotherapy in combination with tamoxifen for node-positive postmenopausal breast cancer patients. J Clin Oncol 1997; 15:1385–1394.

Pritchard KI, Paterson AHG, Fine S, Paul NA, Zee B, Shepherd LE, Abu-Zahra H, Ragaz J, Knowling M, Levine MN, Verma S, Perrault D, Rivkin SE, Green S, Metch B, Cruz AB, Abeloff MD, Jewell WR, Costanzi JJ, Farrar WB, Minton JP, Osborne CK. Adjuvant CMFVP versus tamoxifen versus concurrent CMFVP and tamoxifen for postmenopausal, node-positive, and estrogen receptor-positive breast cancer patients: a Southwest Oncology Group study. J Clin Oncol 1994; 12:2078–2085.

Walde PLD, Bramwell VHC, Polcijak M, Boyd N, Warr D, Norris BD, Bowman D, Armitage GR, Weizel H, Buckman RA, et al. Randomized trial of cyclophosphamide, methotrexate, and fluorouracil chemotherapy added to tamoxifen as adjuvant therapy in postmenopausal women with node-positive estrogen and/ or progesterone receptor-positive breast cancer: a report of the National Cancer Institute of Canada Clinical Trials Group. J Clin Oncol 1997; 15:2302–2311.

C.4. NODE STATUS UNDETERMINED (NX)

Introduction

In recent years, we have witnessed a greater number of clinical situations in which we question the need for axillary lymph node dissection. In addition, the use of neoadjuvant chemotherapy often leaves the lymph-node status uncertain. This issue has become more acute with the aging of the breast cancer population and with pressure on cost reduction.

Case #C.4.1
Goal: To discuss neoadjuvant chemotherapy in a premenopausal woman

DEBORAH L. TOPPMEYER

A 36-year-old woman presents with a 3-cm, infiltrating ductal carcinoma, estrogen-receptor negative, no palpable axillary lymph nodes. She received four cycles of cyclophosphamide/doxorubicin (CA) at which time her disease was clinically undetectable. A lumpectomy, with axillary lymph node examination was performed. No disease was found.

Primary chemotherapy refers to the use of chemotherapy before definite local treatment of breast cancer is performed. Other terms synonymous with primary chemotherapy include "preoperative chemotherapy," "neoadjuvant chemotherapy,'' and ''upfront chemotherapy.'' The role of primary chemotherapy has been explored since the early 1970s, initially to improve local control and survival in women with large breast tumors or inflammatory breast cancer. The use of primary chemotherapy has induced tumor regression in 60–90% of women and has had a significant impact on survival in the treatment of inflammatory breast cancer.

The concept of primary chemotherapy is attractive for several reasons. First, shrinkage of a large tumor can improve the likelihood of successful breast-conservation surgery. Second, the initial response to primary chemotherapy may identify women who will respond better to later chemotherapy. Patients who have a poor initial response may be better served by changing to a non-cross-resistant therapy or be potential candidates for investigational therapies. Third, based on the Goldie-Coldman hypothesis, the potential for eradication of metastatic tumor clones is greater prior to surgery and therefore might improve survival. Theoretically, earlier introduction of non-cross-resistant chemotherapy would prevent the establishment of drug-resistant clones that arise from continued cell growth and somatic mutation.

Five prospective randomized trials have addressed the issue of ''primary chemotherapy.'' The most definitive and largest was the NSABP B-18 trial recently presented in abstract form. A total of 1523 patients were randomized to standard doxorubicin and cyclophosphamide (600 mg/m^2 and 60 mg/m^2, respectively every 21 days) for four cycles prior to or following definitive surgery. Disease-free and overall-survival through 5 years of follow-up were 67% and 80%, respectively, in both groups. Notably, the response rate in the group receiving primary chemotherapy was 80%, with 36% of patients demonstrating a complete response and 44% demonstrating a partial response by standard criteria. As a result, more patients received breast-conserving surgery in the primary chemotherapy group. This difference was statistically significant and was greatest in patients with tumors measuring ≥5.1 cm (8% vs. 22%). In addition, patients with clinically positive lymph nodes who received primary chemotherapy had a lower incidence of pathological involvement of lymph nodes compared to those who received postoperative chemotherapy (41% vs. 57%). Similarly, other studies have demonstrated an increase in breast conservation with the use of primary chemotherapy, but the impact on survival was not clear.

The ability to assess response is an advantage of primary chemotherapy. Several studies have demonstrated that response to chemotherapy predicts for better relapse-free and overall survival. Although the adage that responders fare better than nonresponders is not new, a poor response to chemotherapy may select a population of patients that may benefit from additional non-cross-resistant therapies or participation in clinical trials of new investigational drugs such as MDR modulators in combination with chemotherapy or high-dose therapy protocols. Furthermore, the ability to examine histopathological and molecular markers in the primary tumor before and after chemotherapy and correlate these finding with response is appealing as it provides insight into potential mechanisms of drug resistance. For example, both mutant p53 and *bcl*-2 expression have been correlated with resistance to chemotherapy, and *erb*B2 overexpression may be responsible for resistance to alkylator-based regimens. Exploiting this basic understanding of response will help tailor therapy and strategically target new therapeutic interventions.

In summary, it appears that the greatest benefit from primary chemotherapy is the ability to perform breast conservation in patients where such an approach may be equivocal. There appears to be no difference in disease-free or overall survival. Most significantly, there appears to be no increased rate of ipsilateral breast recurrence. The potential downfall of primary chemotherapy is compromising the ability to prognosticate based on lymph node status and to tailor chemotherapy or enrollment in clinical trials based on this information. Primary chemotherapy is a modality still being explored in clinical trials and efforts should be directed at enrolling patients on these trials if neoadjuvant therapy is to be considered.

BIBLIOGRAPHY

Bonadonna G, et al. Primary chemotherapy in surgically resectable breast cancer. CA Cancer J Clin 1995; 45:227–243.

Fisher B, et al. Effect of preoperative therapy for primary breast cancer on local-regional disease, disease-free survival, and survival: results from NSABP B18. Proc Am Soc Clin Oncol 1997; 16:127a.

Harris L, Swain S. The role of primary chemotherapy in early breast cancer. Semin Oncol 1996; 23(1):31–42.

Jacquillat C, Weil M, Baillet F. Results of neoadjuvant chemotherapy and radiation therapy in the breast-conserving treatment of 250 patients with all stages of infiltrative breast cancer. Cancer 1990; 66:119–129.

Legler C, et al. Primary chemotherapy of resectable breast cancer. Breast J 1995; 1: 42–51.

Mauriac L, et al. Effects of primary chemotherapy in conservative treatment of breast cancer patients with operable tumors larger than 3 cm. Ann Oncol 1991; 2: 347–354.

Powles T, et al. Randomized trial of chemoendocrine therapy started before or after surgery for treatment of primary breast cancer. J Clin Oncol 1995; 13:547–552.

Scholl S, et al. Neoadjuvant versus adjuvant chemotherapy in premenopausal patients with tumors considered too large for breast conserving surgery: preliminary results of a randomized trial: S6. Eur J Cancer 1994; 30A:645–652.

Semiglazov V, et al. Primary (neoadjuvant) chemotherapy and radiotherapy com-
    pared with primary radiotherapy alone in stage IIb–IIIb breast cancer. Ann
    Oncol 1994; 5:591–595.
Swain S, Lippman M. Systemic therapy of locally advanced breast cancer: review
    and guidelines. Oncology 1989; 3:21–28.

Case #C.4.2
Goal: To discuss the utility of node dissection in young women with T1a tumors

THOMAS J. KEARNEY

*A 36-year-old woman presents for evaluation for adjuvant therapy. A
palpable breast mass led to an excisional biopsy of a fibroadenoma.
Adjacent to the fibroadenoma was a 0.3-cm area of invasive breast cancer.
Immunocytochemical determination of hormone receptor status is
technically inadequate.*

This woman has a very small, invasive breast cancer. Since women
with T1a and T1b primary tumors with uninvolved nodes (stage I) have a
low likelihood of distant recurrence, systemic adjuvant therapy is usually
not warranted. However, if this same woman had involved axillary nodes,
she would have stage II breast cancer and adjuvant therapy would be recommended since it would improve her relative survival rate by 25–30%.
Therefore, the results of an axillary dissection would add important prognostic information and would help guide adjuvant therapy. The common
complications of axillary dissection include lymphedema, which affects
15–20% of women, and numbness of the inner aspect of the upper arm,
affecting over 75% of women. Other complications include seroma formation and shoulder dysfunction. Therefore, the decision to perform axillary
dissection rests on weighing the likelihood that useful information will be
obtained against the potential complications.

Reports demonstrate a wide range of axillary node positivity in women
with small cancers. One report suggests that patients with invasive tumors
less then 5 mm have as low as a 4% probability of harboring axillary node
metastases when the primary tumor is nonpalpable. However, other reports
describe rates of 10% or higher. Currently, it is standard to perform axillary
dissection in women with invasive breast cancer. The results of axillary
dissection will guide adjuvant therapy in women with small primary cancers.
Axillary dissection can be avoided in women who present with ductal carcinoma in situ since the rate of positive nodes is about 1%. Similar recommendations can be made for so-called "microinvasive" cancer, which
also has a positive node rate of about 1%. The surgeon must realize that

"microinvasive" cancer has various definitions and should consult directly with the reporting pathologist (see case B.2.8). In addition, certain subtypes of invasive breast cancer such as pure tubular carcinoma can be treated without axillary dissection owing to the low rate of positive nodes. Sentinel node biopsy may be able to replace standard axillary dissection in the future if it proves to be sensitive and reproducible.

The final question in this patient's care concerns the role of radiation therapy to the breast. Multiple prospective studies have shown that lumpectomy with breast radiation is equivalent to modified radical mastectomy in the local treatment of invasive breast cancer. If the patient has clean margins and no suspicious areas of microcalcification on mammography, she should be treated with breast conservation. Several clinical trials have examined the possibility of avoiding radiation after breast-conserving surgery and all have shown higher local recurrence rates in the nonirradiated patients. Even in highly selected patients, local recurrence rates without radiation are unacceptably high. Therefore, standard care for this patient would involve radiation therapy following breast-conserving surgery.

BIBLIOGRAPHY

Albertini JJ, Lyman GH, Cox C, et al. Lymphatic mapping and sentinel node biopsy in the patient with breast cancer. JAMA 1996; 276:1818–1822.

Guiliano AE, Jones RC, Brennan M, et al. Sentinel lymphadenectomy in breast cancer. J Clin Oncol 1997; 15:2345–2350.

Harris JR, Morrow M. Treatment of early-stage breast cancer. In: Harris JR, Lippman ME, Morrow M, et al, eds. Diseases of the Breast. Philadelphia: Lippincott-Raven, 1996; 522–524.

Lin P, Allison D, Wainstuck J. Impact of axillary lymph node dissection on the therapy of breast cancer patients. J Clin Oncol 1993; 11:1536.

Recht A, Houlihan MJ. Axillary lymph nodes and breast cancer. Cancer 1995; 76: 1491–1512.

Silverstein MJ, Gierson ED, Waisman JR, et al. Predicting axillary node positivity in patients with invasive carcinoma of the breast using a combination of T category and palpability. J Am Coll Surg 1995; 180:700–704.

Werner RS, McCormick B, Petrek JA, et al. Arm edema in conservatively managed breast cancer: obesity is a major predictive factor. Radiology 1991; 180:177.

Wong JH, Kopald KH, Morton DL. The impact of microinvasion on axillary node dissection for T1a breast carcinoma: is it indicated? Arch Surg 1990; 125: 1298–1302.

D. Locally Advanced Breast Cancer

Case #D.1
Goal: To discuss the diagnosis of locally advanced breast cancer

MICHAEL H. TOROSIAN

A 33-year-old woman seeks evaluation of a left breast mass. She states that it has been present for approximately 2 years and has slowly increased in size. Physical examination demonstrates a 4-cm, hard, mobile mass with puckering of the overlying skin. There is a hard mass in the axilla, approximately 3 cm in diameter, fixed to the chest wall, and felt to represent matted lymph nodes.

This premenopausal patient has a locally advanced breast carcinoma by clinical presentation. Initial diagnostic evaluation should consist of bilateral mammograms and fine-needle aspiration of both the 4-cm breast mass and the fixed axillary lymph nodes. This initial evaluation should be performed during her first office visit so that the diagnosis can be rapidly established and treatment initiated.

Following confirmation of breast carcinoma with metastasis to the axillary lymph nodes, complete metastatic evaluation should be performed consisting of chest X-ray, bone scan, and liver function tests or computed-tomography scan of the abdomen. Assuming there is no evidence of distant metastatic disease, this patient presents with stage IIIb disease and has a high risk of recurrence. Therefore, the first line of treatment should consist of systemic chemotherapy. Several studies have demonstrated the efficacy of cytoreductive chemotherapy administered to patients with locally advanced breast cancer prior to local or regional therapy (i.e., surgery and radiation therapy). Multimodality treatment typically consists of at least three cycles of neoadjuvant 5-fluorouracil, adriamycin, and cyclophosphamide (FAC) followed by surgery (modified radical mastectomy or lumpectomy and axillary dissection) and/or radiation therapy. Chemotherapy can be administered for three cycles or more until an optimal response has been achieved. The sequence of performing surgery and administering radiation therapy can vary. My preference would be to perform surgery before radiation therapy if the regional lymph nodes become free by the neoadjuvant chemotherapy regimen. Alternatively, radiation therapy would be provided prior to surgery if the axillary lymph nodes remained fixed following systemic therapy.

If evidence of systemic metastasis exists at the time of initial presentation, chemotherapy should be administered followed by complete radiological restaging. If response or stabilization of metastatic disease has occurred with systemic treatment, consideration can be given to total mastectomy for local control. Removal of axillary lymph nodes in the presence of metastatic disease is not indicated and will only increase the risk of upper extremity lymphedema. If disease progression occurs despite first-line chemotherapy, breast surgery is not indicated and either second-line chemotherapeutic agents or bone marrow/autologous stem cell transplantation should be considered.

In summary, this patient presents with a locally and regionally advanced carcinoma. The high risk of locoregional recurrence and systemic metastasis mandates early, aggressive systemic treatment. Rapidly establishing the diagnosis of malignancy and prompt institution of systemic therapy are critically important in the management of this patient.

BIBLIOGRAPHY

Bonadonna G, Valagussa P, Brambilla C, et al. Adjuvant and neoadjuvant treatment of breast cancer with chemotherapy and/or endocrine therapy. Semin Oncol 1991; 15:515.

Fisher B, Rockette H, Ribidoux A, et al. Effect of preoperative therapy for breast cancer (BC) on local-regional disease: first report of NSABP B-18. Proc ASCO 1994; 13:64.

Mauriac L, Durand M, Avril A, et al. Effects of primary chemotherapy in conservative treatment of breast cancer patients with operable tumors larger than 3 cm: results of a randomized trial in a single center. Ann Oncol 1991; 2:347.

Touboul E, Lefranc JP, Blondon J, et al. Multi-disciplinary treatment approach to locally advanced non-inflammatory breast cancer using chemotherapy and radiotherapy with or without surgery. Radiother Oncol 1992; 25:167.

Case #D.2
Goal: To discuss the use of neoadjuvant chemotherapy

LARRY NORTON and TERESA GILEWSKI

A 44-year-old woman is found to have a 7-cm, mobile breast cancer diagnosed by fine-needle aspiration cytology. Four 1.5-cm, mobile lymph nodes are palpable in the right axilla. Metastatic workup is negative. Evaluation by a surgical oncologist suggests that the cancer is "technically resectable" with a modified radical mastectomy.

Approximately 80–90% of large primary breast cancers will respond to preoperative systemic therapy. This has been demonstrated by venerable trials in T3 tumors as well as recent experience with preoperative chemotherapy for operable (T2) lesions. When a cancer would be unresectable without such a response, preoperative chemotherapy is always indicated as it almost always improves the odds of a good surgical result. (Inoperable breast cancer is always fatal. Hence, preoperative chemotherapy in these cases is lifesaving.)

This degree of local response has encouraged some theoreticians to conclude that occult micrometastatic disease should respond as well, translating into survival benefit. The argument was extended to the hypothesis that early use of chemotherapy could kill cancer cells in distant sites before they had time to mutate to drug resistance. However, for operable disease (T2 or smaller), in spite of these theoretical arguments, there is no evidence thus far that preoperative chemotherapy improves overall prognosis. Hence, the decision to use preoperative chemotherapy for operable disease should be based on considerations of convenience, feasibility, and overall therapeutic plan. Since preoperative treatment does downstage the axilla to a small degree, one loses the prognostic significance of number of involved nodes, which might be useful for treatment planning.

This patient is young, indicating that "adjuvant" chemotherapy will be indicated regardless of axillary status. Palpable axillary lymph nodes are not a sure sign of metastatic involvement, but it is likely that she will have positive nodes given the large tumor size. It is also likely that she would be best treated by mastectomy given the size of the lesion, even if the lesion responded to chemotherapy. The role of lumpectomy in this situation remains investigational. If the number of involved nodes would not influence the choice of chemotherapy regimen, then preoperative treatment is reasonable, since it will almost always make the surgeon's task easier. However, if the number of involved axillary lymph nodes would be important for choosing which chemotherapy to use, surgical resection before chemotherapy would make more sense. This decision—preoperative or postoperative chemotherapy—therefore depends in part on local usage patterns for chemotherapy. In both cases postmastectomy, postchemotherapy radiation to the chest wall would be indicated to reduce the odds of local recurrence and, perhaps thereby, decrease the odds of metastatic spread.

BIBLIOGRAPHY

Bonadonna G, Valagussa P, Zucali R, et al. Primary chemotherapy in surgically resectable breast cancer. CA 1995; 45:227–243.

Early Breast Cancer Trialists' Collaborative Group. Effects of radiotherapy and surgery in early breast cancer: an overview of the randomized trials. N Engl J Med 1995; 333:1444–1455.

Fisher B, Brown A, Mamounas E, et al. Effect of preoperative chemotherapy on local-regional disease in women with operable breast cancer: findings from

National Surgical Adjuvant Breast and Bowel Project B-18. J Clin Oncol 1997a; 15:2483–2493.

Fisher B, Brown A, Mamounas E, et al. Effect of preoperative therapy for primary breast cancer (BC) on local-regional disease, disease-free survival (DFS), and survival (S): results from NSABP B-18. Proc Am Soc Clin Oncol 1997b; 16: 127a (abstract).

Fisher B, Wolmark N, Bauer M, et al. The accuracy of clinical nodal staging and of limited axillary dissection as a determinant of histological nodal status in carcinoma of the breast. Surg Gynecol Obstet 1981; 152:765–772.

Goldie JH, Coldman AJ. A mathematical model for relating the drug sensitivity of tumors to their spontaneous mutation rate. Cancer Treat Rep 1979; 63:1727–1733.

Overgaard M, Hansen PS, Overgaard J, et al. Postoperative radiotherapy in high-risk premenopausal women with breast cancer who receive adjuvant chemotherapy. N Engl J Med 1997; 337:949–955.

Perloff M, Lesnick J. Chemotherapy before and after mastectomy in stage III breast cancer. Arch Surg 1982; 117:879–881.

Ragaz J, Jackson SM, Le N, et al. Adjuvant radiotherapy and chemotherapy in node-positive premenopausal women with breast cancer. N Engl J Med 1997a; 337: 956–962.

Ragaz J, Baird R, Rebbeck P, et al. Preoperative (neoadjuvant—PRE) versus post-operative (POST) adjuvant chemotherapy (CT) for stage I-II breast cancer (SI-II BC). Long-term analysis of British Columbia randomized trial. Proc Am Soc Clin Oncol 1997b; 16:142a.

Case #D.3
Goal: To discuss the management of locally advanced breast cancer with a partial response following neoadjuvant chemotherapy

SUSAN A. MCMANUS

A 71-year-old woman completes four cycles of CAF following diagnosis of an inflammatory breast cancer of the left breast. The inflammatory skin changes have resolved, and a palpable axillary node has disappeared. An initial 5-cm, hard, subareolar mass decreased to 2 cm in diameter over the first two cycles and has been unchanged since. Repeat staging workup does not reveal evidence of metastatic disease.

Inflammatory breast carcinoma, which accounts for 1–5% of breast cancer in the United States, is highly aggressive. Regional and distant spread often occur early in the course of the disease. Typically, patients describe a rapid recent increase in the size of the breast, along with breast erythema and pain. Some clinicians attempt to distinguish primary inflammatory carcinoma (simultaneous development of a breast mass and associated inflammatory changes) and secondary inflammatory cancer (inflammatory changes developing in association with a long-standing, untreated cancer). Because these entities behave similarly, however, the distinction is probably not helpful. Although many believe that a skin biopsy demonstrating tumor in the subdermal lymphatics is important to make a diagnosis of inflammatory breast cancer, this is not really necessary. Clinical manifestations of inflammatory carcinoma, even when skin biopsy is not diagnostic, confer the same aggressive course as pathologically demonstrated dermal lymphatic involvement. Either clinical or pathological criteria may be used to establish the diagnosis.

Neoadjuvant chemotherapy is currently recommended for the treatment of inflammatory breast cancer because of the dismal results associated with the initial use of surgery, or surgery combined with radiation therapy. Frequently, a doxorubicin-based regimen is administered for two to four cycles and then a decision is made regarding local treatment. Sixty-two percent of patients respond to neoadjuvant chemotherapy; 49% achieve a partial response and 13% a complete response. When neoadjuvant chemotherapy was followed by surgery and/or radiotherapy, and then additional chemotherapy, 5-year disease-free and overall survival rates were 34% and 40%, respectively. This is compared with 0–10% when either surgery or radiation was used as initial therapy.

Following neoadjuvant chemotherapy, staging studies must be repeated before surgery since 20–30% of patients with inflammatory carcinoma present with distant metastases and more than 70% will have distant metastases within 1 year.

Surgery is recommended following induction chemotherapy. Patients treated with mastectomy and chemotherapy survive longer than those treated with radiation and chemotherapy. Mastectomy is usually recommended because residual carcinoma is found in a large percentage of mastectomy specimens following chemotherapy. Recently, Singletary and others studied whether patients with locally advanced breast cancer were candidates for breast-conserving treatment. However, in this study, only 6% of patients with inflammatory breast cancer achieved breast preservation.

Radiation therapy should be administered following mastectomy and should include the axilla and supraclavicular areas. Care should be taken when irradiating the left breast in patients who have underlying heart disease and/or have had induction chemotherapy with a doxorubicin-based regimen, as these patients will be at higher risk for cardiac damage. Whether or not postoperative high-dose chemotherapy with bone marrow or stem cell support is helpful for patients with inflammatory breast cancer is an unanswered question.

I believe that the most prudent course for this patient is a modified radical mastectomy, followed by radiation to the chest wall, and administration of 4 to 6 more cycles of chemotherapy. Approximately 30% of patients who partially respond to neoadjuvant therapy will live for 5 years or longer. Patients who achieve a complete clinical or pathological response to neoadjuvant chemotherapy appear to do even better.

BIBLIOGRAPHY

Aisner J, Morris D, Elisa EG. Mastectomy as an adjunct to chemotherapy for locally advanced or metastatic breast cancer. Arch Surg 1982; 117:882.

Fein DA, Mendenhall NP, March RDW, Bland KI, Copeland EM III, Million RR. Results of multimodality therapy for inflammatory breast cancer: an analysis of clinical and treatment factors affecting outcome. Am Surg 1994; 60:220–225.

Jaiyesimi IA, Buzdar AU, Hortobagyi G. Inflammatory breast cancer: a review. J Clin Oncol 1992; 10:1014–1024.

Moore MP, Ihde JK, Crow JP, Hakes TP, Kinne DW. Inflammatory breast cancer. Arch Surg 1991; 126:304–306.

Case #D.4
Goal: To discuss the management of locally advanced breast cancer with a complete clinical response following neoadjuvant chemotherapy

VERNON K. SONDAK and JULIE A. WOLFE

A 41-year-old woman completes four cycles of systemic chemotherapy (Adriamycin/Taxol) following diagnosis of an inflammatory cancer of the left breast. The inflammatory skin changes have resolved, a previously palpable axillary node has disappeared, and an initial 5-cm, hard, subareolar mass is no longer detectable. Repeat mammogram is now normal, and a staging workup does not reveal any evidence of metastatic disease.

Inflammatory breast carcinoma is a clinical syndrome characterized by breast warmth, tenderness, erythema, and edema, which may or may not be associated with specific histological findings. The characteristic manifestations of inflammatory breast carcinoma include inflammatory changes of the overlying skin and very indistinct margins of the actual lesion—indeed, the entire breast is often abnormal. Microscopically, the breast skin contains dilated dermal lymphatic channels and a lymphocytic reaction within the dermis surrounding the dilated vascular spaces. The histological hallmark of inflammatory breast cancer, intralymphatic tumor emboli in the dermis, is seen in only about half of clinically diagnosed cases.

Inflammatory breast cancer, with or without documented dermal lymphatic involvement, is classified as stage IIIB disease in the American Joint Committee on Cancer staging schema. Almost all women with inflammatory breast cancer have micrometastases at the time of initial presentation. Surgical intervention alone is of little benefit. Women with inflammatory breast cancer treated by radical mastectomy were shown to have a 60% chance of local recurrence, with no patient alive and disease-free at 5 years. Locoregional control of disease may be improved by adding radiotherapy after mastectomy, but the overwhelming incidence of distant metastases mandates a multimodality approach including aggressive systemic chemotherapy.

The optimum systemic therapy regimen for inflammatory breast cancer has yet to be defined. Most oncologists utilize aggressive multiagent regimens including doxorubicin (Adriamycin). The combination of doxorubicin and paclitaxel (Taxol) has significant activity in metastatic breast cancer and represents a reasonable choice for locally advanced breast cancer, although there is less experience with this combination than with other regimens such as doxorubicin/cyclophosphamide or 5-fluorouracil/doxorubicin/cyclophosphamide. Results with these types of regimens have defined general principles for the multimodality management of inflammatory breast cancer.

Initial treatment with systemic chemotherapy or chemohormonal therapy is continued until maximal clinical response is achieved. The patient is then restaged clinically, radiographically, and—if there is no clinical evidence of residual disease—pathologically. In the current case, the patient has had a clinical complete remission; resolution of the inflammatory skin changes and disappearance of previously palpable and radiologically evident disease. We would now recommend repeat biopsy of the site of initial bulky disease in the breast, in this case the subareolar region. If residual microscopic tumor is identified, the patient should undergo modified radical mastectomy and subsequent chest wall and supraclavicular irradiation (and potentially axillary irradiation if multiple positive nodes or gross extranodal extension of tumor is found after chemotherapy). If the patient is found to have a complete pathological response (i.e., no evidence of even microscopic tumor on rebiopsy), our experience has shown that mastectomy is not necessary and satisfactory local control can be obtained by external-beam radiation encompassing the breast, chest wall, axilla, and supraclavicular fossa. Using a chemohormonal regimen that included 5-fluorouracil, doxorubicin, cyclophosphamide, methotrexate, estrogen, and tamoxifen, we achieved at least a partial response in 84 of 87 patients (97%) with stage IIB and III disease, and 53 of the patients (61%) had a complete clinical response. Upon rebiopsy, 23 of the 53 complete clinical responders were found to be complete pathological responders as well (43% of the complete clinical respond-ers, 26% of the total evaluable patients). Twenty-one of these 23 patients were treated with radiation therapy without mastectomy, with only three local recurrences (14%). This compares quite favorably with the results following mastectomy and postoperative radiation; seven of 54 (13%) re-curred locally in this category. Most significantly, the 5-year disease-free survival for the group as a whole was 44%, and for the subgroup of patients with inflammatory breast cancer, 35% were alive and disease-free after 5 years.

Thus, we believe aggressive, multimodality therapy offers the best chance of long-term disease-free survival, good local control, and a chance for breast conservation in about a quarter of patients.

BIBLIOGRAPHY

Haagenson CD, Stout AP. Carcinoma of the breast: criteria of inoperability. Ann Surg 1943; 118:859–870.

Merajver SD, Weber BL, Cody R, Zhang D, Strawderman M, Calzone KA, LeClaire V, Levin A, Irani J, Helvie M, August D, Wicha M, Lichter A, Pierce LJ. Breast conservation and prolonged chemotherapy for locally advanced breast cancer: The University of Michigan experience. J Clin Oncol 1997; 15:2873–2881.

Case #D.5
Goal: To discuss the management of a woman with unresectable disease following neoadjuvant chemotherapy for a locally advanced breast cancer

MICHAEL REISS

A 39-year-old woman is treated with three cycles of chemotherapy (doxorubicin and cyclophosphamide) for a biopsy-proven, locally advanced left breast cancer. At presentation the tumor was 9 cm, ulcerating the skin, fixed to the chest wall, and associated with palpable axillary adenopathy. The tumor decreased by 40% in diameter in response to the chemotherapy, but remains ulcerated and fixed. Restaging workup does not reveal evidence of metastatic disease.

This patient presented with clinical stage IIIB breast cancer. Stage IIIB identifies the subset of patients with locally advanced breast cancer who have no evidence of metastatic disease, but in whom the primary tumor and regional lymph node metastases are so extensive that the surgeon cannot confidently resect all gross disease and obtain negative resection margins.

Many years ago, Haagensen and Stout identified skin ulceration and fixation of the tumor to the chest wall as markers of inoperability because of the extremely high likelihood of locoregional and systemic recurrences after surgery.

The primary treatment approach should consist of cytotoxic chemotherapy followed by measures aimed at achieving local control. Most published reports using this approach report a high (60–80%) rate of major objective regression of the primary tumor mass and adenopathy. However, clinical complete remissions are achieved in only 10–20% of cases, and pathological complete remissions are even less common. Although very few studies have directly compared the efficacy of mastectomy to radiation therapy or to combined modality treatment in achieving local control, the local control rate of ≥80% in patients treated with the combination of surgical resection and radiation therapy appears to be superior to the results obtained with either of the two modalities used alone.*

Additional adjuvant chemotherapy following surgery has been demonstrated to improve the outcome of patients with IIIB disease, with 5-year survival rates of about 50% and 10-year survival of approximately 30%. A question that is currently being addressed in a large number of studies is whether these results can be improved upon by applying consolidation treatment with dose-intense chemotherapy. Furthermore, pathological staging at the time of mastectomy or lumpectomy following induction chemotherapy has been shown to provide important prognostic information. Thus, a pathological complete response at the site of the primary tumor and axillary lymph nodes identifies a subset of patients with a significantly better prognosis than the finding of residual tumor in the breast and/or metastatic lymph nodes. It will be of interest to determine whether this information can be used to assess the need for and the intensity of further systemic therapy.

In summary, it is clear that this patient would benefit most from achieving a sufficient response to induction chemotherapy to allow gross surgical resection of the primary lesion and axillary lymph nodes. Given the failure to achieve a significant clinical response with doxorubicin and cyclophosphamide, other active agents should be considered, such as taxanes or vinorelbine.

Based on whether or not the patient would achieve a pathological complete remission, one should consider a more or less intensive course of adjuvant chemotherapy followed by consolidation with locoregional radiation therapy. On the other hand, if continued primary chemotherapy fails to

---

*Despite the single-institution study from the University of Michigan group, most would agree that mastectomy remains the standard of surgical care for this group of patients.

achieve a sufficient clinical response to allow the surgeon to perform a mastectomy, salvage treatment with high-dose radiation therapy to 60 Gy would be indicated in an attempt to at least achieve locoregional control, although overall survival would not be affected.

BIBLIOGRAPHY

Haagensen CD, Stout AP. Carcinoma of the breast: criteria of inoperability. Am Surg 1943; 118:859.

Jones S, Winer E, Vogel C, Laufman L, Hutchins L, O'Rourke M, Lembersky B, Budman D, Bigley J, Hohneker J. Randomized comparison of vinorelbine and melphalan in anthracycline-refractory advanced breast cancer. J Clin Oncol 1995; 13:2567–2574.

Michelotti A, Gennari A, Salvadori B, Tognoni A, Tibaldi C, Baldini E, Conte PF. Paclitaxel and vinorelbine in anthracycline-pretreated breast cancer: a phase II study. Ann Oncol 1996; 7:857–860.

Ravdin PM. Taxoids: effective agents in anthracycline-resistant breast cancer. Semin Oncol 1995; 22:29–34.

Weber BL, Vogel C, Jones S, Harvey H, Hutchins L, Bigley J, Hohneker J. Intravenous vinorelbine as first-line and second-line therapy in advanced breast cancer. J Clin Oncol 1995; 13:2722–2730.

Case #D.6
Goal: To discuss the management of a woman who presents with stigmata of a locally advanced breast cancer and biopsy-proven, ipsilateral supraclavicular node metastases

WILLIAM P. PETERS

A 37-year-old woman is diagnosed with an inflammatory, right breast, invasive lobular carcinoma. Fine-needle aspiration of a palpable right supraclavicular node confirms the clinical impression of metastatic disease. Staging workup reveals no other evidence of metastases.

We would classify this patient as having a stage IV breast cancer displaying inflammatory local disease. The prognosis of these patients remains poor despite contemporary therapeutic approaches to the management of patients with advanced inflammatory breast cancer with evidence of metastatic supraclavicular disease. Management would include the use of induction therapy followed by local control measures including surgery and radiation therapy; in the appropriate patient we would consider consolidation with high-dose chemotherapy. The strategy we have often employed in this type of patient is intensive induction therapy with a doxorubicin-based regimen followed by surgical evaluation of the breast, assuming that a clinical complete remission has been obtained with the induction therapy. If surgery demonstrates a pathological complete remission, we generally wait 12–16 weeks before proceeding to high-dose intensification based upon data from our randomized trial that indicates a superior survival when a brief interval occurs between the time of completion of induction therapy and transplant. If, however, the patient has a pathological partial response, our strategy is to proceed with the use of high-dose intensification at an interval of approximately 8 weeks from the time of completion of the induction therapy. Subsequent use of radiation therapy to the chest wall would be considered appropriate, as well as the addition of hormonal therapy if the tumor was hormone responsive at the time of initial diagnosis.

Unfortunately, because of the relative rarity of inflammatory carcinoma, the long-term results of randomized trials with bone marrow transplantation are not currently available. This patient would be classified as having a stage IV disease because of the metastatic disease to the supraclavicular region. The expectation would be that if a complete response is obtained to the induction therapy, a long-term (>5 years) overall survival of 20–40% would be expected, depending on the timing of high-dose therapy. Overall, patients who achieve a partial remission would be expected to have approximately a 20% overall survival at 5 years with a similar disease-free survival frequency.

BIBLIOGRAPHY

Antman KH, Rowlings PA, Vaughan WP, et al. High-dose chemotherapy with autologous hematopoietic stem-cell support for breast cancer in North America. J Clin Oncol 1997; 15:1870–1879.

Klein JL, Peters WP. High-dose chemotherapy with autologous haematopoietic progenitor cell transplantation for adenocarcinoma of the breast.

Peters WP. High-dose chemotherapy with autologous bone marrow transplantation for the treatment of breast cancer: yes. In: DeVita VT, Hellman S, Rosenberg SA, eds. Important Advances in Oncology 1995. Philadelphia: JB Lippincott, 1995:215–229.

Peters WP, Dansey R, Klein J, Berry D. High-dose chemotherapy for high-risk primary breast cancer. In: Salmon S, ed. Adjuvant Therapy of Cancer VIII. Philadelphia: Lippincott-Raven, 1997:117–122.

Peters WP, Ross M, Vredenburgh J, et al. High-dose chemotherapy and autologous bone marrow support as consolidation after standard-dose adjuvant therapy for high-risk primary breast cancer. J Clin Oncol 1993; 11:1132–1143.

Case #D.7
Goal: To discuss the management of locally advanced breast cancer following neoadjuvant chemotherapy and surgery

JAMES F. HOLLAND

An otherwise healthy, 63-year-old woman receives four cycles of CAF for a locally advanced left breast cancer. Restaging workup is negative for metastatic disease. She undergoes left modified radical mastectomy that shows residual DCIS and 0/17 positive axillary lymph nodes.

The four cycles of CAF apparently eradicated the invasive cancer and left this patient whose tumor was T3 with T3 ductal carcinoma in situ. It is conceivable that her axillary nodes had contained metastatic tumor, and that this too has been eradicated, which raises optimism that any micrometastatic systemic disease has met a similar fate. Since there can be no certainty about this, however, one might err, and it is better to err on the side of giving the patient the best chance for cure. In the absence of ER and PR data, or other relevant information such as Her-2-*neu* status, or immunostaining of her lymph nodes for cytokeratin or breast cancer antigen, one must not be overly cautious. The best results in patients with Her-2-*neu*-positive tumors in the CALGB study occurred with four cycles of CAF, with doxorubicin at 60 mg/m^2. If the CAF doses here were at a lower level (six cycles at 40 mg/m^2 or four cycles at 30 mg/m^2 were not equal for Her-2-*neu* tumors), I would add three cycles of doxorubicin as CAF at 60 mg/m^2, or two cycles of doxorubicin alone at 90 mg/m^2 (given as 30 mg/m^{2}day $\times$ 3). This would keep her total dose at approximately 360 mg/m^2. Determination of ventricular ejection fraction would be prudent before the last dose of doxorubicin was given.

When she had completed doxorubicin, either at the original four courses at 60 mg/m^2, or with the supplementation specified, I would consider four courses of paclitaxel. This concept is currently being studied in the CALGB by randomization to taxol after completing four courses of therapy with CA (note the omission of F without a trial to prove its dispensability) at 60, 75, or 90 mg/m^2/cycle. Some of the decision would depend on how robust the patient was at the end of the doxorubicin therapy. I consider her at high risk of relapse, and potentially a patient who has demonstrated by tumor regression a real chance at chemotherapeutic cure.

Even if ER and PR cannot be retrieved, I would give her tamoxifen, since the toxicity is remarkably low and data demonstrate some therapeutic advantage, even in ER-negative women.

This patient is not a candidate for high-dose chemotherapy requiring autologous stem cell transplantation or bone marrow transplantation. I would not use radiotherapy to her chest wall or internal mammary nodes. I believe her risk of relapse on the chest wall alone is low, and if her tumor is eradicated systemically it should also be controlled locally.

BIBLIOGRAPHY

Cancer and Leukemia Group B protocol 9344. Doxorubicin dose escalation with or without taxol in the adjuvant CA regimen for node positive breast cancer. Unpublished.

Muss HB, Thor AD, Berry DA, Kute T, Lin ET, Koerner F, Cirrincione CT, Budman DR, Wood WC, Barcos M. c-*Erb*B-2 expression and response to adjuvant therapy in women with node-positive early breast cancer. N Engl J Med 1994; 330:1260–1266. Erratum. N Engl J Med 1994; 331:211.

E. Local/Regional Recurrences

E.1. CHEST WALL RECURRENCE FOLLOWING MASTECTOMY

Case #E.1.1
Goal: To discuss chest wall recurrences in premenopausal women

SANDRA F. SCHNALL

A 46-year-old woman presents with a 1.8-cm skin nodule overlying her modified radical mastectomy scar, 18 months following completion of adjuvant chemotherapy with CMF. Her initial lesion was a 2.0-cm, infiltrating ductal carcinoma, high grade, ER-/PR-, with extensive lymphatic invasion; lymph nodes were negative. Excision of the recurrence reveals invasion into the pectoral muscle and dermal lymphatic invasion.

A local recurrence of breast cancer after a modified radical mastectomy usually presents as one or more nodules along the chest wall. A majority of patients have only one nodule (62%). The risk of developing a chest wall nodule is increased in patients with positive lymph nodes; the risk of multiple chest wall nodules is increased with the number of positive lymph nodes. Eighty-ninety percent of local recurrences present within 5 years of mastectomy. Twenty-five percent of patients with local recurrences have simultaneous distant disease or develop distant disease within a few months of detection. Almost all patients with chest wall recurrence after mastectomy develop distant metastases. In one study, the 5- and 10-year actuarial rates of relapse were 70% and 93%, respectively.

Local control is of initial importance. Options include surgical resection followed by radiation therapy. Systemic treatment alone (i.e., hormone and/or chemotherapy) is usually not adequate to control these lesions. One should ask whether this patient would have benefited from radiation therapy at initial diagnosis. However, from the data we are given, it did not seem warranted. If, however, the original tumor was close to the chest wall margin or if she had positive lymph nodes, recent data support the role of "adjuvant" radiation therapy.

Unfortunately, despite local aggressive treatment for an isolated recurrence after modified radical mastectomy, most patients develop systemic tumor. The disease-free interval from mastectomy to recurrence is associated with the risk of systemic involvement. Those who relapse in less than 2 years have a median survival of 13 months compared with a median survival of 31 months for those who have a recurrence 2–5 years after surgery. Prior systemic therapy does not appear to affect the outcome in several nonrandomized trials.

Whether to add systemic therapy (i.e., hormonal therapy or chemotherapy) at the time of local recurrence in conjunction with local treatment is unclear. Unfortunately, many variables can influence outcome. With the exception of the use of tamoxifen in hormone-receptor-positive recurrences, the use of chemotherapy or hormonal therapy has not been shown to enhance local control. Although the risk of systemic relapse is high, the optimal timing of the systemic therapy is unknown. Hormone therapy may be a logical approach to systemic treatment as it is known that hormone treatments are more effective in areas of soft tissue and bone. As well, overall toxicity is less than with chemotherapy.

In this patient I would recommend local surgical excision with postoperative radiation therapy. As she was hormone-receptor negative, there is little role for "adjuvant" hormonal therapy. I would also consider referral for evaluation for a stem cell transplant or entrance on a clinical trial. The addition of an anthracycline-based regimen or paclitaxel, although not unreasonable, is not supported by prospective data. In addition, the endpoint of treatment is not clear.

BIBLIOGRAPHY

Borner M, Bacchi M, Goldhirsch A, Greiner R, Harder F, Castiglione M, Jungi WF, Thurlimann B, Cavalli F, Obrecht JP, et al. First isolated locoregional recurrence following mastectomy for breast cancer: results of a phase III multicenter study comparing systemic treatment with observation after excision and radiation. Swiss Group for Clinical Cancer Research. J Clin Oncol 1994; 12: 2071–2077.

Halverson KG, Perez CA, Kuske RR. Local regional recurrence of breast cancer; a retrospective comparison of irradiation alone versus irradiation/systemic therapy. Am J Clin Oncol 1993; 15:93.

Sberizk WJ, Silver B, Henderson IC, et al. The use of radiotherapy for treatment of isolated locoregional recurrence of breast carcinoma after mastectomy. Cancer 1986; 58:1214.

Case #E.1.2
Goal: To discuss "adjuvant" treatment following complete resection of a chest wall recurrence

DEBORAH L. TOPPMEYER

A 47-year-old woman undergoes resection of a pair of adjacent 0.8-cm nodules that arose in her mastectomy scar 30 months after initial treatment of an invasive ductal carcinoma. Pathology is consistent with a recurrence of her breast cancer; margins are negative. The original tumor was 2.7 cm, 1/14 nodes, ER-/PR-. At the time, she received four cycles of adjuvant AC. Staging workup is negative for other sites of disease.

Local recurrence is defined as any reappearance of cancer in the ipsilateral breast, the chest wall, the skin overlying the chest wall, the ipsilateral axillary lymph nodes, the supraclavicular lymph nodes, or the internal mammary lymph nodes. The definition of an isolated or solitary local recurrence is the appearance of breast cancer in these areas in the absence of other disease on routine evaluation for metastases. Depending on the series, the incidence of local recurrence following mastectomy ranges from 5 to 30%. Factors predicting for local relapse are similar to those that predict for distant failure. These include the extent of axillary node involvement, the size of the primary tumor, poor nuclear grade, lack of estrogen receptors, and presence of skin changes over the primary tumor.

The median time to the appearance of clinically overt local-regional recurrences after mastectomy is less than 2 years. Eighty to 90% of local recurrences appear within 5 years. At the time of local-regional failure, 25–30% of patients have previously diagnosed metastatic disease; 25% will be diagnosed with distant disease simultaneously or within several months. Retrospective analyses have shown that the time courses for both local-regional and distant relapses are almost the same. Disseminated disease will almost always follow a local-regional recurrence. For example, in a series of patients with local-regional recurrence treated from 1968 to 1978 at the Joint Center for Radiation Therapy, the 5- and 10-year actuarial rates of freedom from distant metastases were 30% and 7%, respectively.

Several factors determine the prognosis following a local-regional recurrence. The most significant prognostic factor is the disease-free interval following mastectomy. Several studies suggest an improved relapse-free and overall survival for those women whose disease-free interval (DFI) was greater than 2 years. Schwaibold et al. demonstrated a 5-year survival rate of 67% for patients with a DFI greater than 2 years compared to a 30% survival rate in those with a shorter DFI. The number of sites of recurrence appears to have predictive value with the 5-year survival rate being 36–59% in patients with a single recurrence compared to 19% in patients with multiple sites of recurrence. The site of recurrence also appears to influence survival; patients who had chest wall rather than regional node relapse had an improved 5-year survival rate (41% vs. 18%). The ability to secure local control of disease at the time of relapse also impacts on overall survival; patients who have established local control had a 5-year survival rate of 64% versus 35% for those with ineffective control of local disease. The size of the lesion appears to have prognostic significance with the survival rates at 5 years decreasing from 70% in patients with recurring lesions smaller than 2 cm, to 39% in patients with larger lesions. Age, menopausal status, prior adjuvant chemotherapy, and type of mastectomy do not affect prognosis after relapse. The initial stage at diagnosis has more significance through its effect on DFI rather than stage alone (i.e., patients with a higher stage at initial diagnosis tend to have a shorter DFI).

The most common initial manifestation of local recurrence is an asymptomatic nodule in the axilla, in the supraclavicular fossa, or in or under the skin of the chest wall. Approximately 50% of all local recurrences involve only the chest wall or the overlying skin. The axilla alone is involved in approximately 10% of patients. The number of separate nodules initially found on the chest wall is usually small. Most nodules are located in or near the scar of the mastectomy or skin graft, with most others in the skin flaps. Only 50% of patients with local-regional failure present with a solitary local recurrence.

Pretreatment evaluation includes (1) a biopsy of the lesion to establish the diagnosis and to determine the HR status, (2) full restaging to rule out distant metastases, and (3) a computed-tomography (CT) scan of the chest wall since 25–67% of patients with chest wall or nodal recurrences may have additional sites of involvement discovered only on CT evaluation.

The optimal timing and treatment (local or systemic) for local recurrence remains controversial. This particular patient is approximately 3 years from her initial diagnosis and had the chest wall lesions, each measuring <3 cm, completely resected. Her history suggests that she should enjoy a relatively good disease-free and overall survival. However, with the use of limited local excision alone the local relapse is approximately 60–75%. Therefore, radiation therapy should also be administered. CRs ranging from 60 to 97% have been reported; despite these encouraging numbers, 30–40% of patients will still fail locally. Local treatment of patients with no evidence of distant metastases reduces morbidity for many patients and may increase survival times for a few individuals. Specifically, patients with a prolonged initial disease-free interval or other favorable prognostic indicators may benefit from more aggressive local treatment. However, the benefit in this group may be more a function of biologically less aggressive disease than of the actual treatment modality itself. Regardless, effective local treatment, even if not curative, can impact on a patient's quality of life. Furthermore, it may provide a relatively long disease-free interval when no treatment needs to be administered. If definitive local therapy is going to be performed, most physicians use more aggressive radiotherapy to provide optimal local-regional control. Several retrospective analyses demonstrated a greater local failure rate when small fields are used in comparison to larger ones.

Thus, the current recommendations include (1) radiation therapy to the entire site of involvement; (2) elective irradiation of the uninvolved supraclavicular fossa to 4600–5000 cGy; (3) consideration of elective chest wall irradiation to at least 5000 cGy; (4) at least 5000 cGy for completely excised recurrences, and at least 6000 cGy for incompletely excised, small (<3 cm) recurrences; and (5) radiation to the axilla is generally not administered given the high potential of toxicity, i.e., lymphedema, and a relatively low risk of relapse in this area.

Aggressive local therapy is not usually curative. Therefore, the use of multimodality therapy (chemotherapy and radiation therapy) following local recurrence has been explored. Only one randomized prospective study, performed in Switzerland between 1982 and 1991, examined this issue. A total of 167 patients who were ER+ or receptor status unknown were randomized to tamoxifen or observation after complete excision and radiation of a chest wall recurrence. All patients had disease-free intervals of greater than 1 year and three or fewer nodules measuring less than 1 cm. Although, initially the tamoxifen-treated group had a greater relapse-free survival (59% vs. 36%), after 9 years from the time of randomization this difference nearly disappeared. Furthermore, there is no difference in overall survival. Other retrospective and single-arm trials suggest some benefit to the use of systemic chemotherapy, but again, analyses of these data reveal problems with interpretation of the results.

In summary, the recommended treatment for this 47-year-old woman would be complete resection followed by radiation. The addition of chemotherapy for this clinical presentation is not well established. Given that the patient is destined to relapse in the future, it would be appropriate to withhold systemic chemotherapy until this time. Based on the patient's disease-free interval, it is probable that she will enjoy a reasonable disease-free survival uncomplicated by the addition of the toxicities of chemotherapy.

BIBLIOGRAPHY

Aberizk JG, Silver B, Henderson IC, Cady B, Harris JR. The use of radiotherapy for treatment of isolated locoregional recurrence of breast carcinoma after mastectomy. Cancer 1986; 58:1214–1218.

Halverson JJ, Perez RR, Ksuke DM, Farcia JR, Fineberg B. Isolated local-regional recurrence of breast cancer following mastectomy: radiotherapeutic management. Int J Radiat Oncol Biol Phys 1990; 19(4):851–858.

Halverson KJ, Perez CA, Kuske RR, Garcia DM, Simpson JR, Fineberg B. Locoregional recurrence of breast cancer: a retrospective comaprison of irradiation alone versus irradiation and system therapy. Am J Clin Oncol 1992; 15(2): 93–101.

Recht A, Hayes DF. Local-regional recurrence after mastectomy or breast-conserving therapy. In: Harris JR, et al, eds. Breast Diseases. Philadelphia: Lippincott-Raven, 1996:649–668.

Schwaibold F, Fowble BL, Solin LJ, Schultz DJ, Goodman RL. The results of radiation therapy for isolated local regional recurrence. Int J Radiat Onocol Biol
Phys 1991; 21(2):299–310.

Case #E.1.3
Goal: To discuss treatment of chest wall recurrences following mastectomy in postmenopausal women

MICHAEL REISS

*A 67-year-old woman develops a chest wall recurrence 3 years following
a modified radical mastectomy for a 1.7-cm, 2/17 node, ER+ tumor. She
had received adjuvant CMF and was taking tamoxifen at the time of
development of the recurrence. The recurrence, 1.1 cm in diameter, arose
in the mastectomy scar. It was removed with negative margins. It remained
strongly ER+.*

Recurrent breast cancer on the chest wall following mastectomy usually presents as discrete subcutaneous metastases. Most of these (80–90%)
appear within the first 5 years following surgery. Risk factors include young
age, large size of the primary tumor, and the presence of axillary lymph
nodes with metastatic carcinoma. In approximately 50% of cases, the diagnosis of distant MBC precedes or is made simultaneously with the appearance of chest wall metastases. In the remainder of the cases, the chest
wall recurrence usually precedes the appearance of subsequent systemic
MBC. For example, of 90 patients with loco-regional recurrences reported
by Aberizk et al., 19 (30%) were free from systemic relapse at 5 years and
only six (7%) at 10 years.

Having suffered a recurrence on the chest wall after mastectomy, the
patient under consideration is at increased risk for both local recurrence and
systemic MBC. Thus, the clinician is faced with two principal questions: (1)
how to best achieve local control and prevent further locoregional recurrences, and (2) how to avoid systemic relapse. Local control of chest wall
relapses is best achieved with a combination of surgical excision and radiation therapy. Although most chest wall metastases will initially regress
when treated with radiation therapy alone, the subsequent local failure rate
is in the order of 25% at 5 years and close to 40% at 10 years. Conversely,
in patients treated with complete resection of the lesions followed by radiation therapy to at least 50 Gy, the local failure rate can be limited to 5%
or less. If complete resection is not possible, a radiation dose of at least 60
Gy is required to achieve approximately the same degree of local control as
with CMT.

Because approximately 25% of patients who present with a chest wall recurrence are found to simultaneously harbor clinically detectable distant metastases, the patient in our case needs to be properly staged. If no evidence of distant metastases is found, the question is raised whether or not she would benefit from adjuvant systemic therapy at this time. Overall, the likelihood that this patient will develop systemic disease is comparable to that of women who present with a primary breast cancer and ≥ 10 axillary nodal metastases, a scenario in which aggressive adjuvant systemic CCT has been shown to be of significant benefit. The principal predictors of systemic relapse following locoregional recurrence include the disease-free interval and the number of involved axillary nodes at the time of initial presentation. The disease-free interval may simply reflect the intrinsic growth rate of the tumor, while the lymph node involvement reflects its metastatic potential. The influence of the disease-free interval on systemic recurrence and survival is summarized in Table 1.

Given that our patient recurred 3 years after her mastectomy, her predicted survival at 10 years is approximately 36%. In spite of this grave prognosis, surprisingly few studies have been conducted to ascertain the efficacy of systemic therapy following a postmastectomy chest wall recurrence. Most of these were retrospective studies, and the conclusions vary greatly, presumably because of the large number of variables that can influence outcome. Only a single prospective, randomized study has been conducted to determine the value of systemic therapy following local treatment of a chest wall recurrence. All patients in this trial had recurred more than 1 year after their initial surgery, had no more than three tumor nodules that were completely resected, and received 50 Gy to the chest wall. Patients with ER+ tumors were then randomized to receive tamoxifen or to be observed until relapse. The relapse-free survival rate at 5 years was 59% in

Table 1 Overall Survival as a Function of Disease-Free Interval

	Disease-free interval	
	<24 months	≥24 months
Danoff et al.	3 yrs: 39%	3 yrs: 63%
Aberizk et al.	5 yrs: 33%	5 yrs: 58%
	10 yrs: 7%	10 yrs: 36%
Deutsch et al.	5 yrs: 23%	5 yrs: 42%
Patanaphan et al.	5 yrs: 25%	5 yrs: 58%
Magno et al.	5 yrs: 20%	5 yrs: 50%
Schwaibold et al.	5 yrs: 30%	5 yrs: 67%

the tamoxifen group compared to only 36% in the untreated group. However, this difference had disappeared by 8–9 years following randomization, presumably because the control group was given tamoxifen at the time of their second relapse. An attempt at conducting a parallel randomized study of chemotherapy in women with ER-negative tumors failed because of poor accrual. Although there appears to be a therapeutic benefit of dose-intensive chemotherapy in other situations in which patients are at high risk for systemic relapse, no such information is available for women who suffer chest wall recurrences. However, these patients may be eligible for a number of ongoing protocols of intensive chemotherapy for metastatic disease, and they should be presented with this option. Given that the recurrent tumor in our case still expressed hormone receptors, systemic treatment with a second-line hormonal agent should be considered. Megestrol acetate and the non-steroidal aromatase inhibitor anastrazol have been shown to possess similar efficacy in the treatment of MBC following tamoxifen failure. Given anastrazol's extremely favorable toxicity profile compared to that of megestrol acetate, anastrazol could be considered. At the time of systemic relapse, third-line endocrine therapy or systemic chemotherapy should be considered.

BIBLIOGRAPHY

Aberizk WJ, Silver B, Henderson IC, et al. The use of radiotherapy for treatment of isolated local recurrence of breast carcinoma after mastectomy. Cancer 1986; 58:1214.

Borner M, Bacchi M, Goldhirsch A, Greiner R, Harder F, Castiglione M, Jungi WF, Thurlimann B, Cavalli F, Obrecht JP, et al. First isolated locoregional recurrence following mastectomy for breast cancer: results of a phase III multicenter study comparing systemic treatment with observation after excision and radiation. Swiss Group for Clinical Cancer Research. J Clin Oncol 1994; 12: 2071–2077.

Buzdar AU, Jones SE, Vogel CL, Wolter J, Plourde P, Webster A. A phase III trial comparing anastrozole (1 and 10 milligrams), a potent and selective aromatase inhibitor, with megestrol acetate in postmenopausal women with advanced breast carcinoma. Arimidex Study Group. Cancer 1996; 79:730–739.

Danoff BF, Coia LR, Cantor RI, et al. Locally recurrent breast carcinoma: the effect of adjuvant chemotherapy on prognosis. Radiology 1983; 147:849.

Deutsch M, Parsons J, Mittal BB. Radiation therapy for local-regional recurrent breast cancer. Int J Radiat Oncol Biol Phys 1983; 12:2061.

Halverson KJ, Perez CA, Kuske RR, et al. Isolated local-regional recurrence of breast cancer following mastectomy: radiotherapeutic management. Int J Radiat Oncol Biol Phys 1990; 19:851.

Jonat W, Howell A, Blomqvist C, Eiermann W, Winblad G, Tyrrell C, Mauriac L, Roche H, Lundgren S, Hellmund R, Azab M. A randomised trial comparing two doses of the new selective aromatase inhibitor anastrozole (Arimidex) with megestrol acetate in postmenopausal patients with advanced breast cancer. Eur J Cancer 1996; 32A:404–412.

Magno L, Bignardi M, Micheletti E, et al. Analysis of prognostic factors in patients with isolated chest wall recurrence of breast cancer. Cancer 1987; 60:240.

Patanaphan V, Salazar OM, Poussin-Rosillo H. Prognosticators in recurrent breast cancer: a 15 year experience with radiation. Cancer 1984; 54:228.

Schwaibold F, Fowble BL, Solin LJ, et al. The results of radiation therapy for isolated local regional recurrence after mastectomy. Int J Radiat Oncol Biol Phys 1991; 21:299.

Case #E.1.4
Goal: To discuss management of locally diffuse chest wall recurrences following mastectomy

ROBERT S. DIPAOLA

An otherwise healthy, 59-year-old woman presents 18 months following a right modified radical mastectomy with four skin nodules, each 0.3–0.6 cm in diameter, spread over an area 5 cm × 7 cm centered on the midportion of her mastectomy incision. Biopsy of two of the lesions reveals recurrence of her invasive lobular carcinoma. The recurrences are ER−. The original tumor was 1.1 cm in diameter, 0/11 nodes, ER−. No adjuvant therapy was given.

Local recurrence after mastectomy should be managed as metastatic disease; despite any local measure, most patients with chest wall recurrence eventually develop distant metastasis. Chest wall recurrence, therefore, behaves as does systemic recurrence. Treatment with radiation therapy or surgery will often control the local disease, but does not appear to change the outcome of these patients. Most patients develop distant metastases, despite local control. However, local control should be addressed since approximately 50% of these patients will be alive at 5 years and could experience significant morbidity from uncontrolled chest-wall disease.

As a systemic recurrence, chest wall disease can be treated with systemic therapy following local treatment. As support to this approach, a randomized trial comparing tamoxifen therapy to no further therapy after surgery and radiation of chest wall recurrences was completed in 1991. A total of 167 patients who were estrogen-receptor (ER) positive or of undetermined status were enrolled. Patients who were treated with tamoxifen had a longer 5-year relapse-free survival (59 vs. 36%). However, the difference disappeared after 8–9 years and overall survival rates were the same in both groups. Treatment with tamoxifen in patients with ER-positive disease is reasonable after surgical resection and or radiation therapy. However, the result of treatment with chemotherapy for patients who are ER negative, as in this case, is not known. Chemotherapy could be withheld until distant metastases occur. Alternatively, patients with measurable disease such as in this patient would be candidates for clinical trials with new agents. This is an area ripe for clinical investigation.

The plan for this patient includes the options of waiting until symptoms occur, local measures with radiation therapy and/or surgery, and clinical trials. Other options include standard chemotherapy alone, or adjuvant chemotherapy following definitive local control. Clearly, the lack of definite benefit, in terms of survival, of any of these options warrants a detailed discussion with the patient to formulate an informed plan.

BIBLIOGRAPHY

Borner M, Bacchi M, Goldhirsch, et al. First isolated loco-regional recurrence following mastectomy for breast cancer: results of a phase III multicenter trial comparing systemic treatment with observation after excision and radiation. J Clin Oncol 1994; 12:2071.

Case #E.1.5
Goal: To discuss the management of locally aggressive chest wall recurrences following mastectomy

EDWARD OBEDIAN and BRUCE G. HAFFTY

A 34-year-old woman received neoadjuvant chemotherapy (CAF), right modified radical mastectomy, high-dose chemotherapy with stem cell rescue, and chest wall irradiation for an inflammatory right breast cancer. Seven months after completing her therapy, she presents with an extensive right chest wall recurrence of her cancer. Restaging workup is negative. Biopsy confirms the clinical impression of a recurrence.

Inflammatory breast cancer represents 4% of breast cancer cases. It is a clinicopathological diagnosis manifested by erythematous, warm, edematous, and indurated skin associated with dermal lymphatic invasion.

Treatment of inflammatory breast cancer with mastectomy with or without postoperative radiation therapy but without systemic therapy results in an approximately 80% distant failure rate. Therefore, combined-modality therapy including combination chemotherapy has become the standard of care.

Prognostic factors in patients undergoing combined-modality therapy for inflammatory breast cancer include response to induction chemotherapy and clinical involvement of supraclavicular lymph nodes. Patients who have a complete response to induction chemotherapy have an approximately 66% chance of long-term survival compared to 40% for partial responders. The clinical supraclavicular nodal status for the patient in this case was not stated, but if positive would be associated with a worse outcome. Other poor prognostic factors evident in this patient include age < 50, disease-free interval less than 24 months, and large/advanced size of recurrent disease.

Despite this patient's poor prognosis, further treatment with surgery and reirradiation may be effective. If the recurrence is small, then a wide local excision with or without adjuvant systemic therapy may be adequate therapy. In this case, however, the recurrence appears to be extensive. Therefore, consideration should be given to surgical excision with skin grafting and postoperative radiation therapy. This next course of radiation would be targeted to the area of recurrence plus a margin using electrons. Laramore et al. reported local control without soft tissue necrosis in eight of 13 patients undergoing reirradiation with 7 MeV electrons to a total dose of 40–50 Gy.

An investigational approach for this patient would also include reirradiation with hyperthermia. Dragnovic et al. reported a 57% (17/30) complete response rate for reirradiation with hyperthermia for recurrent disease in previously irradiated patients. These patients were treated with 6 or 9 MeV electrons to a total dose of 32 Gy in eight fractions delivered twice weekly and followed by hyperthermia. Of note, 11% of these patients eventually developed ulceration. Seegenschmiedt et al. reported a 41% skin blister/ulceration rate in 13 patients reirradiated for recurrent disease. Perez et al. reported a 65–80% complete response rate with a 25% ulceration rate using reirradiation with 9–16 MeV electrons to total doses of 20–40 Gy given biweekly followed by hyperthermia.

A phase I–II RTOG trial investigating radical radiation plus hyperthermia in 133 patients for recurrent cancer (33 had recurrent breast cancer) reported an 85% complete response rate with a 70% risk of acute thermal blisters and 16% risk of late ulceration or necrosis. In this trial, patients were treated with conventional electron-beam irradiation to 60–70 Gy with hyperthermia delivered biweekly for 6 weeks. This approach may be best suited for previously irradiated patients who are unresectable and symptomatic.

Given this patient's very poor prognosis, consideration should be given not only to reirradiation with or without hyperthermia but also to systemic therapy with hormones and/or chemotherapy.

In summary, this case illustrates a 34-year-old woman with an extensive chest wall recurrence within 2 years of intensive treatment including chemotherapy, mastectomy, autologous stem cell transplantation, and chest wall irradiation for an inflammatory breast carcinoma. Despite a very poor prognosis, restaging workup is negative. Therefore, she may be salvaged, albeit at a higher rate of toxicity, with aggressive combined-modality therapy with surgery, reirradiation with or without hyperthermia, and systemic therapy.

BIBLIOGRAPHY

Dragnovic J, Seydel HC, Sandhu T, et al. Local superficial hyperthermia in combination with low dose radiation therapy for palliation of locally recurrent breast carcinoma. J Clin Oncol 1989; 7:30–35.

Laramore GE, Griffin TW, Parker RG, Gerdes AJ. The use of electron beams in treating local recurrence of breast cancer in previously irradiated fields. Cancer 1978; 41:991–995.

Perez CA, Kuske RR, Emani B, Fineberg B. Irradiation alone or combined with hyperthermia in the treatment of recurrent carcinoma of the breast in the chest wall: a randomized comparison. Int J Hypertherm 1986; 2:179–187.

Scott R, Gillespie B, Perez CA, et al. Hyperthermia in combination with definitive radiotherapy: increased tumor clearance and reduced recurrence rate in extended follow-up. Int J Radiat Oncol Biol Phys 1984; 10:2119–2123.

Seegenschmiedt MH, Brady LW, Rossmeissl G. External microwave hyperthermia combined with radiation therapy for extensive superficial chest wall recurrences. Recent Results Cancer Res 1988; 107:147–151.

E.2.   IN-BREAST RECURRENCE FOLLOWING BREAST-CONSERVING THERAPY

Case #E.2.1
Goal: To discuss the management of an in-breast recurrence following breast-conserving therapy

ROBERT S. DIPAOLA

A 59-year-old woman develops a palpable mass in the lumpectomy site 4 years after lumpectomy, axillary dissection (1/17 nodes), and breast irradiation. The original tumor was ER+, and the patient has been on tamoxifen since the original surgery. Excisional biopsy of the mass demonstrates a 1.2-cm recurrence of the original invasive ductal carcinoma.

Ipsilateral breast tumor recurrence (IBTR) following conservative surgery and radiation therapy occurs in 10–15% of patients. The risk of IBTR is dependent on multiple factors at the time of initial lumpectomy and can be characterized as high (30–40%), moderate (10–20%), and low (5–10%) (Table 1).

Table 1 Risk Factors for Ipsilateral Breast Tumor Recurrence

High	Moderate	Low
Multifocal/multicentric disease or Diffuse microcalcifications	High grade or Lymphatic invasion or Young age	Tumor size <4–5 cm and Low grade and No lymphatic invasion and Negative margins

The standard treatment of IBTR is mastectomy. The overall survival is over 50% with salvage mastectomy. Fowble et al. attempted to identify a subset of patients who might do as well with a less aggressive approach. Of 31 patients who had initially undergone an excisional biopsy for the diagnosis of recurrence, 13 had no residual tumor, nine had residual tumor in one quadrant, seven had residual tumor in two quadrants, one in three quadrants, and one in four quadrants. Therefore, it was difficult to define a subset of patients for whom wide excision alone would be appropriate, given the high rate of tumor present outside the excision area. Attempts at surgical approaches less than mastectomy should be considered investigational.

The benefit from an axillary lymph node dissection (ALD) after IBTR is unknown. The majority of patients who have been treated with lumpectomy have undergone ALD; subsequent dissections will increase morbidity. The incidence of positive axillary nodes at the time of IBTR is high (33–58%). Despite this high incidence, no definite survival benefit is gained by ALD after IBTR, and ALD should only be considered if the information would guide management, either standard therapy or eligibility in a clinical trial.

The benefit of adjuvant therapy following salvage mastectomy for IBTR has not been determined. Its use should be guided based on the predicted risk of future systemic recurrence and the benefits extrapolated from studies of adjuvant therapy at initial presentation. A review of prognostic factors for recurrence after IBTR (Table 2) reveals that many of the same prognostic factors for primary tumors apply in addition to the interval from the original lumpectomy to recurrence.

The case under consideration represents a patient with a small IBTR, with a minimal risk of future systemic recurrence after salvage mastectomy. However, the risk of systemic recurrence after even a small primary (1.2 cm) is at least 10%. If the data on adjuvant therapy for primary tumors can be extrapolated to IBTR, and currently no data can refute—or support—this possibility, the recurrence could be reduced by 30–40% with treatment with adjuvant therapy. Therefore, after salvage mastectomy adjuvant che-

Table 2   Risk Factors for Systemic Recurrence After In-Breast Tumor
Recurrence

Minimal	Intermediate	High
Noninvasive	Size 1–2 cm	Tumor size >2 cm
Small size and LN neg	DFI 2–5 years	DFI <2 years
>5-year DFI	Lymph nodes involved	Aneuploid
Diploid tumor/low SPF		High SPF

DIF = disease-free interval.

motherapy could be considered after a long and thoughtful discussion with
the patient concerning the lack of current data and the potential risk-benefit
ratio. The patient under discussion could also be considered for reconstruction with autogenous tissue, e.g., a TRAM flap.

Editors' comment: Although we tend to think that an IBTR carries a far
better prognosis than a chest wall recurrence, this is not always the case.
For example, in patients who experience an IBTR within 4 years of diagnosis, the risk of subsequent systemic disease approaches 50%.

BIBLIOGRAPHY

DiPaola RS, Orel SG, Fowble BL. Ipsilateral breast tumor recurrence following
    conservative surgery and radiation therapy. Oncology 1994; 8:59–68.
Early Breast Cancer Trialists' Collaborative Group. Systemic treatment of early
    breast cancer by hormonal, cytotoxic, or immune therapy. Lancet 1992; 339:
    1–71.
Fowble B, Solin LJ, Schultz DJ, et al. Breast recurrence following conservative
    surgery and radiation: patterns of failure, prognosis, and pathologic findings
    from the mastectomy specimens with implications for treatment. Int J Radiat
    Oncol Biol Phys 1990; 190:833.

Case #E.2.2
Goal: To discuss the management of an in-breast recurrence following breast-conserving therapy

SUSAN A. MCMANUS

*A 44-year-old divorcée develops a mammographically detected, 0.6-cm,
in-breast recurrence of an invasive ductal carcinoma 28 months after
initial therapy with a lumpectomy (1.7 cm in diameter), axillary lymph
node dissection (0/23 nodes), and radiation therapy. She had also received*

four cycles of adjuvant chemotherapy. Wide margins are obtained (>1 cm)
upon excision of the recurrence. The patient is adamantly opposed to the
recommendation of mastectomy for treatment of the recurrence.

This 44-year-old woman developed a local recurrence after breast-conserving treatment with lumpectomy, radiation therapy, and chemotherapy. One would anticipate a 5–15% local recurrence rate with this approach. In-breast recurrences are devastating to the patient and frustrating to physicians.

Initial evaluation should review the possible reasons for the recurrence. The histopathology of the first and second tumors should be carefully reviewed. Did the initial tumor contain greater or equal than 25% intraductal carcinoma or a positive surgical margin? Was the original tumor either multicentric or multifocal? Studies of local recurrence after breast-conserving treatment point to these three factors as being important predictors of local recurrence. If any of the three was present initially, it is possible that the original lumpectomy was inadequate. If these factors were not present, the cause of the recurrence is less obvious. Examination of the pathology should also compare the histology of the primary tumor and the recurrence. If the histologies are similar, or if factors suggesting inadequate primary surgery are present, this should be treated as a true recurrence, without consideration of further systemic therapy. However, if the histology of the "recurrence" differs from that of the primary tumor, this should be considered a second primary and staged and treated accordingly.

Approximately 10% of patients who present with an in-breast recurrence will have concurrent distant metastases. This is especially true in women who have a recurrence within a short period of time after their original surgery (less than or equal to 2 years). Therefore, a metastatic workup should be performed prior to undertaking local/regional therapy. These studies, if negative, may help reassure the patient that the recurrence is truly local. In addition to the metastatic assessment, careful examination of the ipsilateral axilla, the supraclavicular areas, and the contralateral breast and axilla should be carried out. Bilateral mammography is also indicated. There is a high incidence (30–50%) of positive axillary nodes at the time of diagnosis of a local recurrence. If the axillary examination is clinically negative and an axillary dissection had been previously performed, reexploration of the axilla is not indicated.

The psychosocial impact of a recurrence must be carefully assessed and managed. It is easy to understand why a patient may feel that any treatment will be useless after a local recurrence, especially if it happens shortly after the initial surgery. For the patient presented, the fact that her recurrence occurred more than 2 years after her primary treatment places her in a better prognostic category; this should be reassuring. The fact that her tumor was identified mammographically and measured only 6 mm is also favorable. If the histology is identical to the initial tumor or if this is a new 6-mm tumor, chemotherapy should not be recommended.

Discussion of the options for local/regional control should include presentation of the available data on reexcision versus mastectomy. The term "salvage" mastectomy should be avoided in discussions with the patient and her family as this term connotes a pessimistic view. Discussion of reexcision alone needs to include the recurrence rate, which may approach 40%. Unfortunately, even after mastectomy for an in-breast recurrence, there is a chest-wall recurrence rate of 10–12%. DiPaola et al. were unable to identify a subset of patients in whom a wide excision alone constituted adequate therapy after an in-breast recurrence. Certainly, discussion of mastectomy should include the option of immediate reconstruction. Usually a tranverse rectus abdominis myocutaneous (TRAM) or other autologous flap is preferable because of prior radiation treatment.

Survival data vary depending on the factors that were considered. In Schwartz's series, the interval between diagnosis and recurrence was 4.6 years on average and the 10-year survival was approximately 80%. In Osborne's study, there was a 65% overall survival after treatment for recurrence. If breast conservation is chosen, careful mammographic follow-up every 6 months after lumpectomy is required, as it is likely that a second recurrence would be detected most early as a mammographic abnormality.

BIBLIOGRAPHY

DiPaola RS, Orel SC, Fowble BL. Ipsilateral breast tumor recurrence following conservative surgery and radiation therapy. Oncology 1994; 8:(12):59–67.

Hall A, Fallowfield LJ, A'Hern RP. When breast cancer recurs: a 3-year prospective study of psychological morbidity. Breast J 1996; 2:197–203.

Veronesi U, Marubini E, Delvecchio M, et al. Local recurrences and distant metastasis after conservative breast cancer treatments: partly independent events. J Natl Cancer Inst 1995; 87(1):19–27.

Case #E.2.3
Goal: To discuss the management of an in-breast recurrence following limited therapy of an invasive breast cancer in an elderly woman

JAY K. HARNESS

An 84-year-old woman was treated with a negative margin lumpectomy and tamoxifen 3 years ago for a 2.1-cm, hormone-receptor-positive, invasive ductal carcinoma. At the time her cancer was diagnosed, she was recuperating from a myocardial infarction. While still on tamoxifen she develops an in-breast recurrence 5 cm away from the original lumpectomy scar. Her cardiac status is stable; she is asymptomatic and on no cardiac medications currently.

This case of an in-breast recurrence in an elderly woman who was initially treated with lumpectomy plus tamoxifen without radiation raises several interesting points. One of the most important is the tendency to modify the surgical management of elderly women with breast cancer. Two important studies by August and co-workers, from the University of Michigan, and Wanebo and colleagues, from Brown University, have noted several differences in breast cancer diagnosis and treatment of elderly women. They and other investigators have found in women over 65: (1) fewer receive standard therapy for breast cancer (appropriate use of either lumpectomy, radiotherapy, axillary dissection, or mastectomy); (2) initial diagnosis at more advanced stage; (3) lower intensity of screening mammograms; (4) increased use of lumpectomy without axillary dissection; and (5) increased use of limited breast excision plus tamoxifen. While there is some controversy about the biology of breast cancer in the elderly, age- and stage-related survival is not different in elderly patients compared to their younger counterparts. The only exception may be in women aged 39 and younger, who appear to have a worse prognosis.

There are several different types of in-breast recurrences after breast-conserving therapy. First, there are recurrences at the site of the initial cancer, which typically appear underneath the scar of the previous excision. Second, there are recurrences within the same quadrant of the initial tumor, which may represent evolution of in situ or multifocal disease present at the time of the initial therapy. Third, there are recurrences in another quadrant of the breast, which may represent new primaries or synchronous primaries with slower doubling times. Finally, the rarest type of recurrences are radiation-induced malignancies that occur within the field of whole-breast radiation.

Eighty percent to 90% of in-breast recurrences within 2–7 years of primary treatment are located (as in this case) within 5 cm of the primary tumor. No information is given in this case to whether the recurrence is in the same or adjacent quadrant. Also no information is given about the original or the most recent mammograms.

The clinical pathway for in-breast recurrence calls for a staging evaluation to rule in or rule out distant metastases. If no distant metastases are found, a mastectomy is recommended. If distant metastases are found, chemotherapy or tamoxifen therapy is recommended. I do not know many medical oncologists who would recommend chemotherapy for an 84-year-old patient!

There are two fundamental roles for axillary lymph node dissection in breast cancer. The foremost is the staging of the disease, which not only may predict prognosis, but may also be used to govern adjuvant therapy. The second role is to resect lymph nodes that may harbor palpable or microscopic disease, which in turn helps local/regional control and helps to decrease axillary recurrences. If the axilla was not previously staged, the only role of an axillary dissection now would be to stage the patient, suggest adjuvant therapy, or remove palpable disease. Even if the nodes were positive, it would not affect subsequent therapy since chemotherapy should not be used and the recurrence occurred in the face of tamoxifen therapy. The tamoxifen therapy should be discontinued. It appears that this patient's underlying medical condition is stable and that she is now a candidate for more standard forms of surgical therapy of her recurrence.

There are two primary options for treatment of this patient's in-breast recurrence. First, of course, is a total mastectomy, which could easily include the level I lymph nodes around the tail of Spence. The second option is a repeat lumpectomy (with negative margins), followed by whole-breast radiotherapy (which she had not previously received). My recommendation would be total mastectomy. It would be the most efficient form of therapy. If the patient refused, then I would recommend lumpectomy and whole-breast radiotherapy.

Editors' comment: It is easy to fall into the trap of recommending less than standard therapy for patients based solely on their age. The dismissal of the use of chemotherapy may be hasty.

BIBLIOGRAPHY

August DA, Rea T, Sondak VK. Age-related differences in breast cancer treatment. Ann Surg Oncol 1994; 1:15–52.

Dunser M, Haussler B, Fuchs H, Martgreiter R. Lumpectomy plus tamoxifen for the treatment of breast cancer in the elderly. Eur J Surg Oncol 1993; 19:529–531.

Kennedy MJ, Abeloff MD. Management of locally recurrent breast cancer. Cancer 1993; 71(7):2395–2409.

Osborne MP, Simmons RM. Salvage surgery for recurrence after breast conservation. World J Surg 1994; 18:93–97.

Wanebo HJ, Cole B, Chung M, et al. Is surgical management compromised in elderly patients with breast cancer? Ann Surg 1997; 225(5):579–589.

Case #E.2.4
Goal: To discuss an in-breast recurrence in the tail of the breast in a young woman

SUSAN A. MCMANUS

A 32-year-old female fashion model presented 18 months ago after noticing a lesion "under her arm." Examination revealed a 2.0-cm lesion in the tail of the right breast. An excisional biopsy revealed an 1.8-cm, infiltrating ductal carcinoma, of medium grade, hormone receptor negative. The lesion was in the tail of the breast and was amenable to an axillary lymph node dissection through the same incision. All lymph nodes were negative. She underwent adjuvant chemotherapy followed by radiation therapy (5000 rads to the whole breast with a 1000-rad boost to the area of the lesion). She returns 18 months later with a palpable lesion at the most lateral margin of her breast. Excision of the lesion reveals recurrence of her infiltrating ductal carcinoma. The margin is positive. She requests breast conservation.

I would begin by discussing with the patient the implications of her recurrence. It is alarming to a young patient to suffer a recurrence less than 2 years following aggressive treatment for stage I breast cancer. It has been noted by Veronesi and others that young age appears to be an independent risk factor for recurrence of breast cancer in women. Careful evaluation of the patient may reveal that her initial tumor had an extensive intraductal component, was multifocal or multicentric, or was treated with an excision that failed to achieve adequate margins.

This recurrence will require local/regional treatment after restaging. Prior to surgery, bilateral mammograms should also be obtained. The local/regional management should be either mastectomy or wide local excision of the tumor. If the initial lesion in the tail of the breast was lateral to the pectoralis major muscle, a mastectomy would remove tissue that has little or nothing to do with the area of the local recurrence. However, since management of a patient with breast cancer following lumpectomy would normally include breast irradiation, and since this patient has already received a full course of radiation, mastectomy remains the standard approach to this patient's local recurrence. Alternatively, a wide local excision down to the chest wall could remove the old incision with an ellipse of skin. The defect could be filled with autologous tissue such as a latissimus flap. This approach would allow for local control and spare her the mastectomy that she wishes to avoid. If the more standard treatment, mastectomy, is used, this patient would be an excellent candidate for a tranversus rectus abdominis myocutaneous (TRAM) reconstruction. With either surgical approach, the axilla, if possible, should be palpated intraoperatively to permit evaluation of any remaining lymph nodes.

The prognosis of a patient with an in-breast recurrence is dependent in part on the timing of the recurrence. Patients who recur less than 2 years after primary therapy, like this patient, are at much higher risk for developing distant metastases. An early in-breast recurrence may be regarded as a marker for distant disease. In contrast, patients who recur 5 years or more after initial surgery have an excellent prognosis. In a study by Osborne et al., the average length of time to recurrence was 4.6 years; in this patient population there was an 82% long-term survival rate. The long-term survival rate for young women who recur within 2 years of initial therapy may be as low as 45%. For this reason, some recommend that patients in this subgroup receive systemic therapy. In DiPaola's series, local recurrence was associated with a 5-year survival rate of 79%.

BIBLIOGRAPHY

DiPaola RS, Orel SG, Fowble BL. Ipsilateral breast tumor recurrence following conservative surgery and radiation therapy. Oncology 1994; 8(12):59–67.

Fisher B, Anderson S, Fisher ER, et al. Significance of ipsilateral breast tumor recurrence after lumpectomy. Lancet 1991; 338:327–331.

Kurtz JM, Jacque-Mier J, Amalric R, et al. Why are local recurrences after breast conserving therapy more frequent in young patients? J Clin Oncol 1990; 8: 591–598.

Osborne MP, Simmons RM, et al. Salvage surgery for recurrence after breast conservation. World J Surg 1994; 18:93.

E.3. AXILLARY LYMPH NODE RECURRENCE

Case #E.3.1
Goal: To discuss the management of an axillary recurrence of a breast cancer following axillary dissection

EDWARD OBEDIAN and BRUCE G. HAFFTY

A 61-year-old woman develops a 2-cm mass in her left axilla 14 months after undergoing a modified radical mastectomy for a 2.2-cm, invasive lobular carcinoma, ER−, with 1/9 positive nodes. She received adjuvant CMF postoperatively. Negative margin biopsy of the axillary mass reveals recurrence of her original cancer. Staging workup is negative.

Risk factors for a local-regional recurrence after mastectomy include clinical, pathological, and treatment-related factors. Although this patient did not have significant risk factors for local regional relapse post mastectomy, up to 15% of patients with early-stage operable breast cancer may experience local-regional relapse following modified radical mastectomy. Other risk factors for local-regional recurrence not manifest in this patient include age <40, large size of primary tumor ≥5 cm, four or more involved nodes, positive surgical margins of resection, pectoral fascia involvement, and less extensive surgery.

This patient presents with an isolated axillary recurrence after mastectomy. Several prognostic factors for disease-free or overall survival following local regional relapse have been reported. The most important factors appear to be the disease-free interval and the initial pathological stage of the patient. Patients with an initial large tumor and pathologically involved lymph nodes have worse prognoses than patients with small, node-negative tumors. Patients who develop recurrent disease within 2 years of initial treatment have significantly decreased survival rates compared to patients recurring more than 2 years after treatment.

The management of an isolated axillary recurrence after mastectomy involves surgery and radiation therapy. Before treatment, however, a chest computed-tomography scan will help determine the extent of disease and may identify previously unsuspected disease. This patient underwent an excisional biopsy of the axillary recurrence. This will serve as good cytoreduction of the tumor burden and may improve local control. However, after excision alone, local recurrences are seen in 50–75% of cases. Therefore, consideration could be given to a repeat axillary node dissection as in the case of an isolated axillary recurrence after conservative management and radiation therapy.

Radiation therapy for an axillary nodal recurrence after excisional biopsy involves irradiation of the chest wall and supraclavicular regions. After a regional nodal failure, 25–40% of patients will subsequently recur in the chest wall if chest wall irradiation is not employed. Elective axillary radiation may not be necessary if a more extensive nodal dissection is performed; this may result in significant morbidity and axillary relapses with repeat dissection are relatively rare. Omitting elective supraclavicular radiation, however, results in subsequent supraclavicular relapse rates of 15–30%. This patient should be treated to a total dose of at least 5000 cGy using tangential fields to the chest wall matched to a supraclavicular field if more extensive axillary surgery is performed. If the dissection is not performed, or if extensive disease is noted at the time of dissection, axillary radiation may be considered.

The role of chemotherapy after an isolated axillary recurrence after mastectomy is unclear. However, since the majority of patients with an isolated local-regional recurrence will ultimately develop metastatic disease, chemotherapy is also potentially beneficial. Chemotherapy alone is less effective than radiotherapy alone in achieving local control. There are no prospective randomized trials comparing radiotherapy alone to radiotherapy combined with chemotherapy in this setting. Therefore, it is unclear whether the addition of chemotherapy to radiotherapy will confer a survival advantage to patients with isolated local-regional recurrence after mastectomy. Adjuvant hormonal therapy may also benefit patients with regional recurrence after mastectomy if they are receptor positive, have not previously received hormonal therapy, or have had a long disease-free interval (>6 months) on hormonal therapy.

In summary, this patient presents with an isolated axillary recurrence after mastectomy. Poor prognostic features in this patient are a short disease-free interval (<24 months) and initial node-positive and ER-negative tumor. She is at high risk for local-regional recurrence. Therefore, a repeat axillary dissection should be considered and she should undergo radiation therapy to the chest wall and supraclavicular nodal regions. Although she has no evidence of metastatic disease, she is also at high risk for the subsequent development of distant metastases and may benefit from adjuvant systemic therapy. Unfortunately, prospective data regarding adjuvant systemic treatment in this setting are currently unavailable.

BIBLIOGRAPHY

Fisher B, Redmond C, Fisher ER, Bauer M, Wolmark N, Wickerham L, Deutsch M, Montague E, Margolese R, Foster R. Ten-year results of a randomized clinical trial comparing radical mastectomy and total mastectomy with or without radiation. N Engl J Med 1985; 312:674–681.

Forrest ADM, Stewart HJ, Roberts MM. Simple mastectomy and axillary node sampling in the management of breast cancer. Ann Surg 1982; 196:371–378.

Fowble B, Schwaibold F. Local-regional recurrence following definitive treatment for operable breast cancer. In: Fowble B, Goodman RL, Glick JH, Rosato EF, eds. Breast Cancer Treatment: A Comprehensive Guide to Management. St Louis: Mosby-Year Book, 1991:373–402.

Halsted WS. The results of operations for the cure of cancer of the breast performed at the Johns Hopkins Hospital from June 1889 to January 1894. Med Class 1938; 3:441–474.

Halverson KJ, Perez CA, Kuske RR, et al. Isolated local-regional recurrence of breast cancer following mastectomy: radiotherapeutic management. Int J Radiat Oncol Biol Phys 1990; 19:851–858.

Case #E.3.2
Goal: To discuss the management of an axillary recurrence of a breast cancer following axillary dissection

EDWARD OBEDIAN and BRUCE G. HAFFTY

A 44-year-old woman develops a palpable axillary mass 22 months after undergoing lumpectomy, axillary dissection, and radiation therapy for a 0.5-cm, estrogen-receptor-positive, node-negative (0/19) medullary carcinoma. No systemic chemotherapy or hormonal therapy was administered. Excisional biopsy of the mass reveals a 1.4-cm ER recurrence that arose in an axillary lymph node; margins are negative. Staging workup is negative.

Regional-node failure following conservative surgery and radiation most commonly occurs in the axilla with or without a simultaneous breast recurrence. This patient presents with an isolated axillary nodal recurrence after conservative management. Most of these occur within 5 years, and the median interval for an isolated axillary relapse is approximatley 15 months.

The usual approach to an isolated axillary failure is repeat axillary dissection. Since this patient has only undergone an excisional biopsy, further surgery may be considered. Based on experience from the University of Pennsylvania, repeat axillary dissection should provide about a 91% chance of ultimate regional control: of 11 patients undergoing a repeat axillary dissection, only one developed a subsequent axillary recurrence; whereas one of two patients treated with excisional biopsy recurred in the axilla. In a report by Dewar et al. the treatment of an isolated axillary recurrence with radiation and chemotherapy resulted in regional control in only one of four patients.

In a series by Recht et al., the salvage rate with gross total excision and/or radiation therapy for an isolated axillary failure was 61%. However, irradiation of a dissected axilla must be weighed against the associated increased risk of arm edema as well as possibly brachial plexopathy, sarcomas, and shoulder restriction. Radiation therapy (RT) to the axilla without surgery is associated with a 4% risk of arm edema at 6 years compared to 6% in patients with only a level I or I/II dissection versus 36% in patients with a complete axillary dissection. There is little data regarding the risk of arm edema after a repeat axillary node dissection with radiation.

One question in the management of this patient would be whether she would benefit from mastectomy. However, this patient has no evidence of recurrence in the breast. Therefore, provided both physical examination and mammography are negative, mastectomy is not necessary in the management of an isolated axillary recurrence.

Having suffered an axillary nodal recurrence, the patient is at increased risk not only for locoregional recurrence but also for systemic disease. Unfortunately, there are no prospective data evaluating the role of adjuvant systemic therapy in this setting. Based on the relatively high rate of ultimate systemic metastasis, however, systemic therapy may be considered in this case. If the recurrence were estrogen-receptor positive, hormonal therapy should be strongly considered. Other pathological factors, such as S-phase fraction, tumor grade, lymph vascular invasion, and ploidy, may also help in the decision-making process regarding systemic treatment.

Survival rates following regional nodal recurrence after conservative surgery and radiation are variable depending on the location of the relapse and prior surgical and or radiation treatment to the region. Unlike patients with supraclavicular recurrences, those with isolated axillary recurrences have a relatively favorable prognosis. This result is consistent with data from the NSABP B-04 trial in which a group of clinically node-negative mastectomy patients did not undergo axillary dissection until subsequent relapse in the axilla. In that trial, the patients who underwent a salvage axillary node dissection at the time of an isolated axillary relapse had equivalent overall survival, disease-free survival, and distant-disease-free survival rates compared to mastectomy patients undergoing axillary dissection at the time of mastectomy.

In summary, this case depicts a premenopausal woman who is post an excisional biopsy of an isolated axillary recurrence within 2 years of conservative surgery and radiation therapy. She is at high risk for local and distant relapse. Therefore, she would best be served by a repeat axillary node dissection as opposed to axillary RT; adjuvant systemic therapy should also be considered.

BIBLIOGRAPHY

Clark RM, Wilkinson RH, Miceli PN, MacDonald WD. Breast cancer: experiences with conservation therapy. Am J Clin Oncol 1987; 10:461–468.

Clarke DH, Le MG, Sarrazin D, Lacombe M, Fontaine F, Travagli J, May-Levin F, Contesso G, Arriagada R. Analysis of local-regional relapse in patients with early breast cancers treated by excision and radiotherapy. Experiences of the Institut Gustave-Roussy. Int J Radiat Oncol Biol Phys 1985; 11:137–145.

Delouche G, Bachelot F, Premont M, Kurtz JM. Conservation treatment of early breast cancer: long term results and complications. Int J Radiat Oncol Biol Phys 1987; 13:29–34.

Dewar JA, Sarrazin D, Benhamou E, et al. Management of the axilla in conservatively treated breast cancer: 592 patients treated at Institut Gustave-Roussy. Int J Radiat Oncol Biol Phys 1987; 13:475–481.

Fisher B, Redmond C, Fisher ER, Bauer M, Wolmark N, Wickerham L, Deutsch M, Montague E, Margolese R, Foster R. Ten-year results of a randomized clinical trial comparing radical mastectomy and total mastectomy with or without radiation. N Engl J Med 1985; 312:674–681.

Fowble B, Schwaibold F. Local-regional recurrence following definitive treatment for operable breast cancer. In: Fowble B, Goodman RL, Glick JH, Rosato EF, eds. Breast Cancer Treatment: A Comprehensive Guide to Management. St. Louis: Mosby-Year Book, 1991:373–402.

Fowble B, Solin LJ, Schultz DJ, Goodman FL. Frequency, sites of relapse and outcome of regional node failures following conservative surgery and radiation for early breast cancer. Int J Radiat Oncol Biol Phys 1989; 17:703–710.

Haffty BG, Fischer DB, Fischer JJF. Regional nodal irradiation in the conservative management of breast cancer. Int J Radiat Oncol Biol Phys 1989; 17:703–710.

Harris JR, Recht A, Amalric R, Calle R, Clark RM, Reid JG, Spitalier JM, Vilcoq JR, Hellman S. Time course and prognosis of local recurrence following primary radiation therapy for early breast cancer. J Clin Oncol 1984; 2:37–41.

Larson D, Weinstein M, Goldberg I, et al. Edema of the arm as a function of the extent of axillary surgery in patients with stage I–II carcinoma of the breast treated with primary radiotherapy. Int J Radiat Oncol Biol Phys 1986; 12:1575–1582.

Leung S, Otmezguine Y, Calitchi E, Mazeron JJ, leBourgeois JP, Perquin B. Local regional recurrences following radical external beam irradiation and interstial implantation for operable breast cancer-a twenty three year experience. Radiother Oncol 1986; 5:1–10.

Pierquin B, Mazeron J, Glaubiger D. Conservative treatment of breast cancer in Europe: report of the groupe Europeen du Curietherapie. Radiother Oncol 1986; 6:187–198.

Recht A, Pierce SM, Abner A, Vicini F, Osteen RT, Love SM, Silver B, Harris JR. Regional nodal failure after conservative surgery and radiotherapy for early-stage breast carcinoma. J Clin Oncol 1991; 9:988–996.

F.   Metastatic Disease

Introduction

Metastatic breast cancer presents as the initial manifestation of the disease in 7% of patients, and will eventually develop in 5–25% of stage I, 30–60% of stage II, and 60–80% of stage III patients. To date, all patients with metastatic disease who achieve a clinical remission will eventually relapse. The use of high-dose chemotherapy with autologous stem cell rescue is receiving considerable attention in these patients. We have chosen to divide the management of metastatic breast cancer into three categories; those who present with stage IV disease, those who relapse after adjuvant treatment, and those who experience subsequent responses after initial treatment for metastatic disease. We have further divided our decision analyses based on the presence of visceral-predominant disease, in contrast to disease involving bone or soft tissues.

F.1.   STAGE IV AT PRESENTATION

Case #F.1.1
Goal: To discuss the management of a premenopausal ER+, non-visceral-predominant patient

JAMES F. HOLLAND

A 32-year-old woman presents with low back pain. Physical examination reveals a 2.0-cm mass in the right breast; her bone scan is positive at L5. Biopsy of breast reveals ER+, infiltrating ductal carcinoma of moderate grade. The tumor is diploid/ high S phase.

Breast cancer at age 32 is more virulent than in postmenopausal women, but a positive bone scan for a single lesion is an inadequate basis on which to accept the hot spot as a metastasis. Although plain films may be indicative, a computed-tomography (CT) scan has more sensitivity to display a bony lesion. Magnetic resonance imaging is even more sensitive in showing tumor tissue in the vertebra. If imaging studies are positive, a blind biopsy of the posterior iliac crest marrow is a simple medical oncological procedure and will often be positive. If that biopsy is negative, a CT-guided, interventional radiological needle biopsy of the vertebral body or an orthopedic biopsy is necessary. Hemangioma of the vertebral body is a benign lesion that can mimic metastasis.

If the biopsy is positive in the skeleton, treatment for the disease should include tamoxifen and chemotherapy. If the breast biopsy were an excision, even if the tumor touched the excision margin microscopically (but not grossly), this patient does not need additional surgery, but rather eventually

323

radiotherapy to breast and axilla. As she will receive chemotherapy in any event, axillary dissection is unnecessary. The type of chemotherapy for a 32-year-old with metastatic disease is not without controversy. Some would point to the response in terms of long-term disease-free survival following high-dose chemotherapy with autologous stem cell rescue. Induction chemotherapy with a powerful regimen would be a part of the prelude. Where possible she should enter a national or cooperative group study so that evaluation of this approach can at last be made scientifically. For patients who decline such therapy (or whose resources, personal preference, or insurance determine their exclusion) a combination regimen of powerful drugs is appropriate. We have used a sequential combination of the Cooper regimen (CMFVP) for 4 months, followed by high-dose doxorubicin given for four cycles. Similar results have been obtained with CAF given at doxorubicin 40 mg/m^2 $\times$ 6 cycles or doxorubicin 60 mg/m^2 given $\times$ 4 cycles together with cyclophosphamide and fluorouracil by Cancer and Leukemia Group B, and probably by the Hudis/Norton regimen of doxorubicin, paclitaxel, and cyclophosphamide.

Laparoscopic oophorectomy might be considered later if the patient progresses on tamoxifen, because occasional responses have been reported.

Radiation to the breast and axilla can be delayed until impact on the systemic disease has been achieved. As the breast and axillary tumor, if any, are also exposed to the antiestrogen and chemotherapy, it is not as if they were left untreated. Radiotherapy to L5 would be appropriate if pain persisted despite chemotherapy and an osteoclast inhibitor such as pamidronate. A back brace can also be useful.

If the skeletal disease is explained by a cause other than breast cancer, conventional wisdom would recommend completion of the lumpectomy and axillary node sampling of levels I and II. It is premature to adopt the sentinel node approach until comparative trials have been completed. Since this patient is a candidate for adjuvant chemotherapy in any event, with a high-S-phase 2-cm tumor, and probability of unresectable micrometastatic disease (portending relapse) of at least 20%, which is too high to accept at age 32, I would offer her chemotherapy and tamoxifen as outlined above (without the high-dose option) followed by radiation to the breast and axilla. Radiotherapy can eradicate cancer in the breast and axilla, and is, in fact, the primary therapeutic modality in many clinics in France.

The timing of when to start the tamoxifen has been controversial, with reluctance on the part of some to begin simultaneously with chemotherapy for fear of slowing cellular growth and compromising the chemotherapeutic effect. The NSABP has started tamoxifen concurrently with the chemotherapy, however, and patients on those studies also have benefited from other good chemotherapy regimens. It is unlikely that this question will ever be deemed important enough to merit the size of a comparative trial it would take to settle it.

BIBLIOGRAPHY

Bhardwaj S, Holland JF, Norton L. An intensive adjuvant sequenced chemotherapy regime for breast cancer. Cancer Invest. 1993; 11:6–9.

Fisher B, Osborne CK, Margolese RG, Bloomer WD. Neoplasms of the breast. In: Holland JF, Frei E III, Bast RC JR, Kufe DW, Morton DL, Weichselbaum RR, eds. Cancer Medicine, 4th ed. Baltimore: Williams & Wilkins, 1997.

Holland JF, Bhardwaj S, Norton L. "We may be lost, but we're sure makin' good time." Cancer Invest 1994; 12:270–272.

Hudis C, Seidman A, Raptis G. Fennelly D, Gilewski T, Baselga J, Theodoulou M, Sklarin N, Moynahan M, Surbone A, Currie V, Lebwohl D, Uhlenhopp M, Crown J, Norton, L. Sequential adjuvant therapy: the Memorial Sloan-Kettering experience. Semin Oncol 1996; 23:58–64.

Case #F.1.2
Goal: To discuss the management of premenopausal, ER−, stage IV disease at presentation

WILLIAM P. PETERS

A 40-year-old woman, with a negative past medical history, presents with a "swollen left breast"; examination confirms the presence of a 2-cm breast mass, as well as freely movable, palpable, axillary lymph nodes. Chest X-ray reveals multiple discrete nodules in both lung fields. You recommend lumpectomy followed by CAF chemotherapy with an eye toward transplantation. After four cycles, she has experienced a partial response. What would you recommend next?

This is a patient with previously untreated metastatic breast cancer. Despite the relatively limited disease, the long-term prognosis for a patient with metastatic breast cancer remains poor with conventional-dose therapy. Among patients who are treated with chemotherapy such as cyclophosphamide, cisplatin, and 5-fluorouracil, CAF, or even with more contemporary regimens including taxanes, progression-free survival at 5 years would be expected to be in the range of no more than 5–8%.

Critical to the management of the patient would be confirmation that the pulmonary lesions represent breast cancer and a biopsy of these lesions would be considered at our institution as part of the initial workup. We have seen patients referred for transplant procedures in this setting who have lesions on computed-tomography scan in the previously untreated setting being declared metastatic cancer but in which tissue diagnosis has demon-strated fungal or other nonmalignant diseases.

Assuming this 40-year-old patient was interested in an aggressive ap-proach, we would recommend the use of an intensive induction regimen such as doxorubicin and taxol followed by a high-dose consolidation with CPB and autologous stem cell support. Assuming the induction therapy and transplant had rendered her disease-free in the lungs, management would include subsequent resection of the dominant breast mass, clearing of ob-vious carcinoma in the axilla, followed by posttransplant radiation to the breast and chest wall.

BIBLIOGRAPHY

Antman KH, Rowlings PA, Vaughan WP, et al. High-dose chemotherapy with au-tologous hematopoietic stem-cell support for breast cancer in North America. J Clin Oncol 1997; 15:1870–1879.

Klein JL, Peters WP. High-dose chemotherapy with autologous haematopoietic pro-genitor cell transplantation for adenocarcinoma of the breast.

Peters WP. High-dose chemotherapy with autologous bone marrow transplantation for the treatment of breast cancer: yes. In: DeVita VT, Hellman S, Rosenberg SA, eds. Important Advances in Oncology 1995. Philadelphia: JB Lippincott, 1995:215–229.

Peters WP, Dansey R, Klein J, Berry D. High-dose chemotherapy for high-risk pri-mary breast cancer. In: Salmon S, ed. Adjuvant Therapy of Cancer VIII. Phil-adelphia: Lippincott-Raven, 1997:117–122.

Peters WP, Ross M, Vredenburgh J, et al. High-dose chemotherapy and autologous bone marrow support as consolidation after standard-dose adjuvant therapy for high-risk primary breast cancer. J Clin Oncol 1993; 11:1132–1143.

Case #F.1.3
Goal: To discuss the management of postmenopausal, ER+, stage IV disease at presentation (visceral predominant)

MICHAEL REISS

A 68-year-old woman presents with a breast mass and bone pain. Evaluation confirms that the patient has metastatic breast cancer (MBC) that expresses estrogen and progesterone receptors (ER/PgR+). The computed-tomography scan of the abdomen reveals multiple lesions within the liver compatible with metastases.

Recommendations on how to best treat patients with metastatic breast cancer (MBC) are dependent on the extent and locations of metastatic lesions, the length of the disease-free interval, whether or not the tumor cells express ER and/or PgR, and the patient's performance status. Staging studies provide an estimate of total tumor burden and whether or not the tumor involves vital organs (for example, lung parenchyma or liver). The time that has elapsed between diagnosis of the primary tumor and the appearance of metastatic lesions (disease-free interval) presumably reflects the growth rate of the tumor. The extent of involvement of vital organs as well as the tumor growth rate determines the immediacy of the threat to the patient's life. This is particularly important in the management of MBC because we have a choice of two types of systemic treatment with radically different mechanisms of action: cytotoxic chemotherapy (CCT), which has immediate activity but can be associated with significant toxicity, and endocrine therapy, which has a delayed onset of action, but is significantly less toxic than CCT. Thus, in the clinical setting of a rapidly growing breast cancer associated with a large tumor burden that involves vital organs, treatment with CCT should be initiated as soon as possible. On the other hand, patients who present many years after their initial diagnosis with low-volume MBC that does not involve viscera may be safely treated with endocrine therapy. Patient age and performance status play a secondary role in treatment decisions: patients with a poor performance status, particularly if they are elderly, are likely not to tolerate intensive CCT as well as younger women with excellent performance status.

The case under consideration raises several questions. First, complete staging should be performed and should include a bone scan as well as a computed-tomography (CT) scan of the chest and upper abdomen to accurately assess the extent and location of metastatic deposits. Patients who present with bone pain will usually display evidence of MBC on radionuclide bone scans. However, one should keep in mind that positive bone scans reflect osteoblastic activity adjacent to tumor foci rather than tumor itself. Most skeletal lesions develop by direct extension from metastatic deposits to the bone marrow. Thus, early marrow metastases will not be detected by bone scans. Similarly, purely lytic skeletal lesions that fail to induce osteoblastic activity will often not be detected by bone scans. Newer imaging modalities, such as positron emission tomography or magnetic resonance imaging, which can detect tumor against the background of normal bone marrow, have a higher sensitivity and may eventually supplant radionuclide bone scanning as the staging modality of choice.

Second, the patient is found to harbor MBC at the time of her initial presentation. Thus, we cannot estimate the growth rate of her tumor, as she may have had asymptomatic metastases for many years. Moreover, we are not informed about her performance status, nor about the extent of her liver metastases. If the liver lesions visualized by CT scanning represent the only putative evidence of MBC, the differential diagnosis should include benign etiologies, such as simple cysts or hemangiomata. Cysts can be identified by ultrasound. Radiolabeled red cell scans or CT scanning using a hemangioma protocol allow one to differentiate between benign hemangiomas and cancer metastases. Occasionally, for example in the case of a single liver lesion of unclear significance in the absence of other sites of metastatic disease, the diagnosis of MBC will need to be confirmed by performing a percutaneous liver biopsy under CT or ultrasound guidance.

Assuming that, in the case under discussion, the patient is found to have multiple skeletal and liver metastases, which are limited in size and number and express ER and PgR, the question is raised whether she would derive the greatest benefit from endocrine therapy or CCT. The drug of choice for the initial endocrine therapy of MBC is the antiestrogen tamoxifen. Although it is often stated that endocrine therapy is less effective against visceral metastases, particularly if these involve the liver, the literature fails to support this view. Most of the early studies evaluating the efficacy of tamoxifen against MBC were conducted in patients who had been heavily pretreated. Thus, one should be cautious in extrapolating from these results to the scenario of newly diagnosed MBC. Moreover, a compilation of early studies of the use of tamoxifen in patients with MBC demonstrated that an overall response rate of 35% was achieved, independent of the dominant site of metastatic involvement, including the liver.

It should also be noted that the early studies of tamoxifen were conducted in the era before the expression of ER/PgR was routinely determined. We now know that the response rate of breast tumors to endocrine therapy increases as a function of the level of expression of hormone receptors by the tumor cells. Thus, patients whose cancers are known to express hormone receptors are more likely to benefit from tamoxifen than an average response rate of 35% would suggest. On the other hand, only 10–15% of patients whose tumors are known to express low or undetectable levels of ER and PgR benefit from endocrine therapy.

In summary, in patients with hormone-receptor negative MBC, CCT would be the treatment of choice. In contrast, patients whose tumors express hormone receptors are candidates for endocrine therapy. Because of the time required for endocrine therapy to exert its maximal effect, i.e., at least 6–8 weeks, the decision whether or not to use endocrine therapy should be based on an assessment of whether the disease is immediately life-threatening rather than on the organ sites of involvement per se.

BIBLIOGRAPHY

Beex L, Pieters G, Smals A, Koenders A, Benraad T, Kloppenborg T. Tamoxifen versus ethinyl estradiol in the treatment of postmenopausal women with advanced breast cancer. Cancer Treat Rep 1981; 65:179–185.

De Lena M, Brambilla C, Jirillo A. Tamoxifen efficacy in advanced breast cancer previously treated with endocrine and cytotoxic therapy. Tumori 1980; 66: 339–348.

Mouridsen H, Palshof T, Patterson J, Battersby L. Tamoxifen in advanced breast cancer. Cancer Treat Rev 1978; 5:131–141.

Case #F.1.4
Goal: To discuss the management of ER−, non-visceral-predominant, stage IV disease at presentation in a postmenopausal woman

JOSEPH AISNER

A 59-year-old woman presents with low back pain and weakness in the right leg. Your evaluation reveals a breast mass, which is confirmed by biopsy as invasive ductal carcinoma. ER/PR−. A bone scan is positive at L3.

Patients who present with metastatic breast cancer present a special problem in management. The approach in this setting should be divided into several steps; the first step is to determine whether there is any eminent problem that might threaten the life or function of this patient. Thus, brain metastases producing neurological symptoms, hypercalcemia, organ function impairment, bone instability, and evidence of epidural spinal cord compression are all instances that represent relative medical emergencies requiring intervention for the immediate threat before proceeding to definitive therapy for the metastatic breast cancer. Thus, in this patient who exhibits back pain, and leg weakness with the bone scan positive at L3, there is a very high likelihood of epidural spinal cord compression. Prospective studies at the Albany Medical College showed that patients with a defined diagnosis of cancer who presented with back pain and showed radiological evidence of abnormalities had a 90% likelihood of epidural spinal cord compression. This represents a medical emergency since once there is neurological impairment, there is rapid loss of neurological function, some of which is often irretrievable. Thus, in this setting the patient should receive steroids and a magnetic resonance imaging (MRI) scan of the entire spine. This is likely to provide immediate definition of the extent of cord compression. Once the extent of cord compression is defined (by specific views of positive areas seen on the MRI), the patient should be referred to radiotherapy for immediate radiation to prevent progression of the neurological dysfunction. During the time in which radiation therapy has been started, the remainder of the staging evaluation can proceed.

After completion of the radiation therapy to the immediate threat (epidural spinal cord compression) and completion of the staging to define extent of disease, this patient is a candidate for chemotherapy. In the absence of hormone receptors, hormonal manipulations are unlikely to produce any response and should be skipped. Standard therapy in this case would consist of combination chemotherapy, although the specific regimen will vary. Because of irradiation to the spine, I would prefer to allow 2 weeks of rest before initiating chemotherapy. Among the many regimens that might be offered, cyclophosphamide, Adriamycin (CA), cyclophosphamide, Adriamycin, and flurouracil (CAF), Adriamycin followed by CMF, and Adriamycin plus paclitaxel are the most commonly used. The appropriate choice of regimen depends in part on the experiences of the physician and the expectations of the patient.

Despite the enthusiasm for high-dose therapy with stem cell rescue, there is little evidence at present to suggest that this approach offers any improvement in long-term disease-free or overall survival. Recent analyses of an unselected stage IV population suggest that the criteria used to select patients for high-dose therapy with stem cell rescue chooses those patients most likely to do best, but has little impact on the overall outcome of the population in general. Prospective studies have not validated the role of high-dose therapy in this setting and its routine use outside of studies should be discouraged.

BIBLIOGRAPHY

Aisner J, Abrams JS. The treatment of metastatic breast cancer. In: Wise E, ed. Breast Cancer: Controversies in Management. New York: Futura Publishing Co, 1994:459–478.

Rahman Z, Frye D, Buzdar A, et al. A retrospective analysis to evaluate the impact of selection process for high dose chemotherapy (HDCT) on the outcome of patients (PT) with metastatic breast cancer (MBC). Proc Am Soc Clin Oncol 1995; 14:95 (abstract 78).

Rodichok LD, Harper GR, Ruckdeschel JC, et al. Early diagnosis of spinal epidural metastases. Am J Med 1981; 70:1181–1188.

Ruckdeschel JC, Patterson SG, Cutherberson DD, et al. Rapid cost-effective diagnosis of spinal cord compression: scanning MRI as the initial diagnostic test. Proc Am Soc Clin Oncol 1997; 16:418a (abstract 1496).

Case #F.1.5
Goal: To discuss the management of brain metastases as initial presentation of breast cancer

MAX S. WICHA

A 42-year-old woman is referred to you after her primary physician diagnosed brain metastases after a workup for headache. She has a past medical history of hypertension, which has been well controlled on diuretics. Computed-tomography scan of the brain reveals a single right parietal lobe lesion that enhances with contrast without a shift in midline structures. Examination of the breast reveals a 3.2-cm lesion of the right breast.

The two main objectives in deciding on the best approach to this patient involve obtaining a correct diagnosis and proceeding with appropriate treatment. The issue of diagnosis concerns both the breast lesion and the brain lesion. First, the 3.2-cm lesion in the right breast should be biopsied to ascertain whether this is indeed a breast malignancy. In addition, since subsequent treatment decisions will be influenced by the extent of systemic disease, I would recommend getting a metastatic workup, including a chest and abdominal computed-tomography (CT) scan. A contrast-enhanced magnetic resonance imaging of the brain is also indicated as this technique is more sensitive than CT scan and may reveal other occult metastasis.

The major decision concerns the role of resection and/or radiation therapy of the solitary lesion in the brain. In deciding on the proper course, one must consider both the need to obtain a tissue diagnosis and the therapeutic considerations. Breast cancer is a relatively frequent contributor to brain metastases, second only to lung cancer, comprising approximately 15% of brain metastases from primary tumors. However, the brain lesion might represent a primary brain tumor as well as benign conditions such as a cerebral infarct. A recent study indicated that 11% of solitary lesions turned out to be something other than brain metastases. Half of these nonmetastatic lesions were primary brain tumors. The other half were infections. Obtaining tissue is the only way to distinguish these possibilities. Although one could perform a stereotactic biopsy to obtain tissue, it is also important to consider the therapeutic benefits of resection plus radiation therapy versus radiation therapy alone. There have now been two randomized studies that examine the role of surgery in addition to whole-brain radiation therapy compared to radiation therapy alone for single brain lesions. The first, a study by Patchell et al. from the University of Kentucky, examined 48 patients with active systemic cancer and a single brain metastasis treated with surgical resection combined with whole-brain radiation therapy, 36 Gy and 12 fractions, compared to whole-brain radiation therapy alone. They demonstrated that the median time to recurrence in the surgery and radiation therapy arm was more than 59 weeks compared to 21 weeks in patients treated with whole-brain radiation therapy alone. There was also an advantage in quality of life in the surgical arm compared to the radiation therapy arm. These results were essentially confirmed by a second randomized trial by Noordijk et al., who demonstrated an advantage in overall survival for those patients undergoing surgical resection and whole-brain radiation therapy as compared to whole-brain radiation therapy alone (median 10 months vs. 6 months). The greatest difference in survival was found for patients with limited extracranial disease and age under 60 years. On the basis of these studies it is currently recommended that in young patients with limited systemic disease and a single metastasis, surgical resection followed by radiation therapy is the preferred choice compared to radiation therapy alone.

Another option is the more recently developed technique of radiosurgery in which high doses of radiation therapy are utilized to ablate the tumor utilizing highly focused beams of stereotactically directed radiation. This approach might be reasonable if the patient was found to have more widely disseminated disease at the time of metastatic workup. However, a disadvantage of this approach is the lack of surgical confirmation of metastasis and the current lack of studies showing that radiosurgery is equivalent to surgery in such a patient.

In summary, in the absence of demonstrating other metastasis in this patient, I would recommend surgical resection of the primary breast cancer and brain metastasis followed by whole-brain radiation therapy.

BIBLIOGRAPHY

Cairncross JG, Kim JH, Posner JB. Radiation therapy for brain metastases. Ann Neurol 1980; 7:529.

Markesbery WR, Brooks WH, Gupta GD, et al. Treatment for patients with cerebral metastases. Arch Neurol 1978; 35:754.

Noordijk EM, Vecht CJ, Haaxma-Reiche H, et al. The choice of treatment of single brain metastasis should be based on extracranial tumor activity and age. Int J Radiat Oncol Biol Phys 1994; 29:711.

Patchell RA, Tibbs PA, Walsh JW, et al. A randomized trial of surgery in the treatment of single metastases to the brain. N Engl J Med 1990; 322:494.

F.2. FIRST DISTANT RECURRENCE

Case #F.2.1
Goal: To discuss treatment of first relapse in an estrogen-receptor-positive visceral-predominant, asymptomatic patient

DANIEL F. HAYES

A 62-year-old white woman presents 4 years after a diagnosis of stage II infiltrating ductal carcinoma of the left breast (1.5-cm lesion, estrogen receptor positive/progesterone receptor negative, diploid low S, 5/16 positive lymph nodes). She was initially treated with adjuvant CMF followed by tamoxifen, which she has taken ever since. Her physician was following her CA27.25 which has increased fivefold. A metastatic workup revealed abnormalities on the bone scan and on computed-tomography scan of the liver. A biopsy of the liver revealed adenocarcinoma consistent with her breast primary. The patient remains totally asymptomatic. Laboratory results are remarkable only for a slightly elevated alkaline phosphatase.

This patient represents the unusual circumstance of presentation of multiple metastatic sites in the absence of symptoms. Her disease was detected by a rising tumor marker. Most patients who are followed with circulating tumor markers do not benefit from this approach.

Will this patient be better treated because of the earlier diagnosis? It is very unusual that a patient with multiple bone metastasis will be asymptomatic. Indeed, it suggests that perhaps she has relatively slow-growing disease. Such a consideration might lead the clinician to consider treating this patient with an alternative hormone therapy after discontinuation of her tamoxifen. Indeed, she has many features suggestive of a relatively high likelihood of response to hormone therapy (ER positivity, long disease-free interval on tamoxifen, and principally bone disease).

The most important question is whether or not the presence of hepatic metastasis is a contraindication to another hormonal therapy. Although it is true that patients with visceral metastasis are less likely to respond to hormone therapy than those without visceral metastasis, this does not imply that all patients with visceral metastasis are refractory to hormone therapy. Many clinicians feel that the choice between chemotherapy and hormone therapy rests on the predicted rapidity of response. However, the real issue is whether a patient who would have responded to chemotherapy if it was used first is placed at a disadvantage by a trial of hormone therapy. A reduced response to chemotherapy is likely only in that small subgroup of patients with rapidly progressing visceral disease in whom the clinician will only get one chance at any type of therapy. In that particular situation, the best available chemotherapy is the treatment of choice. However, in most patients with relatively slow-growing disease in which there is not significant visceral organ dysfunction, it is reasonable to try a course of hormone therapy. If it is successful, then the patient will be well palliated with few side effects. If it is not, then the patient can be treated with chemotherapy with roughly the same likelihood of response as if the chemotherapy had been given upfront. If this patient's liver function tests are not substantially elevated (greater than 2–3 times normal), if her total bilirubin is less than 1.5, and if her computed-tomography scan suggests less than 20–30% replacement, I personally would feel comfortable offering this patient a second hormonal maneuver. I would most likely choose the aromatase inhibitor anastrazole as second-line hormone therapy. However, if the patient had truly slow-growing disease and was only minimally symptomatic, I might recommend a trial of tamoxifen withdrawal therapy. Up to 15–20% of patients who have previously responded to tamoxifen may benefit from such a maneuver. If we were to assume that the patient is refractory to hormone therapy, the choice of first-line chemotherapy appears to be one that can be made pragmatically. Recently reported randomized trials suggest that single-agent doxorubicin (A) and single-agent paclitaxel (T) are equally as effective as combination AT for patients with newly diagnosed, hormone-refractory metastatic breast cancer. Other studies have also suggested similar outcomes for comparison of various chemotherapeutic regimens including single-agent docetaxol and combination CMF. In all of these studies, with relatively minor variations, response rates, time to progression, and overall survival appear to be similar regardless of how the patients are treated. Thus, the selection of chemotherapeutic regimens for individual patients is really a "dealer's choice."

It would be preferable to treat this patient with effective therapy in a prospective clinical trial. She could participate in studies of new hormone or chemotherapy treatments. Given that she has not yet been treated with standard, known effective chemotherapy, it would seem inappropriate to offer this patient treatment in a phase I study in which a truly novel therapy is first being tested in the clinic. However, it is not inappropriate to offer this patient the chance to participate in a phase I trial of known effective drugs that are being tested in novel schedules or doses, or in a clinical study in which a novel therapy is being coadministered with an agent that is known to be effective. Obviously, this decision must be individualized on a case-by-case basis.

Finally, is high-dose chemotherapy (HDC) requiring stem cell support appropriate? After 15 years of clinical research, this question still remains unanswered. It is clear that HDC does not result in substantial benefit to patients who have progressed through standard hormone and chemotherapies. Furthermore, the toxicity of HDC in such patients is extraordinary. On the other hand, many uncontrolled pilot studies have suggested that approximately 20% of patients with metastatic breast cancer who initially respond to induction therapy and achieve a complete response after HDC will remain progression free for 1–2 years following HDC. Of course, these patients are highly selected and comparison to the routine metastatic breast cancer experience is inappropriate. Only two randomized trials of HDC in metastatic disease have been reported. One of these studies suggests a benefit for HDC in patients with metastatic breast cancer, but this study is small, the regimen used is not generally considered conventional, and the control arm does not appear to be faring as well as might have been expected. In the second trial, patients who achieved a complete response to induction chemotherapy were randomly assigned to observation with transplant at the time of subsequent progression versus immediate HDC and bone marrow transplant. As expected, the group of patients who received immediate HDC had a longer time to progression. Enigmatically, the overall survival of the group in the observation arm is superior. There are many explanations for this unexpected finding. These include a false-positive observation by chance, kinetic differences in the two populations, damage to the immune system, and so forth. However, it is difficult to determine whether this study provides useful clinical information for the average patient as it is not determined whether HDC is superior to standard chemotherapy. Other randomized trials are nearing completion, and it is hoped that definitive answers will soon be available.

BIBLIOGRAPHY

Bezwoda W, Seymour L, Dansey R. High-dose chemotherapy with hematopoietic rescue as primary treatment for metastatic breast cancer: a randomized trial. J Clin Oncol 1995; 13:2483–2489.

Bishop J, Dewar J, Tattersall M, Smith J, Oliver I, Ackland S, et al. Taxol alone is equivalent to CMFP combination chemotherapy as front-line treatment in metastatic breast cancer. Proc Am Soc Clin Oncol 1997; 16:153a.

Chan S, Friedrichs K, Noel D, Duarte R, Vorobiof D, Piner T, et al. A randomized phase III study of taxotere versus doxorubicin in patients with metastatic breast cancer who have failed an alkylating containing regimen: preliminary results. 1997.

Cummings FJ, Gray R, Davis TE, Tormey DC, Harris JE, Falkson G, et al. Adjuvant tamoxifen treatment of elderly women with stage II breast cancer. Ann Intern Med 1985; 103:324–329.

Hayes DF, Henderson IC, Shapiro CL. Treatment of metastatic breast cancer: present and future prospects. Semin Oncol 1995; 22:5–21.

Paridaens R, Bruning P, Klijn J, Gamucci T, Biganzoli L, Van Vreckem A, et al. An EORTC crossover trial comparing single-agent Taxol and doxorubicin as first- and second line chemotherapy in advanced breast cancer. Proc Am Soc Clin Oncol 1997; 16:154a.

Peters W, Jones R, Vredengburgh J, Shpall E, Hussein A, Elkordy M, et al. A large prospective randomized trial of high-dose combination alkylating agents with autologous cellular support as consolidation for patients with metastatic breast cancer achieving complete remission after intensive doxorubicin-based induction therapy. Proc Am Soc Clin Oncol 1996; 15:121a.

Sledge G, Neuberg D, Ingle J, Martino S, Wood W. Phase III trial of doxorubicin vs. paclitaxel vs. doxorubicin + paclitaxel as first line therapy for metastatic breast cancer: An Intergroup trial. Proc Am Soc Clin Oncol 1997; 16:1a.

Case #F.2.2
Goal: To discuss first recurrence in a non-visceral-predominant, ER+, postmenopausal patient

DANIEL F. HAYES

A 67-year-old woman presents with new bone pain. She had been on tamoxifen for 8 years following mastectomy for an T2N1M0 estrogen-receptor-positive/progesterone-receptor-negative breast cancer. She developed the first evidence of bone disease 2 years ago, when you switched her to Megace and again she enjoyed a complete remission. She has no complicating medical problems.

Treatment of patients with metastatic disease is both "bad news" and "good news." Unfortunately, routinely available therapies rarely, if ever, result in long-term disease-free survival (in other words, few, if any, patients with metastatic breast cancer are cured of their disease). The good news is that metastatic breast cancer can be well palliated with careful and judicious application of a series of systemic and local therapies including hormone therapy, chemotherapy, radiation, and surgery. Recently, the availability of several new systemic agents has added considerably to the clinician's ability to treat patients with metastatic breast cancer. These include both new hormonal treatments and new chemotherapeutic agents.

This patient clearly has hormonally responsive breast cancer. She has several features that are highly suggestive of an increased likelihood of responding to hormone therapy, including her age (an older postmenopausal woman), her long disease-free interval between initial diagnosis and subsequent recurrence (8 years), the presence of estrogen receptor positivity, the lack of visceral disease, and perhaps most importantly, the dramatic response to megestrol acetate (Megace).

This patient is very likely to respond to yet a third hormonal maneuver. I would estimate the odds of her responding to a third hormonal maneuver to be at least 50%, if not 75%. As most hormone therapies are associated with substantially fewer side effects and complications than chemotherapy, the use of hormone therapy for palliation is preferred when it is likely to be effective. In the past, third-line hormonal treatment included the use of either aminoglutethamide, pharmacological doses of estrogen, or androgens. However, over the last several years, several agents that selectively inhibit aromatase activity in both distant tissues and perhaps in tumor tissues themselves have become available. Prospective randomized trials have demonstrated that these agents are as effective as megestrol acetate and perhaps may even provide prolonged responses and improved overall survival. Furthermore, they are as well, if not better, tolerated as megestrol acetate. Thus, these drugs have rapidly become the drugs of choice for patients in whom tamoxifen is no longer effective. There is also evidence that, like aminoglutethamide, aromatase inhibitors may be effective after megestrol acetate. Thus, if this patient is not eligible for any of the ongoing clinical trials involving new aromatase inhibitors, I would, without hesitation, offer her the only approved aromatase inhibitor in the United States, anastrazole (Arimidex). Of interest, several other aromatase inhibitors are being developed, some of which appear to have higher affinity or slightly different mechanisms of action. Moreover, clinical trials are now being started in the United States of a new agent that selectively and almost irreversibly blocks the estrogen receptor. This agent, (Faslodex), appears to have no estrogenic activity, unlike tamoxifen. In preclinical and early phase II trials, this drug appears to have a wider therapeutic range than tamoxifen, yet its side effect profile appears to be nearly as favorable. It is expected that this drug will be added to the series of hormonal therapies that already exist.

The question is raised by the primary oncologist as to whether the patient should have been treated more aggressively earlier, and whether chemotherapy should be offered to her now. I believe this patient has been treated appropriately. There have been and continue to be substantial data published regarding the benefits of tamoxifen in a postmenopausal, 60-year-old, node-positive, ER-positive patient. Furthermore, when she had her initial mastectomy, few, if any, data suggested that the addition of chemotherapy to tamoxifen was preferable to tamoxifen alone (although there were randomized trials open at that time). Although one might have questioned whether she would have benefited from high-dose chemotherapy with bone marrow transplant at the time of her first recurrence, there are no prospective randomized data to suggest that a hormonally sensitive, postmenopausal patient benefits from such an approach. Indeed, only a single randomized trial has suggested any benefit for high-dose chemotherapy versus standard doses of chemotherapy in metastatic disease. The results of this small and somewhat unconventional study have yet to be reproduced or confirmed. Therefore, it is hard to imagine any approach that would have resulted in better palliation in this patient or in improved survival. Personally, I do not initiate chemotherapy in a patient with metastatic disease until she is clearly hormone refractory. The issue of hormone refractoriness is subjective and must be decided jointly by both the patient and her physician. A complete response to megestrol acetate followed by a 2-year remission-free interval strongly suggests that this patient remains highly hormonally responsive, and therefore is very likely to benefit from ongoing hormonal therapy.

Editors' comment: We would not expect this patient's response to third-line hormonal therapy to be as high as suggested. As a general rule, response to second-line hormonal therapy after an initial response followed by relapse decreases by 30–50%.

BIBLIOGRAPHY

Bezwoda W, Seymour L, Dansey R. High-dose chemotherapy with hematopoietic rescue as primary treatment for metastatic breast cancer: a randomized trial. J Clin Oncol 1995; 13:2483–2489.

Buzdar A, Jonat W, Howell A, Jones S, Blomqvist C, Vogel C, et al. Anastrozole, a potent and selective aromatase inhibitor, versus megestrol acetate in postmenopausal women with advanced breast cancer: results of overview analysis of two phase III trials. J Clin Oncol 1996a; 14:2000–2011.

Buzdar A, Smith R, Vogel C, Bonomi P, Keller A, Favis G, et al. Fadrozole HCL (CGS-16949A) versus megestrol acetate treatment of postmenopausal patients with metastatic breast cancer. Cancer 1996b; 77:2503–2513.

DeFriend D, Howell A, Nicholson R. Investigation of a new pure antiestrogen ICI 182780 in women with primary breast cancer. Cancer Res 1994; 54:408–414.

Early Breast Cancer Trialists' Collaborative Group T. Systemic treatment of early breast cancer by hormonal, cytotoxic, or immune therapy: 133 randomised trials involving 31,000 recurrences and 24,000 deaths among 75,000 women. Lancet 1992; 339:1–15, 71–85.

Fawell S, White R, Hoare S. Inhibition of estrogen receptor-DNA binding by the "pure" antiestorgen ICI 164,384 appears to be mediated by impaired receptor dimerization. Proc Natl Acad Sci USA 1990; 87:6883–6887.

Hayes DF, Henderson IC, Shapiro CL. Treatment of metastatic breast cancer: present and future prospects. Semin Oncol 1995; 22:5–21.

Howell A, DeFriend D, Robertson J. Pharmacokinetics, pharmacological and anti-tumor effects of the specific anti-oestregen ICI 182780 in women with advanced breast cancer. Br J Cancer 1996; 74:300–308.

Case #F.2.3
Goal: To discuss first recurrence in a non-visceral-predominant, ER+, postmenopausal patient

ROBERT S. DIPAOLA

A 67-year-old woman presents with recurrent breast cancer in new bone sites. She had been on tamoxifen for 8 years following mastectomy for a T2N1M0 estrogen-receptor-positive/progesterone-receptor-negative breast cancer

This represents a typical patient with metastatic breast cancer to bone while on tamoxifen following initial mastectomy.

The management of patients with metastatic disease is based on certain basic principles. Hormonal therapy can produce good disease control with minimal side effects. An initial decision to use hormonal therapy or chemotherapy should be based on the likelihood of hormonal response. Factors that predict a response to hormonal therapy include ER positivity, site of metastasis (soft tissue, bone > visceral), prior response to hormonal therapy, or disease-free interval of more than 36 months before recurrence. This patient with an ER positive tumor, bone metastases, and a long disease-free interval would be an excellent candidate for a second line hormonal agent such as megesterol acetate. Once this patient is unresponsive to hormonal therapy, the use of systemic chemotherapy could be considered to control disease. Additionally, if this patient develops visceral disease that is imminently lethal, such as liver metastasis, the initial use of chemotherapy with a quicker onset of action would be the best choice.

BIBLIOGRAPHY

Epstein RJ. The clinical biology of hormone-responsive breast cancer. Cancer Treat Rev 1988; 15:33.

Case #F.2.4
Goal: To discuss the "flare" reaction with hormonal therapy

WILLIAM N. HAIT

A 56-year-old woman with a history of stage II breast cancer, initially treated 7 years earlier with CMF adjuvant chemotherapy, presents with new low-back pain. A bone scan is consistent with metastatic disease. You start her on tamoxifen and she returns 4 weeks later with worsening pain. A repeat bone scan shows increased intensity of the previous hot spots and a questionable new lesion in the calvarium. Magnetic resonance imaging of the spine shows no evidence of spinal cord compression.

I would continue this patient on tamoxifen and would follow her clinically, at least by phone, weekly until a return visit is scheduled. This decision to continue tamoxifen is based on two assumptions: first, that her worsening pain and bone scan represents a flare reaction to tamoxifen and second, that in fact her initial tumor was HR positive. The 7-year disease-free interval is one indication that her original tumor was HR positive. I would immediately retrieve her tissue blocks and have them stained for both ER and PR, since the response to tamoxifen is proportional to the expression of either of these receptors. Ten to 15% of breast cancer patients experience a flare reaction when started on hormonal therapy, as manifested by increased uptake of the sentinel lesions observed on bone scan. This is presumed to be due to the reactivity of healing bone. A small number of patients also experience pain. Coleman et al. studied 53 patients receiving systemic therapy for bone metastases from breast cancer. In 15/16 patients with healing of the lytic lesions documented by X-ray, there was a worsening of the bone scan after 3 months of treatment. The worsening was seen not only in the initial lesions, but also by the appearance of new lesion. By 6 months, however, the bone scans were improved and no new lesions were seen. These changes were attributed to a "flare" in osteoblastic activity in response to succesful treatment and bone remodeling and was confirmed by a transient rise in osteocalcin and alkaline phosphatase-B1. The authors suggested that this flare might be a harbinger of a good response since it was seen in only 5/23 nonresponders.

BIBLIOGRAPHY

Coleman RE, Mashiter G, Whitaker KB, et al. Bone scan flare predicts successful systemic therapy for bone metastases. J Nucl Med 1988; 29:1354.
Plotkin P, Lechner JJ, Jung WE, et al. Tamoxifen flare in advanced breast cancer. JAMA 1978; 240:2644.

F.3. SUBSEQUENT RECURRENCES

Case #F.3.1
Goal: To discuss the interpretation of a metastatic site that is discordant, in terms of hormone receptors, from the primary

MAX S. WICHA

A 45-year-old premenopausal woman presents following bone marrow transplantation for metastatic, ER/PR strongly positive, primary, infiltrating ductal carcinoma. Biopsy of an enlarged cervical lymph node reveals carcinoma consistent with the breast primary. However, hormone receptors are now negative. Repeat assays on the original and recurrence are done by both immunohistochemistry and biochemical methods and yield the same results, a positive primary and a negative recurrence.

This case is an example of discordance between hormone receptors in primary breast cancer and in subsequent metastases. A number of studies have addressed the issue of discordant ER/PR receptors in primary and metastatic sites in both metachronous as well as asynchronous recurrences. Two large studies included patients with systemic adjuvant treatment showing discordant rates in estrogen receptor status in 19–40% of metastases compared to the primary tumor. Earlier studies utilized biochemical assays of tissue, which can give spurious results due to contamination by nonmalignant cells. A recent study showed results from carefully matched samples in 50 patients who had not received adjuvant therapy. Estrogen receptor (ER) and progesterone receptor (PR) status was determined immunohistochemically from histologically representative frozen and fixed paraffin-embedded tissue. In addition, ER status was ascertained by mRNA in situ hybridization. It was found that hormone receptor status of the recurrent tumor differed from that of the primary tumor in 36% of cases. Discordant cases were always due to loss of either ER, PR, or both. Receptor-negative primary tumors were always accompanied by receptor-negative recurrences. Of significance, among 27 patients with ER-positive primary tumors, loss of ER was a significant predictor ($p = 0.0085$) of a poor response to subsequent endocrine therapy. Only one of eight patients with lost ER expression responded to tamoxifen therapy, whereas the response rate was 74% for patients whose recurrent tumors had retained ER expression.

On the basis of these studies, the above patient would best be treated with chemotherapy rather than additional hormone therapy, since the chances of response to hormone therapy would be extremely low. Since this patient has already undergone bone marrow transplantation, it is likely that she has had standard chemotherapy but might be a candidate for chemotherapy with taxol, navelbine, gemcitabine, or an investigational agent.

BIBLIOGRAPHY

Hull DF, Clark GM, Osborn CK, et al. Multiple estrogen receptor assays in human breast cancer. Cancer Res 1983; 43:413–416.

Kuukasjarvi T, Kononen J, Helin H, Holli K, Isola J. Loss of estrogen receptor in recurrent breast cancer is associated with poor response to endocrine therapy. J Clin Oncol 1996; 14(9):2584–2589.

Rasmussen BB, Kamby C. Immunohistochemical detection of estrogen receptors in paraffin sections from primary and metastatic breast cancer. Pathol Res Pract 1989; 185:856–859.

Case #F.3.2
Goal: To discuss visceral-predominant, hormone-receptor-negative disease

JOSEPH AISNER

A 41-year-old woman experienced her first recurrence with metastatic breast cancer 2 years ago. Her adjuvant chemotherapy was CMF; she recurred 2 years later with three pulmonary nodules and achieved a clinical complete remission on CAF × 6 cycles. She has remained clinically free of disease for 1 year but now returns with pulmonary and liver metastases. Examination reveals a slightly enlarged liver; there is no jaundice or signs of pleural or pericardial effusions. Her performance status is ECOG 1. You plan to start her on paclitaxel but she seeks a second opinion at the university cancer center.

This patient had a 2-year disease-free period following CMF adjuvant chemotherapy, and then achieved a complete clinical remission on six cycles of CAF. The second disease-free period lasted 1 year, after which the patient presents with pulmonary and liver metastases. This patient now presents with visceral dominant disease, and is an appropriate candidate for third-line therapy. However, several issues need to be defined with respect to therapeutic options.

First, patients who present with metastatic disease often have disease in multiple sites. The purpose of any treatment for metastatic disease should be (1) to achieve comfort; (2) to achieve function, and (3) if the above two are achieved, to maintain this as long as possible. To that extent the patient's chemistries should be reviewed to see if there is any suggestion of bone metastases, calcium imbalance, or disturbances of hematopoiesis. I would favor obtaining a bone scan with careful analysis of any bone-scan-positive areas to assess whether there is any threat to the stability of the axial skeleton. Irradiation of any lesions that have any degree of bone loss helps to prevent any disabling bone fractures, and this would likely take precedence over any third-line therapy. Similarly, a careful analysis of the neurological function and ophthalmological examination, can be useful in assessing whether the patient should undergo brain scans to assess for brain metastases. Radiation in this setting can be used to prevent complications such as bone fractures, progressive central nervous system metastases, or impending obstructions of visceral organs such as bronchi.

Assuming that these issues were considered and evaluated and there was no need for immediate radiotherapy, then the next step is to decide which therapeutic approach would be most likely to help. Taxol clearly has activity in breast cancer and is likely to be the most active agent in this setting. However, there is compelling evidence that patients who enjoy relatively long responses to prior therapy such as CMF or CAF may be candidates for retreatment with the same regimen. Thus, one alternative to treatment with taxol would be to restart CAF to see whether any additional response could be achieved. Alternatively, Taxol can be used as a single agent, or as a basis for combination with other agents including doxorubicin. The latter is still reasonable since this woman experienced a year of progression-free survival. Finally, several new agents, including the camptothecins, Navelbine, and Gemcitabine, are currently under testing to define their role. Additional approaches, such as the use of monoclonal antibodies directed against Her-2-*neu* in combination with chemotherapy, are also being tested in women whose disease was found to express Her-2-*neu* antigen. Thus, this patient has several possible options using both conventional and investigational approaches.

Duration of chemotherapy for recurrent and metastatic disease has to be determined. There is surprisingly little data to define the duration of optimal therapy for patients who achieve complete response. Furthermore, there is no evidence that chemotherapy beyond six cycles improves either long-term survival or quality of life. Thus, it is perfectly reasonable, and my usual practice, to discontinue CAF after six cycles. The decision for discontinuing therapy, however, is often based on the level of response. Thus, if the patient has achieved complete response within four cycles, I would routinely go to six and stop. If the patient's disease continues to respond at the sixth cycle, I would be inclined to continue until the patient has no further evidence of disease regression for two cycles, or there are toxicity limitations, bearing in mind the limitation of the doxorubicin dosage.

Editors' comment: The search for asymptomatic sights of disease so that treatment can be applied in a prophylactic manner is somewhat controversial.

Although the yield of these tests is low, they may be improved in the setting of higher prevalence of the problem.

BIBLIOGRAPHY

Aisner J, Abrams JS. The treatment of metastatic breast cancer. In: Wise E, ed. Breast Cancer: Controversies in Management. New York: Futura Publishing Co, 1994:459–478.

Coates A, Gebski V, Stat M, et al. Improving quality of life during chemotherapy for advanced breast cancer. A comparison of intermittent and continuous treatment strategies. N Engl J Med 1987; 317:1490–1495.

Dickson RB, Lippman ME. Cancer of the breast. In: DeVita VT, Hellman S, Rosenberg SA, eds. Cancer: Principles and Practice of Oncology, 5th ed. Philadelphia: Lippincott-Raven, 1997:1604–1605.

Muss H, Case I, Richards F, et al. Interrupted v. continuous chemotherapy in patients with metastatic breast cancer. N Engl J Med 1991; 325:1342–1348.

Case #F.3.3
Goal: To discuss hormone-receptor-positive, non-visceral-predominant disease in a premenopausal woman

SANDRA F. SCHNALL

A 38-year-old woman presents with increased bone pain 6 months after completing a course of paclitaxel for bone recurrence of a hormone-receptor-positive, infiltrating ductal carcinoma. Her adjuvant treatment was CAF × 6. A repeat bone scan shows new metastatic lesions. She has no signs of spinal cord compression.

Bone metastasis present a significant problem for many women with breast cancer. Osseous involvement often presents with pain, difficulty ambulating, and impaired quality of life. Certain tumors exhibit "osteotropism" with a high risk of bone metastasis (i.e., breast cancer, lung cancer, prostate cancer).

Treatment options for bony metastasis are often aimed at relieving pain, preventing pathological fractures, and enhancing quality of life. As metastatic breast cancer is incurable, the majority of treatment goals aim at obtaining effective palliation with minimal toxicity. Patients with breast cancer who develop bone-only metastatic disease may have longer survivals than those with concurrent visceral and/or visceral-only metastasis.

This patient developed (presumed) bone-only metastasis after adjuvant therapy with CAF. She subsequently received paclitaxel for her bone recurrence. She then developed progressive disease 6 months after completing the course of salvage chemotherapy.

Treatment options, at this juncture, are somewhat dependent upon her symptoms. Radiation therapy is often effective in alleviating pain to some degree in up to 90% of patients. However, in patients with multiple sites of bony metastases, radiation therapy may not be as effective, as several sites may need to be targeted. Therefore, other options to consider would be hormonal therapy, further salvage chemotherapy, radionuclide intervention, or bisphosphonates.

Hormonal therapy for metastatic breast cancer is felt to be most effective in lesions involving the soft tissue and bone. However, the role of hormonal therapy in premenopausal women is somewhat controversial. At some level, ovarian ablation may be of benefit in the premenopausal woman, especially the patient with bone-predominant disease. Ovarian ablation may be obtained by an oophorectomy, tamoxifen, or other hormone analogs. Some physicians are concerned that tamoxifen may cause stimulation of ovarian steroidogenesis in premenopausal women. However, others have shown that tamoxifen may be safely used in premenopausal women, without adverse side effects or stimulation of tumor growth.

Other treatments that may be used in conjunction with hormone therapy may be the bisphosphonates, such as Pamidronate. Bisphosphonates have been used to stabilize bone mineralization and theoretically inhibit bone reabsorption. Although Pamidronate does not usually confer a survival advantage, it does decrease the risk of hypercalcemia, bone fractures, and other skeletal events.

Therefore, in this patient who is estrogen/progesterone-receptor positive I would proceed (if she truly has bone-only disease) with a hormone manipulation, such as tamoxifen with concurrent Pamidronate. If she has progressive tumor in a greater than 6-month period, I would consider alternative hormone intervention. If, however, she has relatively hormone-refractory tumor (i.e., relapse in 3–6 months), I would consider alternative chemotherapy (i.e., vinorelbine, phase I agents, etc.). If painful bony events are a predominant symptom, one could consider the role of strontium 89 as a radionuclide intervention.

BIBLIOGRAPHY

Henderson CI. New treatments for breast cancer. Semin in Oncol 1996; 23(4):506–528.

McGuire WL, Clark GM. Prognostic factors and treatment decisions in axillary node negative breast cancer. N Engl J Med 1992; 326:1756–1761.

Perez JE, Machiavell IM, Leone BA, et al. Bone only versus visceral only metastatic pattern in breast cancer: analysis of 150 patients. Am J Clin Oncol 1990; 13:294.

Case #F.3.4
Goal: To discuss non-visceral-predominant, ER+, postmenopausal disease

DANIEL F. HAYES

A 62-year-old woman presents with a chest wall recurrence of chest wall disease, 1 year after treatment of her initial chest wall recurrence with excision, radiation, and tamoxifen. Physical examination reveals multiple skin nodules, the largest measuring 1.5 cm. She is asymptomatic aside from the local discomfort. A metastatic workup is negative.

The most feared consequence of having breast cancer is the risk of death. However, many patients with recurrent, metastatic breast cancer can be palliated by judicious use of a series of treatments, including surgery, radiation therapy, hormone therapy, and chemotherapy. Nonetheless, although all metastatic breast cancer is bad news, perhaps the two most feared complications other than mortality are uncontrolled local disease and refractory, metastatic disease to the bone.

Of those patients who are destined to develop recurrent disease, 30% of first recurrences are on the chest wall or within regional lymph nodes only. Another 15–30% of first recurrences include chest wall and/or regional lymph nodes in addition to other distant sites. Several clinical series have suggested that most patients who develop a local-regional recurrence will go on to suffer distant metastatic disease. However, 10–15% of patients who suffer local-regional recurrence can be rendered disease-free and do not develop distant recurrence over the next 5–10 years. Features that predict a favorable, prolonged, progression-free interval after local-regional recurrence include a long disease-free interval from the primary diagnosis to first recurrence, single nodules that can be totally excised, and other general features that are associated with favorable prognoses in metastatic disease (low cellular turnover rate, estrogen receptor positivity, etc.). Rapid recurrence of multiple nodules on the chest wall after initial treatment, especially within an irradiated field, are predictive of both a high risk of distant recurrence and uncontrollable local disease.

Almost every study of newly diagnosed patients with breast cancer demonstrates that more aggressive local therapy at the time of initial diagnosis results in fewer local recurrences. However, few, if any, of these studies actually follow patients to the point of determining whether a patient has *uncontrollable* local disease. Only a single study has reported the ultimate risk of uncontrolled local disease in patients who are randomly assigned to adjuvant radiation therapy versus observation after mastectomy. In this series, the risk of long-term uncontrollable metastasis is decreased by almost 50% by the use of adjuvant chest wall radiotherapy. However, this series is small, and the incidence of ultimately uncontrollable metastasis in both groups appears higher than one would expect from most clinical experiences. Thus, although the risk of chest wall recurrence is roughly parallel to the risk of distant recurrence, and although one can decrease the risk of local recurrence with adjuvant chest wall radiation therapy in patients who are at high risk, it is not clear that irradiating all patients after mastectomy will ultimately reduce the odds of long-term, uncontrollable local disease.

Once a patient has a local recurrence, the clinician should take into consideration the various features that will predict whether the patient already has or is likely to soon have distant metastatic disease. If these are favorable, many patients may be well treated with local therapy only. There is only a single randomized study of adjuvant systemic therapy after chest wall recurrence. The results of this small study suggest that adjuvant tamoxifen after mastectomy in ER-positive patients prolongs the time to subsequent local recurrence, but may not impact on distant recurrence or mortality. It would seem reasonable to offer adjuvant tamoxifen if the patient is hormone receptor positive and has not previously become refractory to tamoxifen. If the patient has had a long disease-free interval on tamoxifen, it would not be unreasonable to apply other means of hormone therapy, such as an aromatase inhibitor. The benefits of adjuvant chemotherapy in patients who have had local recurrence are simply unknown. In patients who have documented distant metastases, or who have chest wall recurrence after prior treatment for chest wall recurrence, treatment decisions should be similar to those that would be made for any patient with distant metastatic disease. However, this still leaves the patient at substantial risk for ultimate uncontrollable local disease. Some authors have advocated performing a total excision of the chest wall in selected patients. There are scattered case reports of patients who have been rendered disease-free for prolonged periods after this procedure, but it is quite morbid and most patients would probably not consider this approach an acceptable alternative.

A few studies have suggested that other means of local therapy may, on occasion, result in palliation in patients whose disease has recurred within irradiated fields. These would include photodynamic therapy and/or hyperthermia. However, both are highly specialized techniques that require sophisticated equipment. Furthermore, these therapies are not appropriate for all patients, depending on the size of the required field to be treated.

In summary, this patient presents a particularly worrisome scenario. One might try an alternative hormone therapy, but the relatively short disease-free interval (less than 1 year) after her initial recurrence suggests that this patient may be refractory to other hormone therapies. Alternative local therapies such as chest wall excision, photodynamic therapy, and hyper-thermia might all be considered but the expected results are all less than satisfactory. It seems a shame to expose this patient to the side effects of systemic chemotherapy to treat local disease. However, such an approach is probably her best opportunity for palliation. Unfortunately, I suspect that even this approach is also destined for failure and that this patient may well suffer the misery of *uncontrollable* local breast cancer, perhaps even leading to carcinoma *en cuirasse*, a condition in which the patient's thorax becomes circumferentially involved with diffuse, subcutaneous, infiltrating breast can-cer. This condition, usually refractory to any form of therapy, may result in bleeding, infection, and even restrictive pulmonary defects.

BIBLIOGRAPHY

Borner M, Bacchi M, Goldhirsch A, Greiner R, Harder F, Castiglione M, et al. First isolated locoregional recurrence following mastectomy for breast cancer: re-sults of a phase III multicenter study comparing systemic treatment with ob-servation after excision and radiation. J Clin Oncol 1994; 12:2071–2077.

Harris J, Morrow M. Treatment of early-stage breast cancer. In: Harris J, Lippman M, Morrow M, Hellman S, eds. Diseases of the Breast. Philadelphia: JB Lip-pincott, 1996:487–547.

Hayes DF, Kaplan W. Evaluation of patients after primary therapy. In: Harris J, Lippman M, Morrow M, Hellman S, eds. Diseases of the Breast. Philadelphia: JB Lippincott, 1996:627–645.

Recht A, Hayes DF, Eberlein T, Sadowsky N. Local-regional recurrence after mas-tectomy or breast conserving therapy. In: Harris J, Lippman M, Morrow M, Hellman S, eds. Diseases of the Breast. Philadelphia: JB Lippincott, 1996: 649–667.

Rutqvist L. Adjuvant radiation therapy versus surgery alone in operable breast can-cer: long-term follow-up of a randomized clinical trial. Radiother Oncol 1993; 26:104–110.

G. Surveillance/Follow-up

Introduction

The follow-up of patients with breast cancer is a poorly defined area that has come under particular scrutiny with the advent of managed care. The major issues to be considered in the management of patients include the likelihood of detecting changes that if acted upon would change the course of the disease; the psychosocial benefits gained or lost from being in close contact with the oncologist; and finally, the coordination of care between the team of doctors, nurses, and social workers required for the optimum management of breast cancer patients.

Case #G.1
Goal: To discuss the follow-up of an uncomplicated, low-risk patient

SANDRA F. SCHNALL

A 43-year-old woman with stage I breast cancer (T1N0M0; ER/PR−) has been treated with lumpectomy and four cycles of CA chemotherapy. She is about to complete radiation therapy and returns to the medical oncologist for a follow-up visit. She feels "a little tired" but otherwise well. Physical examination reveals redness of the irradiated breast, without other findings. She wants to know how frequently she should see you and whether she should also keep appointments for follow-up with her surgeon and radiation oncologist.

Patients diagnosed with breast cancer are routinely followed to detect recurrences at an early stage. Some physicians have advocated that if recurrence is detected early, while the tumor burden is low, there is a higher likelihood of achieving either disease control or extended survival. This has motivated the use of surveillance studies, including laboratory data and radiographic tests. Until recently, no definitive guidelines have been established for posttherapy follow-up of stage I and stage II breast cancer. Clearly, patients require careful follow-up and observation, but the benefit of long-term follow-up is less well established.

Screening mechanisms should be focused during a time when the chance of relapse is greatest. Although, risk for relapse may vary by cell type and other prognostic parameters, the peak risk of recurrence for infiltrating carcinomas is in the first 2−3 years after diagnosis.

Screening by organ site is dependent upon the most common pattern of spread. The most common sites for breast cancer to recur are local regional areas (i.e., chest wall or regional nodes) and bone; less common sites are the liver, lung, and CNS. Bone scanning to detect relapse is not useful, as only one in nine women will have an asymptomatic bony recurrence. Similarly, surveillance hepatic ultrasound is not sufficiently sensitive for detection of early liver metastasis.

Routine laboratory data, such as a CBC and liver function tests, have little effect on detection of early relapse or influencing survival. Serum markers, such as CEA, CA15-3, and CA27.29, are of little value in determining the differential diagnosis of metastatic lesions, as up to 20% of patients will have benign breast changes with elevations of CEA or CA15-3, making the predictive value of these tests low.

In November 1997, the American Society of Clinical Oncology published recommended breast cancer surveillance guidelines. They include a routine history and physical every 3–6 months for the first 3 years after primary therapy and then every 6–12 months for the next 2 years and then annually. They recommend that all women perform monthly breast self-examinations indefinitely. A mammogram is recommended yearly for any woman with a prior diagnosis of breast cancer. However, women treated with breast-conserving surgery and postoperative radiation should receive their first posttreatment mammogram approximately 6 months after completion of radiation therapy and then annually or as indicated. Evaluation by all the involved physicians in the treatment of breast cancer should be coordinated so as not to duplicate care. It is therefore recommended that subsequent care be done through one primary physician who will follow the patient as above.

Editors' comment: We recommend that, whenever possible, routine follow-up be done in a multidisciplinary setting by the team of physicians caring for the patient.

BIBLIOGRAPHY

Hayes DF, Kaplin W. Evaluation of patients after primary therapy. In: Harris J, Littman M, Morrow M, Hellman S, eds. Diseases of the Breast. Philadelphia: Lippincott-Raven, 1996:629–647.

Pedrazzini A, Gelber R, Isley M, et al. First repeat bone scan in the observation of patients with operable breast cancer. J Clin Oncol 1986; 4:389–394.

Recommended breast cancer surveillance guidelines. J Clin Oncol 1997; 15:2149–2156.

Case #G.2
Goal: To discuss the use of tumor markers

DANIEL F. HAYES

A 63-year-old woman, post modified radical mastectomy for a T2N1M0 infiltrating ductal breast cancer, hormone receptor positive, is currently receiving her second year of tamoxifen. You have been following tumor markers and document a doubling of her CA125 and CA27.29. She is asymptomatic. Physical examination is unrevealing.

The general public and most physicians have widely accepted the concept that early diagnosis and treatment of breast cancer will result in better outcomes. This has certainly been demonstrated in regard to primary, surgically treatable breast cancer. The concept of early systemic therapy for breast cancer is embodied in adjuvant treatment. Unfortunately, once detectable metastases have occurred, systemic treatment does not appear to substantially prolong survival, although it does provide palliation.

Circulating tumor markers might be useful in one of many situations. One of these might be to monitor patients after primary, local, and adjuvant systemic treatment for evidence of impending relapse. Indeed, several studies demonstrate that two classes of circulating tumor markers, carcinoembryonic antigen (CEA) and the protein product of the *MUC*-1 gene (e.g., CA15-3 and CA27.29), are reasonably sensitive and reliable indicators of relapse. Accumulated data suggest that approximately 40–50% of those patients who are destined to recur will have a rising CEA and/or MUC-1 protein product prior to recurrence. If appropriately stringent cutoff points are used, the median lead time between an elevated marker and the appearance of detectable and/or symptomatic disease is approximately 6 months. Thus, the positive predictive value of a continuously rising marker (predictive that the patient will suffer recurrence within the next 12 months) is well over 90%. Likewise, the negative predictive value (that a patient with a nonrising marker does not have recurrence) is also quite high. But, of course, that depends on the patient's odds of recurrence in the first place. For example, the negative predictive value will be higher for a node-negative patient than a node-positive patient.

Therefore, although we can detect impending recurrence, should we? Recently, the American Society of Clinical Oncology convened a Tumor Marker Expert Panel to establish practice guidelines for the use of tumor markers. While the use of circulating tumor markers was recommended for selected patients with established metastatic disease to monitor their clinical course, the Expert Panel did not recommend serial tumor markers to detect impending relapse in an asymptomatic patient who is otherwise free of detectable recurrent disease. Although no randomized trials have been reported in which patients have either been followed closely with tumor marker results or observed without obtaining these tests, two randomized trials have been published in which patients have been followed closely with serial radiographic analysis (chest X-ray, bone scan, liver imaging) versus simple clinical visits. All patients had routine mammography. In both of these studies, although there was a slight lead time in diagnosis in the patients who were more intensively followed, overall survival of the two groups was identical. These data are consistent with several retrospective studies that suggest that survival after treatment of asymptomatic patients with detectable metastases (presumably early metastases) is no better than that for patients who are not treated until they develop symptomatic metastases.

In summary, there appear to be several possible reasons for detecting early metastases:

1. Early treatment of impending symptomatic metastases might improve survival. There is little, if any, evidence that this is the case with currently available therapies for breast cancer.

2. Early detection and treatment of patients with impending metastases might improve palliation. It is difficult to argue that any treatment of asymptomatic patients will improve their current palliation. No studies have been performed in which the concept of "upfront palliation" has been tested. One might argue that upfront palliation might delay subsequent symptoms and especially subsequent clinical disasters, such as rapidly progressive visceral disease, bone fracture, or spinal cord compression. Again, no data exist to support any of these potential benefits, and furthermore, it is unlikely that any of these three situations would be preceded by a substantial lead time provided by increasing tumor markers.

3. Patients (and physicians) might derive emotional benefit from negative results at a time when the patients are otherwise free of recurrent disease. Because the odds of recurrence at any given clinic visit for an asymptomatic breast cancer patient are so low, especially if she had a good prognosis initially, it is true that the negative predictive value of any of these tests is quite high. However, the negative predictive value of providing an asymptomatic patient reassurance in the absence of tumor marker results is also quite high. Moreover, as there is little clinical utility in knowing about a rising marker, one must be concerned that, in fact, an asymptomatic patient's well-being is jeopardized by the knowledge that she has impending relapse coupled with the relative inability to do anything about that.

Nonetheless, on occasion, both patient and physician prefer to follow the patient with circulating tumor markers. Although the positive predictive value of a rising marker is reasonably high, the clinician should be certain to rule out other causes of elevated tumor markers. These include the occurrence of other new primary cancers that might produce either CEA and/or MUC-1 protein products (for example, a new breast cancer or cancers of the gastrointestinal tract, female genital or urinary tract, and lung). Some benign conditions may also increase circulating tumor marker levels, most commonly benign inflammatory diseases of the liver (hepatitis) and of the gastrointestinal tract (inflammatory bowel disease, ulcerative colitis). However, these conditions are usually clinically quite obvious and rarely are the cause of a rising marker in a patient who has previously had breast cancer.

I would not have recommended obtaining tumor markers in this patient, for the reasons I have stated. Now that they are known, I would be certain she does not have one of the nonmetastatic breast cancer causes of a rising tumor marker. For example, given that she has a rising CA125, one must be certain she does not have new ovarian cancer. However, elevated CA125 levels have been reported to be common in women with breast cancer. Now that she has rising markers, one must have a long discussion with the patient regarding whether she would wish to continue on her current therapy (which is probably failing) or change to an alternative therapy, such as an aromatase inhibitor, which might also have few side effects.

BIBLIOGRAPHY

ASCO Expert Panel T. Clinical practice guidelines for the use of tumor markers in breast and colorectal cancer: report of the American Society of Clinical Oncology Expert Panel. J Clin Oncol 1996; 14:2843–2877.

Chan D, Beveridge R, Muss H, Fritsche H, Hortobagyi G, Theriault R, et al. Use of Truquant BR radioimmunoassay for early detection of breast cancer recurrence in patients with stage II and stage III disease. J Clin Oncol 1997; 15: 2322–2328.

GIVIO Investigators. Impact of follow-up and testing on survival and health-related quality of life in breast cancer patients: a multicenter randomized controlled trial. JAMA 1994; 271:1587–1593.

Hayes DF. Tumor markers for breast cancer: current utilities and future prospects. In: Hayes DF, ed. Hematology/Oncology Clinics of North America: Tumor Markers in Adult Solid Malignancies. Philadelphia: WB Saunders, 1994: 485–506.

Hayes DF, Bast R, Desch CE, Fritsche H, Kemeny NE, Jessup J, et al. A tumor marker utility grading system (TMUGS): a framework to evaluate clinical utility of tumor markers. J Natl Cancer Inst 1996; 88:1456–1466.

Hayes DF, Henderson IC, Shapiro CL. Treatment of metastatic breast cancer: present and future prospects. Semin Oncol 1995; 22:5–21.

Hayes DF, Kaplan W. Evaluation of patients after primary therapy. In: Harris J, Lippman M, Morrow M, Hellman S, eds. Diseases of the Breast. Philadelphia: JB Lippincott, 1996:627–645.

Nyström L, Rutqvist LE, Wall S, Lindgren A, Lindqvist M, Rydén S, et al. Breast cancer screening with mammography: overview of Swedish randomised trials. Lancet 1993; 341:973–978.

Perey L, Hayes D, Tondini C, van Melle G, Bauer J, Lemarchand T, et al. Elevated CA125 levels in patients with metastatic breast carcinoma. Br J Cancer 1990; 62:668–670.

Rosselli Del Turco M, Palli D, Cariddi A, Ciatto S, Pacini P, Distante V. Intensive diagnostic follow-up after treatment of primary breast cancer: a randomized trial. JAMA 1994; 271:1593–1597.

Case #G.3
Goal: To discuss the use of tumor markers in the management of metastatic disease

LARRY NORTON and TERESA GILEWSKI

A 38-year-old woman who is post lumpectomy, radiation, and CAF × 6 for a stage II breast CA (T2N1M0) ER/PR. Two months ago she was found to have an elevated CA 15-3 and CA125 and new bony metastases. She was started on Taxol 1 month ago. Repeat tumor markers drawn in your office today have increased by 50%. You deliver a second cycle of paclitaxel and a repeat CA 15-3 and 125 remains abnormal.

CA 125 is often elevated in metastatic breast cancer, but is not the best marker, since both CEA and CA 15-3 are more sensitive and specific. An elevated CA 125 in the setting of stage IV disease, however, can be useful for monitoring response to therapy. One must be sure that an occult ovarian cancer is not the cause of the elevated CA 125. Pelvic sonography or computerized axial tomography is sometimes used for this purpose. If the CA 125 is elevated, the other tumor markers (plus alkaline phosphatase) should also be assessed. Assuming that the bone lesions are breast cancer (biopsy material would be most helpful in this regard), and that no other lesions are available for assessing response, the markers as a whole should tend to decrease as the lesions respond to systemic therapy.

In addition, sudden but transient increases in markers may be documented at the time of initiation of a therapy that is later proven to be effective. Such "biochemical flares," however, are always short-lived, so a persistently climbing CA 125 through 2 months of paclitaxel therapy is of concern. We should be more concerned if the CEA, CA 15-3, or alkaline phosphatase also rose, particularly if they were accompanied by increasing osseous symptoms such as pain. If the lesions are asymptomatic, however, and other markers are normal or falling, or if there is objective evidence of response by radiographic imaging, an isolated rise in the CA 125 should not be interpreted as unequivocal evidence of progressive disease. In other words, while a rising tumor marker is always a cause for special scrutiny, our interpretation of marker results cannot be divorced from the overall clinical picture.

BIBLIOGRAPHY

Bast RC, Klug TL, St John E, et al. A radioimmunoassay using a monoclonal antibody to monitor the course of epithelial ovarian cancer. N Engl J Med 1983; 309:883.

Kiang DT, Greenberg LJ, Kennedy BJ. Tumor marker kinetics in the monitoring of breast cancer. Cancer 1990; 65:193–199.

Tumor Marker Expert Panel. Clinical practice guidelines for the use of tumor markers in breast and colorectal cancer. J Clin Oncol 1996; 14:2843–2877.

H. Special Situations

H.1. MALE BREAST CANCER

Case #H.1.1
Goal: To discuss the management of male breast cancer

KEVIN R. FOX

A 67-year-old man presents with a new, palpable, 1.8-cm mass in the left breast just superior to the areolar border. It is hard, mobile, and non-tender. The axillary lymph nodes are clinically negative. An excisional biopsy reveals an infiltrating ductal carcinoma, ER/PR+; axillary node dissection reveals three of 10 positive lymph nodes.

Breast cancer in men is an uncommon disease accounting for fewer than 1% of all breast cancer cases or approximately 1000 cases per year in the United States. Predisposing causes for breast cancer in men are not well understood. Sufficient evidence exists in family studies to suggest some familial risk, although the majority of cases in any "high-risk" family will necessarily be female. The genetics of breast cancer suggests a heightened risk of breast cancer in male carriers of mutations of the *BRCA*-2 gene, when such mutations are discovered in the setting of a "high-risk" family. The lifetime risk of developing breast cancer may be as high as 10% in such men. Little else can be said regarding the epidemiology of male breast cancer. Associations between breast cancer and orchitis, Turner's syndrome, hyperestrogenemia, undescended testes, androgen insufficiency, and radiation exposure have been described.

The histological nature of male breast cancer is almost always ductal. Invasive lobular cancers occur very rarely. Male breast cancer tends to be hormone-receptor positive more often than in women, with receptors demonstrated 70–80% of the time.

The diagnosis of breast cancer in men is usually made after the clinical finding of a painless breast mass, as was the case in our patient. The differential diagnosis usually includes cancer and gynecomastia. Fine-needle aspiration alone may not be reliable. Surgical biopsy should thus be relied upon for diagnostic purposes, and hormone receptor studies should always be performed. The percentage of newly diagnosed patients with concurrent metastatic disease at presentation may be up to three times greater in men (30%) than in women, and evaluation for metastases with chest X-ray, bone scan, and liver function tests should be considered routine.

Treatment paradigms in male breast cancer typically follow those outlined for women, with a few variations. For example, the local-regional management of male breast cancer is usually a modified radical mastectomy. The proximity of the male breast tissue to the pectoralis muscles results in a greater proportion of cases with muscle invasion. As a result, surgical excision of a portion of or all of the muscle may be required. The role of breast-conserving surgery and adjunctive radiotherapy has not been explored adequately in men and cannot be recommended.

The role of postmastectomy radiation therapy in male breast cancer is not well defined. Radiation therapy should be employed for tumors with positive or close deep surgical margins, for lesions that invade the pectoralis muscle, and in patients with extensive lymph node involvement (>3).

The prognosis of male patients with breast cancer is most closely related to tumor size and number of positive lymph nodes, as is the case with women. Adjuvant systemic therapy recommendations should follow those outlined for women, as adequate data from controlled clinical trials have not been obtained in men. Our patient is known to have three positive lymph nodes and positive hormone receptors and thus should receive adjuvant tamoxifen for 5 years. However, there now exist ample data from clinical trials in older, node-positive, receptor-positive women to suggest a benefit in both disease-free and overall survival if doxorubicin-based chemotherapy is used in conjunction with tamoxifen, and this approach should be considered superior to tamoxifen alone. I would therefore favor treating this patient, after mastectomy, with a 12-week course of doxorubicin/cyclophosphamide chemotherapy, provided his cardiac function is normal and his overall medical condition permits, and would follow chemotherapy with 5 years of tamoxifen using standard doses.

Editors' comment: We would recommend postoperative radiation therapy in this patient. Although there are no prospective randomized trials in male breast cancer, because of the three positive lymph nodes, we estimate the patient's risk of local regional recurrence to be as high as 30%. Traditionally, radiation oncologists have been inclined to apply criteria for radiation more liberally in male patients because of the limited breast tissue.

BIBLIOGRAPHY

Elder S, Nash E, Abrahamson J. Radiation carcinogenesis in the male breast. Eur J Surg Oncol 1989; 15:274.

Erlichman C, Murphy K, Elkhaim T. Male breast cancer: a 13-year review of 89 patients. J Clin Oncol 1984; 2:903.

Patel H, Buzdar A, Hortobagyi G. Role of adjuvant chemotherapy in male breast cancer. Cancer 1989; 64:1583.

Case #H.1.2
Goal: To discuss the management of male breast cancer

WILLIAM N. HAIT

A 38-year-old man presents with a painful lesion of the right breast. He is treated with a 10-day course of antibiotics without change in the lesion. A fine-needle aspiration of the lesion reveals infiltrating lobular carcinoma, ER+. The remainder of the examination is unremarkable.

I would immediately question the diagnosis, since infiltrating lobular carcinoma would be reportable in males. Therefore, I would recommend a mammogram and a repeat biopsy using a Tru-cut or other technique to obtain a greater amount of tissue to make a definitive diagnosis. Assuming that the diagnosis is truly a malignancy, and that the histology is infiltrating ductal, the patient should undergo a modified radical mastectomy. The adjuvant treatment follows recommendations for women with breast cancer and therefore depends on tumor size, lymph node status, receptor status, and to a lesser extent, the DNA and proliferative indices. Given the young age of the patient and the hormone receptor positivity, I would recommend the use of adjuvant chemotherapy, e.g., doxorubicin plus cyclophosphamide for four cycles, perhaps followed by four cycles of paclitaxel, followed by 5 years of tamoxifen. Adjuvant radiation would depend on the ability to obtain clean margins, the size of the tumor, and the number of positive lymph nodes.

BIBLIOGRAPHY

Fisher B, Brown AM, Dimitrov NV, et al. Two months of doxorubicin-cyclophosphamide with and without interval reinduction therapy compared with 6 months of cyclophosphamide, methotrexate, and fluorouracil in positive-node breast cancer patients with tamoxifen-nonresponsive tumors: results from the NSABP B-15. J Clin Oncol 1990; 8:1483–1496.

Fisher B, Dignam J, Bryant J, et al. Five versus more than five years of tamoxifen therapy for breast cancer patients with negative lymph nodes and estrogen receptor-positive tumors. J Natl Cancer Inst 1996; 88:1529–1542.

Holleb A, Freeman H, Farrow J. Cancer of the male breast. NY State Med J 1968; 68:836.

H.2. PAGET'S DISEASE

Case #H.2.1
Goal: To discuss the management of Paget's disease

KIRBY I. BLAND and DANIEL S. KIM

A 56-year-old woman presents with a 6-month history of nipple irritation with pruritus and occasional bleeding. Cytological analysis of a smear of an associated serosanguineous discharge reveals malignant cells. Bilateral mammograms reveal multiple subareolar calcifications in the involved breast.

Velpeau in 1856 was the first to describe the crusting, bleeding, and ulceration of the nipple associated with Paget's disease. However, in 1874, Sir James Paget was the first to associate the characteristic skin changes with the subsequent development of breast cancer.

Paget's disease of the nipple is the presenting sign of breast cancer in 0.5–4.3% of all cases. The peak incidence is during the sixth and seventh decades, with a median age of 56 years. The lesion presents as a chronic, eczematous eruption of the nipple. It is classically unilateral, well delineated, often slightly infiltrated, and exudative or scaly. Tiny vesicles may erupt, heal, and recur with occasional serous or bloody discharge. The lesion usually starts on the nipple and spreads to the areola and rarely to the surrounding skin. Itching and soreness are present in 25% of cases. This woman's age and presentation are classic. The 6-month duration of symptoms prior to presentation is also consistent with the literature.

Paget's disease should be considered as a presentation of breast cancer rather than a type of breast cancer because the underlying malignancy is variable. The patient may have no underlying malignancy, which occurs in 10% of patients, ductal carcinoma in situ (DCIS), and/or an invasive cancer. Therefore, the evaluation of the underlying process is of most importance in treatment and prognosis.

The histogenesis of the Paget's cell, although controversial, has two main hypotheses: epidermotrophism and intraepithelial carcinomatous metaplasia. The epidermotrophic theory suggests that Paget's cells are ductal carcinoma cells that have migrated along basement membranes of the underlying duct to the nipple epidermis. The intraepithelial carcinomatous metaplasia theory postulates that Paget's cells are transformed malignant keratinocytes organized as in situ carcinoma. Immunohistochemical evidence supports the epidermotrophic theory and this theory is generally favored.

Paget's is usually associated with extensive DCIS and rarely (10% or less) presents with disease limited to the nipple and areola. A palpable mass should raise the suspicion of an underlying invasive carcinoma. At this stage, lymph node metastases are seen in one-half to two-thirds of patients.

The Paget cell, a large, pale, vacuolated cell in the rete pegs of the epithelium, is pathognomonic of Paget's disease. The differential diagnosis includes eczema, nipple duct adenoma, Bowen's disease, and most commonly, malignant melanoma. Identification of low-molecular-weight cytokeratin and C-*erb*B2 offers the highest sensitivity and specificity for the Paget's cells. The diagnostic workup begins with a thorough physical examination. Mammography is essential, particularly in the absence of a palpable mass, to detect subclinical mass lesions or microcalcifications. Cytological analysis of discharge or scrapings may be helpful as seen in this patient. Confirmation is obtained by full-thickness nipple biopsy, and we would also perform a needle localization biopsy of the subareolar calcifications.

The gold-standard treatment of Paget's is a modified radical mastectomy, and we would offer this treatment to this patient if her breast biopsy revealed invasive carcinoma with or without DCIS. We would also offer her adjuvant therapy based on the histological grade, margins, nodal involvement, and estrogen and progesterone receptor status of the invasive neoplasm. If the biopsy reveals only DCIS, we would perform a segmentectomy followed by radiotherapy, based on the early results of the National Surgical Adjuvant Breast and Bowel Protocol (NSABP) B-17. In other words, we would treat the underlying lesion no differently than if it had presented without nipple changes.

This also means that the same controversies regarding conservation therapy apply. The use of wide local excision with or without radiation therapy if the underlying lesion is DCIS may be answered by the B-17 trial of the NSABP. The controversy specific to Paget's disease and breast conservation pertains to limited nipple and areola excision when disease appears limited to the nipple. There is not enough evidence to support limited nipple and areola excision given the high incidence of underlying DCIS and/or invasive carcinoma.

This woman's development of Paget's disease has led to an earlier detection of her underlying disease and may have improved her prognosis. Paget's disease of the nipple does not negatively alter the prognosis of the underlying carcinoma. If the disease is limited to the nipple, it is considered carcinoma in situ and has a 90–100% 5-year survival rate.

Editors' comment: A recent collaborative study by Pierce et al. (*Cancer*, 1997) demonstrated acceptable local regional control in Paget's disease with wide local excision and radiation therapy.

BIBLIOGRAPHY

Bland KI, Vezeridis MP, Copeland EM. Breast. In: Schwartz SI, Daly JM, Galloway
    AC, Fischer JE, eds. Principles of Surgery, 7th ed. New York: McGraw-Hill,
    1998:533–599.
Fisher ER, Costantino J, Fisher B, et al. Pathologic findings from the National Sur-
    gical Adjuvant Breast and Bowel Project (NSABP) protocol B-17. Cancer
    1995; 75:1310–1319.
Jamali FR, Ricci A, Deckers PJ. Paget's disease of the nipple-areola complex. Surg
    Clin North Am 1996; 76:365–381.
Lagios MD, Page DL. In situ carcinoma of the breast: ductal carcinoma in situ,
    Paget's disease, lobular carcinoma in situ. In: Bland KI, Copeland EM, eds.
    The Breast: Comprehensive Management of Benign and Malignant Diseases,
    2nd ed. Philadelphia: WB Saunders, 1998:261–283.

H.3.   AXILLARY NODAL ADENOCARCINOMA OF UNKNOWN PRIMARY

Case #H.3.1
Goal: To discuss the management of adenocarcinoma of unknown primary presenting in the axillary lymph nodes

KEVIN R. FOX

*A 47-year-old woman presents with a palpable lymph node in the left
axilla. Excisional biopsy reveals metastatic adenocarcinoma of unknown
primary. A chest X-ray is negative, as are the remainder of the physical
examination and bilateral mammograms.*

The presence of adenocarcinoma in the axilla of a young woman must
be assumed to be breast carcinoma unless proven otherwise. Although other
adenocarcinomas of lung, stomach, and pancreas could theoretically present
in the axilla, such an event is decidedly uncommon. Whether one should
bother to evaluate the pancreas and stomach with appropriate radiographs is
not a subject of general agreement in patients such as this, and some authors
feel that the search for a "primary" tumor need not extend beyond a simple
chest X-ray. I see little harm in performing an abdominal computed-tomography scan and upper gastrointestinal series before embarking upon treatment for breast cancer, provided that the search for a breast primary has
been appropriately thorough.

The evaluation of our patient, who has an adenocarcinoma presenting
in the axilla, presumably in an axillary node, has already included a normal
physical examination and normal mammograms. At this point, she should

be considered a candidate for contrast-enhanced magnetic resonance imaging (MRI) scanning of the ipsilateral breast. Most MRI centers are not equipped with appropriate technical and expert tools for such breast-specific evaluation and referral to a center with experience in this regard should be sought. Our own center has been able to detect occult primary lesions in nearly 75% of patients who are clinically and mammographically normal. In such patients, we have then employed MRI-guided excisional biopsy to confirm the diagnosis and have followed a treatment course identical to patients whose diagnoses were rendered by more conventional means. When the diagnosis is confirmed, the patient will then undergo reexcision as necessary to obtain clear surgical margins as well as a level I and II axillary node dissection. Breast-conserving irradiation and adjuvant systemic therapy are given as in conventionally diagnosed patients. Whether this approach will achieve local control rates consistent with traditional breast conservation approaches remains to be seen. Of course, if the MRI scan suggests multifocal carcinoma, or if adequate surgical excision cannot be done, we recommend a modified radical mastectomy.

If MRI breast imaging is not available or if an MRI was obtained and was unrevealing, we must revert to a more conventional approach to the axillary carcinoma of presumed breast origin. The standard treatment under these circumstances is the modified radical mastectomy, which will succeed in revealing the occult primary lesion at pathological examination in approximately 60% of cases.

The use of primary radiation therapy in the absence of a detectable breast primary has been used as an alternative to mastectomy. The number of reported patients treated in this way is small. The incidence of in-breast recurrence has been approximately 10%.

If one chooses neither mastectomy nor radiation therapy, one should anticipate the eventual appearance of the breast primary at least 40% of the time. Therefore, this approach cannot be recommended.

It has been our institutional policy to recommend mastectomy to patients with undetectable primary lesions. We recommend breast-conserving therapy only to those patients whose MRI-detected primary lesions can be excised with an acceptable cosmetic result. In all instances, a formal axillary node dissection should be done. Recommendations for postoperative therapy (both systemic and radiotherapeutic) are best made when the actual number of positive axillary lymph nodes is elucidated. Finally, if hormone receptor analyses have not been performed on the original excised node, such analyses should be requested on paraffin-embedded sections.

The prognosis of patients with occult breast primary lesions and axillary presentations is felt to be somewhat better than that of patients presenting in a more typical fashion. In spite of this tendency, prudence suggests that recommendations for adjuvant systemic therapy in these patients should follow the same guidelines as proposed for breast cancer patients in general. Our patient, who is of premenopausal age and whose tumor is hormone-receptor-negative should receive a standard course of adjuvant therapy with a regimen such as CMF or a 3-month course of doxorubicin/cyclophosphamide following definitive measures of local-regional control. If her formal axillary node dissection reveals more than 10 involved axillary nodes, then consideration should be given to a more intensive therapeutic regimen, including high-dose chemotherapy and autologous stem-cell transplantation.

Editors' comment: The importance of a careful review of the histology of the unknown primary cannot be underestimated. The presence of hormone receptors would add further credence to the breast as the site of origin.

BIBLIOGRAPHY

Baron P, Moore M, Kinne D, et al. Occult breast cancer presenting with axillary metastases: updated management. Arch Surg 1990; 125:210.

Campana F, Fourquet A, Ashby MA. Presentation of axillary lymphadenopathy without detectable breast primary (T0N1b breast cancer): experience at Institute Curie. Radiother Oncol 1989; 15:321.

Ellerbroeck N, Holmes F, Singletary E. Treatment of isolated axillary metastases in patients with an occult primary consistent with breast. Int J Rad Oncol Biol Phys 1989; 17(Suppl):178.

Rosen P, Kimmel M. Occult breast carcinoma presenting with axillary lymph node metastases: a follow-up study of 48 patients. Hum Pathol 1990; 21:518.

H.4. LESS COMMON HISTOLOGIES

Case #H.4.1. Colloid Carcinoma
Goal: To discuss the management of colloid carcinoma

MICHAEL H. TOROSIAN

A 34-year-old woman presents with a biopsy-proven, 8-mm colloid carcinoma of the right breast detected on routine physical examination. Biopsy margins are negative. There is no palpable regional adenopathy.

Colloid carcinoma, also called mucinous carcinoma, is typically a slow-growing tumor with a better prognosis than routine infiltrating ductal carcinoma. Other variants of invasive breast carcinoma exhibiting improved prognosis compared to infiltrating ductal carcinoma include medullary, tubular, and papillary carcinomas. The histological features of colloid carcinoma include islands of tumor cells within a sea of mucin under low-power microscopy. Higher magnification shows nests of tumor cells that are generally uniform in appearance. The presence of an 8-mm colloid carcinoma implies a low-grade malignancy and an excellent prognosis.

The incidence of regional lymph node metastasis in this patient should be less than 5%. However, in the small subset of premenopausal patients with colloid carcinoma found to have axillary lymph node metastases, the recommendations for postoperative systemic therapy are drastically different than in the majority of patients found to be node negative. Therefore, in this premenopausal patient with a small colloid carcinoma, my recommendation is to perform a level I lymph node dissection. A level I lymph node dissection allows histological evaluation of the most lateral lymph nodes in the axilla and minimizes the risk of postoperative lymphedema. The standard axillary dissection performed for patients with typical infiltrating carcinomas includes removal of level I and II axillary lymph nodes. By removal of only level I axillary lymph nodes in this patient, additional collateral lymphatic flow is maintained to minimize the risk of subsequent lymphedema.

Two points deserve consideration in patients with colloid carcinoma or other carcinomas of low-grade histology. In postmenopausal patients in whom chemotherapy will not be administered regardless of the axillary node status, axillary lymph node dissection should not be performed. Axillary lymph node dissection should be reserved for those patients in whom the pathological findings will alter systemic therapy. Second, the technique of sentinel lymph node biopsy in breast cancer patients is currently under investigation and would be an excellent alternative to formal axillary dissection in patients with low-grade breast carcinomas. This technique involves injecting the site of the primary tumor with a blue dye (often in combination with a radioactive tracer). The sentinel lymph node(s) represents the initial site of metastasis from the breast region involved by the primary tumor. The sentinel lymph node is identified by making a small axillary incision and then visualizing the blue-stained and/or radioactive lymph node. Removal of this lymph node has reliably predicted axillary lymph node metastasis in preliminary clinical studies. Further investigation is required before this technique is accepted as standard surgical practice.

In summary, this patient presents with a small, low-grade breast carcinoma. Surgical management of the axilla in this situation depends on the age and menopausal status of the patient as these factors determine her subsequent clinical management.

Editors' comment: Although we agree with the expert's assessment that formal level I and II axillary lymph node dissection is generally unnecessary in women with clinically node-negative, good-prognosis histologies (tubular, colloid, papillary, and medullary), we do not support performance of a more limited level I only dissection. This operation may understage 10–15% of the time. We prefer an all-or-nothing approach; if node information is important, perform a formal lymphadenectomy. The sentinel technique described will likely make this point mute. As the technique is perfected, it is probable that almost all women with breast cancer will first undergo sentinel node biopsy, with formal level I and II dissection reserved for those patients whose sentinel node(s) contain metastatic tumor.

BIBLIOGRAPHY

Cady B, Stone M, Wayne J. New therapeutic possibilities in primary invasive breast cancer. Ann Surg 1993; 183:338.

Giuliano A, Kirgan D, Guenther J, et al. Lymphatic mapping and sentinel lymphadenectomy for breast cancer. Ann Surg 1994; 220:391.

Morrow M. The role of axillary node dissection in breast cancer management. Contemp Oncol 1994; 4:16.

Silverstein M, Gierson E, Waisman J, et al. Axillary lymph node dissection for T1a breast carcinoma: is it indicated? Cancer 1994; 73:664.

Case #H.4.2. Medullary Carcinoma
Goal: To discuss the management of medullary carcinoma

JAY K. HARNESS

A 63-year-old woman undergoes biopsy of a mammographically detected breast mass revealing a 2.1-cm medullary carcinoma. Margins are negative. The tumor is cytologically high grade. Axillary lymph node dissection demonstrates 0/17 nodes.

Medullary carcinoma of the breast is a term that has been used for decades to describe a large, solid tumor with a papillary or fleshy gross appearance. On gross inspection, a smaller medullary carcinoma can be confused with a fibroadenoma.

Medullary carcinomas are unusual tumors constituting fewer than 5–7% of breast cancers in centers with large experiences. Patients with medullary carcinoma tend to be relatively young with 40–60% of patients under 50 years. Bilaterality has been reported in as many as 18% of patients. Fewer than 10% of these neoplasms contain detectable estrogen or progesterone receptors. Medullary carcinoma is relatively uncommon in elderly patients. The intense lymphohistiocytic response in and about the tumor is often associated with benign enlargement of the ipsilateral axillary lymph nodes and often contributes to erroneous clinical staging of disease.

It is generally agreed that it is necessary to follow strictly defined morphological criteria if the diagnosis of medullary carcinoma is to be predictive of a favorable prognosis. In 1977, Ridolfi et al. more precisely defined medullary breast carcinoma by grouping several histological criteria. This work allowed a more reproducible classification of medullary carcinoma, which also demonstrated its better prognosis. For a tumor to be classified as medullary carcinoma it should have all of the following definitive characteristics:

1. A lymphoplasmacytic reaction that involves the periphery and is diffusely present in the substance of the tumor. The lymphoplasmacytic infiltrates are often a mixture of lymphocytes (peripherally) and plasma cells (centrally).
2. Microscopic circumscription of the border of the infiltrating carcinoma. The edge of the tumor should have a smooth, rounded contour that appears to push aside rather than infiltrate the breast.
3. A syncytial pattern (one in which the tumor growth is arranged in broad, irregular sheets or islands) in which borders of individual cells are indistinct.
4. Poorly differentiated nuclear grade and high mitotic rate.

Other features that may be found in medullary carcinoma include intraductal carcinoma at the periphery of nearly half of these tumors, necrosis within zones of syncytial epithelial growth, and metaplastic changes (in a minority of tumors).

Medullary carcinoma is one of the fastest-growing carcinomas of the breast. High nuclear grade and high mitotic index correlate with DNA aneuploidy and high S-phase fraction. Paradoxically, in medullary carcinomas, DNA aneuploidy and high S-phase fractions have not been associated with poor outcomes as is the case in other infiltrating ductal carcinomas.

The size of the primary tumor and axillary nodal status are significant determinants of survival for patients with medullary carcinoma. While this group of patients tends to have a lower incidence of axillary metastasis, a tumor size of 3 cm or less is a very important prognostic indicator. Patients with tumors 3 cm or less have reported 10-year survival rates of approximately 90%. When the same group of smaller tumors is also node negative, 10-year survival rates of 97% have been reported.

Mastectomy is the most frequently reported modality of primary treatment of medullary carcinoma. No large series exist on lumpectomy with adjuvant whole-breast radiotherapy, although local recurrence rates following lumpectomy and radiation therapy have been reported to be acceptable. Few reports exist on the use of adjuvant chemotherapy for this entity. Since most of these tumors are ER negative, there appears to be little justification to recommend the use of tamoxifen.

This case describes a patient with an excellent prognosis based on the tumor size of 2.1 cm and lymph node negativity (T2N0). A completion mastectomy would offer this patient a 95% 10-year disease-free survival. If the patient is motivated for breast conservation, the issue of ipsilateral breast recurrence needs to be considered. Recurrences tend to occur early in the clinical course of patients with medullary carcinoma, with very few women having recurrences 5 years or more after diagnosis.

I would favor breast conservation in this patient provided adjuvant whole-breast radiotherapy was included in the treatment regimen. Her resection margins were negative and radiotherapy may be of benefit when used as an adjuvant given its success as primary treatment of medullary carcinoma as reported in small series. Additional trials of patients treated by lumpectomy and radiotherapy for less advanced medullary carcinoma will be needed to determine the effectiveness of breast conservation in the management of medullary carcinoma. Unfortunately, it may take a long time to accrue sufficient numbers of patients given the low frequency of this type of infiltrating breast carcinoma.

BIBLIOGRAPHY

Cook DL, Weaver DL. Comparison of DNA content, S-phase fraction and survival between medullary and ductal carcinoma of the breast. Am J Clin Pathol 1995; 104(1):17–22.

Pedersen L, Zedeler K, Holck S, et al. Medullary carcinoma of the breast. Prevalence and prognostic importance of classical risk factors in breast cancer. Eur J Cancer 1995; 31A(13–14):2289–2295.

Rapin V, Contesso G, Mouriesse H, et al. Medullary breast carcinoma. A reevaluation of 95 cases of breast cancer with inflammatory stroma. Cancer 1988; 61:2503–2510.

Reinfuss M, Stelmach A, Mitus J, et al. Typical medullary carcinoma of the breast: a clinical and pathological analysis of 52 cases. J Surg Oncol 1995; 60(2):89–94.

Ridolfi R, Rosen P, Port A, et al. Medullary carcinoma of the breast. A clinicopathologic study with 10 year follow-up. Cancer 1977; 40:1365–1385.

Case #H.4.3. Anaplastic Carcinoma
Goal: To discuss the management of anaplastic carcinoma

MICHAEL H. TOROSIAN

A healthy, 71-year-old woman presents for an opinion regarding adjuvant therapy following modified radical mastectomy for a 2.4-cm anaplastic carcinoma of the breast; 2/21 lymph nodes were positive.

Anaplastic breast carcinoma is an aggressive, rapidly growing cancer associated with a poor prognosis. Anaplastic breast carcinomas typically exhibit high histological grade, high nuclear grade, aneuploidy, and high S-phase fraction, and are usually hormone receptor negative. These tumors have a high propensity to metastasize to regional lymph nodes and distant sites.

Because of the aggressive nature of these tumors, complete radiological staging is indicated at the time of presentation. Chest X-ray, bone scan, and computed-tomography scan of the abdomen should be performed to identify pulmonary, skeletal, and hepatic and intra-abdominal metastases, respectively. In this case, definitive surgical treatment consisted of modified radical mastectomy with two of 21 axillary lymph nodes being positive for regional metastatic disease.

Radiation therapy is not indicated in this patient as she has undergone modified radical mastectomy for local/regional control. Indications for radiation therapy following mastectomy include involvement of four or more axillary lymph nodes, extracapsular extension of carcinoma in the involved axillary lymph nodes, or microscopically positive margins of surgical resection.

Adjuvant therapy in postmenopausal, node-positive, hormone-receptor-negative patients remains controversial. Results from existing clinical trials lack consistency for defining a standard treatment recommendation. However, in this 71-year-old patient with an aggressive carcinoma and high risk of recurrence and metastasis, combined chemohormonal therapy should be considered. MUGA cardiac scanning should be performed to determine cardiac ejection fraction if an adriamycin-containing regimen is being considered. Although tamoxifen should theoretically have little effect on outcome in patients with hormone-receptor-negative tumors, several large clinical trials demonstrate efficacy when treating postmenopausal patients with tamoxifen alone and when combined with polychemotherapy regimens. Clinical trials are currently underway to determine the optimal chemohormonal regimen for this challenging group of patients.

BIBLIOGRAPHY

Early Breast Cancer Trialist Collaborative Group. Systemic treatment of early breast cancer by hormonal, cytotoxic, or immune therapy. Lancet 1992; 339(1):71.

Falkson HE, Gray RG, Wolberg WH, et al. Adjuvant trial of 12 cycles of CMFPT followed by observation or continuous tamoxifen versus 4 cycles of CMFPT in postmenopausal women with breast cancer: an Eastern Cooperative Oncology Group phase III study. J Clin Oncol 1990; 8:599.

Goldhirsch A, Belber R. Adjuvant chemo-endocrine therapy or endocrine therapy alone for postmenopausal patients: Ludwig studies III and IV. In: Senn HJ, Goldhirsch A, Gelber RD, et al, eds. Recent Results in Cancer Research. Adjuvant Therapy of Primary Breast Cancer. Berlin Heidelberg: Springer-Verlag Berlin Heidelberg, 1989:153–162.

Taylor SG, Knuiman MW, Sleeper LA, et al. Six-year results of the Easter Cooperative Oncology Group trail of observation versus CMFP versus CMFPT in postmenopausal patients with node-positive breast cancer. J Clin Oncol 1989; 7:879.

Case #H.4.4. Secretory Carcinoma
Goal: To discuss the features and treatment of secretory carcinoma

JAY K. HARNESS

A 23-year-old woman undergoes left breast biopsy for a palpable mass. Pathology demonstrates a 1.4-cm secretory carcinoma. Margins are negative.

Secretory carcinoma of the breast is one of the rarest types of invasive breast cancer. To date, fewer than 100 cases have been reported in the world's literature. It was first described in children under the name of juvenile carcinoma by McDivitt and Stewart in 1966. While secretory carcinoma is the most common variant of breast cancer in children, this tumor more commonly occurs in adults. A 1980 study from the Armed Forces Institute of Pathology had 19 patients with a median age of 25 years (range 9–69 years). This carcinoma has been reported in adult women up to age 73 and in girls at or before age 5. Secretory carcinoma has also rarely occurred in both boys, usually younger then 10 years of age, and men, often in their 20s.

Most patients present with a painless, well-circumscribed mass that may have been present for years. A subareolar tumor is the most common location in prepubertal children and males because most of their breast tissue is localized to this region. Subareolar lesions have been associated with nipple discharge.

These well-circumscribed cancers may occur in any quadrant of the breast. No evidence of a hormonal abnormality has been described that would explain the secretory properties of these tumors. Secretory carcinoma has not been associated with pregnancy. Secretory breast carcinoma has been seen in association with other conditions including juvenile papillomatosis and gynecomastia.

The gross and microscopic pathology of these tumors is interesting. Most tumors are 3 cm or less in diameter, firm, and well circumscribed. Rarely, the tumor has infiltrative margins. These tumors vary in color from shades of white to gray, or tan to yellow.

Secretory carcinoma is a form of ductal carcinoma. The intraductal growth pattern is most commonly papillary or cribriform. The borders are well circumscribed microscopically. The most characteristic feature of the tumor is very prominent intra- and extracellular secretions. In most cells there are prominent intracytoplasmic lumina filled with globoid homogeneous secretions of different tinctorial quality, from pale basophilic to intensely eosinophilic. The nuclei are small, round, and cytologically low-grade. The secretions are often vacuolated or bubbly, reacting positively for mucin and with PAS reaction.

Given the rarity of this form of breast cancer, it is not easy to give a clear statement on prognosis or the optimal form of therapy. In general, the majority of patients have a low-grade clinical course resulting in a good prognosis. Axillary lymph node involvement has been described in both adults and children. Rates of axillary spread vary considerably in published reports. Most series report on five or fewer patients. The rate of axillary involvement averages under 20% and rarely are more than three lymph nodes involved. Slow growth and delayed recurrence are characteristic of many of these tumors. Death from systemic metastases is rare.

The most common form of treatment reported in the literature is mastectomy. Local excision is the preferred initial treatment in children. It is necessary to obtain negative margins, which may require a wider excision in postmenarcheal children and adults. The role of adjuvant whole-breast radiation therapy and systemic adjuvant chemotherapy is unclear as so few patients have been treated with these modalities. Reports on estrogen and progesterone receptor status, as well as flow cytometric analysis, are too few in number to allow any firm conclusions. It appears that diploid DNA content and low S-phase fraction are the usual findings.

The case presented for discussion is that of a 23-year-old woman with a 1.4-cm secretory carcinoma excised with negative margins. If there is no palpable axillary adenopathy, it is hard to justify an axillary dissection since there does not appear to be a role for adjuvant chemotherapy even if the nodes were positive. Systemic failure is rare with this disease.

In making management recommendations, local/regional control of secretory carcinoma is an important factor. Enlarged axillary lymph nodes would justify a level I and II axillary dissection to control disease in the axilla. Slow growth and late recurrence of this tumor mean that long-term follow-up of 20 years or more is necessary to determine the biological behavior in individual patients. Local recurrence within the breast would warrant mastectomy.

The treatment of secretory carcinoma of the breast should be tailored to the circumstances of the individual patient. Some patients may want mastectomy to decrease their concerns about ipsilateral recurrence. Others, with small tumors and negative margins after lumpectomy, may be happy with diligent long-term follow-up.

I would favor the latter approach if the patient was willing.

BIBLIOGRAPHY

Krausz T, Jenkins D, Grontoft O, et al. Secretory carcinoma of the breast in adults: emphasis on late recurrence and metastasis. Histopathology 1989; 14:25–36.

McDivitt RW, Stewart FW. Breast carcinoma in children. JAMA 1966; 195:388–390.

Oberman HA. Secretory carcinoma of the breast in adults. Am J Surg Pathol 1980; 4:465–470.

Rosen PP, Carnor ML. Secretory carcinoma of the breast. Arch Pathol Lab Med 1991; 115:141–144.

Serour F, Gilad A, Kopolovic J, Krispin M. Secretory breast cancer in children and adolescence: a report of a case and review of the literature. Med Pediatr Oncol 1992; 20:341–344.

Tauassoli FA, Norris HJ. Secretory carcinoma of the breast. Cancer 1980; 45:2404–2413.

Tranimura A, Konaka K. Carcinoma of the breast in a 5 year old girl. Acta Pathol Jpn 1980; 30:157–160.

H.5.   PHYLLODES TUMOR

Case #H.5.1. Phyllodes Tumor
Goal: To discuss the features and mangement of phyllodes tumors

VERNON K. SONDAK and JULIE A. WOLFE

A 34-year-old woman undergoes excision of a presumed fibroadenoma. Pathology reveals a 4.1-cm, intermediate-grade, malignant phyllodes tumor.

Phyllodes tumors—previously referred to as cystosarcoma phyllodes —are rare, sometimes malignant tumors that share clinical and pathological features with fibroadenomas. Phyllodes tumors are about 2–4.4% as common as fibroadenoma. They are most often diagnosed in the fourth decade, 10–20 years older than for fibroadenomas. Like fibroadenomas, phyllodes tumors arise in the stromal elements of the breast but have epithelial components as well. As in the present case, phyllodes tumors are frequently mistaken clinically for fibroadenomas, and occasionally for breast cancers (the diagnosis is rarely made preoperatively). Compared to fibroadenomas, phyllodes tumors tend to be larger, faster growing and somewhat less well circumscribed. Indeed, these tumors are named "phyllodes" (leaf-like) as their histological margins usually show long projections that extend into the surrounding breast parenchyma. On mammography, a phyllodes tumor may appear as large, well-circumscribed lesion similar to a fibroadenoma, or as an ill-defined, noncalcified mass that may be lobulated. Ultrasound may suggest a nonspecific hypoechoic mass or fluid-filled clefts within a solid mass.

The term "cystosarcoma phyllodes" was abandoned because only about one-quarter of phyllodes tumors are malignant. Although occasional cases of phyllodes tumor can be difficult to classify as either benign or malignant, in most cases the pathologist can discriminate based on standard features of cellular atypia and pleomorphism, the number of mitoses per high-powered field, the presence or absence of spontaneous necrosis, evidence of infiltrating margins, and the degree of stromal overgrowth. It is helpful for the pathologist to assign to malignant lesions a histological grade using a staging system similar to that used for soft tissue sarcomas, as was done in the present case.

Treatment is tailored to the histological findings, but includes a wide excision in all cases. At least 20% of these tumors will recur within the breast after narrow excision. Recurrences usually have the same histological appearance of the initial tumor but may be more aggressive, including transition to malignancy in a previously "benign" lesion.

Mastectomy is not required as the initial treatment for benign or malignant phyllodes tumors, provided an adequately wide excision (generally taking at least 2-cm margins of normal breast tissue) can be performed with a cosmetic result acceptable to the patient. Axillary dissection is not employed except in the rare event of documented regional spread, which occurs in less than 5% of cases. Postoperative radiation is considered after adequate excision in patients with intermediate- or high-grade malignant lesions, but generally not for low-grade and never for benign tumors. Local recurrence of a phyllodes tumor previously excised with a 2–3-cm margin should generally be treated with mastectomy; radiation should be considered postoperatively for recurrence of a malignant lesion initially treated with wide excision alone. No definite role for adjuvant chemotherapy has been established in breast sarcomas of any histology, including malignant phyllodes tumors. Generalizing from current standards in the treatment of nonbreast soft tissue sarcomas, adjuvant chemotherapy is generally reserved for patients with high-grade sarcomas greater than 5 cm in maximal diameter or intermediate-grade sarcomas greater than 8–10 cm. Utilizing these criteria, few patients with phyllodes tumors should be considered for such treatment.

Although approximately 25% of phyllodes tumors have histological features of malignancy, metastases only occur in about 6% of cases. Metastatic disease usually occurs in the lungs, followed less often by spread to bones, liver, and other sites. Treatment of metastases is similar to that of sarcomas originating elsewhere in the body: resection of isolated metastases where feasible and systemic chemotherapy for unresectable disease. Among 67 reported cases of metastatic disease, the average survival time after diagnosis of metastases was 30 months. The longest survival period was 14.5 years.

In summary, we would recommend wide reexcision without mastectomy, followed by postoperative radiation. Axillary node dissection would not be indicated in the absence of clinical evidence of nodal involvement. A baseline chest X-ray and chest computed-tomography scan would be useful because of the potential for later pulmonary metastases. We would follow the patient at least twice yearly after the completion of treatment, with physical examinations and chest X-rays at each visit and with bilateral mammograms annually. It is worth noting that these recommendations would be essentially the same for most other intermediate-grade breast sarcomas, even if not of the phyllodes type.

BIBLIOGRAPHY

Kessinger A, Foley JF, Lemon HM, Miller DM. Metastatic cystosarcoma phyllodes: a case report and review of the literature. J Surg Oncol 1972; 4:131–147.
Petrek JA: Phyllodes tumors. In: Harris JR, Lippman ME, Morrow M, Hellman S, eds. Diseases of the Breast. Philadelphia: Lippincott-Raven, 1996:863–869.

H.6.   CNS METASTASES

Case #H.6.1
Goal: To discuss the management of a solitary brain metastasis

ROBERT S. DIPAOLA

A 43-year-old woman, 2 years post adjuvant chemotherapy with CAF for stage II, estrogen-receptor-negative breast cancer, presents with headache and diplopia. A CT scan is consistent with a solitary metastasis to the right frontal cortex. The remainder of the metastatic workup is negative. She denies fever, chills, stiff neck, recent travel, or history of HIV.

The initial management of a CNS mass depends on the certainty of the diagnosis. If uncertainty exists, a biopsy must be obtained. Reasons for uncertainty include a history of breast cancer with a low risk of recurrence and the inability to differentiate between menigiomas, brain abscesses, or infarcts on initial radiographic studies. Patients with a low risk of recurrence include those patients who are stage I, characterized by no axillary lymph node involvement and a small (<2 cm) primary mass. Such patients have less than a 10% risk of recurrence in their lifetime and, therefore, have a greater chance that a solitary metastasis is secondary to another disease process or malignancy. For example, patients with carcinoma of the breast have a higher incidence of cerebral meningioma, which may look similar to a solitary brain metastasis on computed-tomography (CT) scan.

In this regard, magnetic resonance imaging (MRI) should be performed in all patients prior to surgery, since an MRI is superior to a CT scan in distinguishing masses such as meningioma from cancer and may demonstrate smaller additional lesions that could not be discerned by the CT scan. However, the accuracy of the MRI should not be overestimated. Although some degree of certainty can be obtained, the gold standard for diagnosis of a solitary brain lesion is biopsy. Prior studies have demonstrated that CT or MRI is incorrect in diagnosing a solitary brain metastasis in a patient with breast cancer 11% of the time. Therefore, some degree of uncertainty exists if a treatment decision is made without biopsy.

In addition to being diagnostic, resection of a solitary metastasis followed by radiation therapy is therapeutic. A randomized study conducted at the University of Kentucky Medical Center assessed the efficacy of surgical resection of brain metastases in 48 patients. Overall survival was significantly longer in the group that had surgery followed by radiation in comparison to patients who received radiation alone. The authors also concluded that only patients with a life expectancy of at least 2 months would benefit from surgery, since the median length of time that performance status was maintained at pretreatment levels was about 2 months in patients treated with radiotherapy alone. Therefore, the resection of a solitary brain metastasis should be considered in a patient with minimal or controllable metastatic disease. Patients with progressive uncontrolled metastatic disease would not likely live long enough to derive a benefit from this procedure.

Considering both the diagnostic and therapeutic benefits, the resection of a solitary brain metastasis followed by radiation therapy in this case would be appropriate. Resection followed by radiation therapy is likely to be beneficial even in the presence of visceral metastasis elsewhere, given the likelihood of control with systemic therapy.

Chemotherapy alone, in contrast to local therapy with surgery and radiation as treatment for a solitary metastasis, traditionally has had little role. Therefore, the use of systemic therapy should be to control systemic disease. However, recent data suggest that chemotherapy can cross the blood-brain barrier when metastases are present. Rosner et al. described 100 patients with brain metastases initially treated with systemic chemotherapy. The response rate was 50% with a median duration of remission of 10 months for complete responders and 7 months for partial responders. Additional data suggest that hormonal therapy is also effective in the treatment of brain metastases in patients whose tumors express the estrogen receptor.

Editors' comment: An alternative strategy for patients with solitary brain metastases is stereotaxic radiosurgery followed by whole-brain irradiation. This may be consider in lieu of surgical resection.

BIBLIOGRAPHY

Early Breast Cancer Trialists' Collaborative Group. Systemic treatment of early breast cancer by hormonal, cytotoxic, or immune therapy. Lancet 1992; 339: 1–71.

Mehta D, Khatib R, Patel S. Carcinoma of the breast and meningioma: association and management. Cancer 1983; 51:1937.

Patchell RA, Tibbs PA, Walsh JW, et al. A randomized trial of surgery in the treatment of single metastasis to the brain. N Engl J Med 1990; 322:494.

Pors H, von Eyben FE, Sorensen OS, et al. Long-term remission of multiple brain metastases with tamoxifen. J Neuro-Oncol 1991; 10:173–177.

Rosner D, Nemeto T, Lane W. Chemotherapy induces regression of brain metastasis in breast carcinoma. Cancer 1986; 58:832–839.

Case #H.6.2
Goal: Evaluation and treatment of postmenopausal women relapsing with brain metastases

JOSEPH AISNER

A 65-year-old woman, 7 years post adjuvant treatment for breast cancer with tamoxifen for stage II hormone-receptor-positive disease, presents with headache and diplopia. A CT scan of the head is consistent with metastatic disease. The remainder of the metastatic workup is negative.

Patients with malignant disease who develop brain lesions, even many years after the initial diagnosis, must be considered to have metastases from the original primary until proven otherwise. Careful history, physical examination, and detailed analysis of risk factors are important in order to consider other causes, including new primaries (with brain metastases), metastatic infectious lesions, or meningiomas.

In addition to considering metastases from the primary breast cancer, a detailed history reveals whether the patient was a smoker. Women who continue to smoke after breast-sparing surgery and breast (or chest wall) irradiation are at a slightly increased risk of developing lung cancer. In the absence of fevers, chills, and recent infections, infectious lesions would be unlikely. Finally, women with breast cancer have an increased incidence of meningioma, and careful review of the location of the lesion often provides greater likelihood of defining the most likely etiology.

The number and size of intracranial lesions can also help distinguish between some of the possibilities. Multiple ring-enhancing lesions seen in patients with prior breast cancer tend to predict for metastases from the primary source. A biopsy is desirable to validate the diagnosis; however, a biopsy may depend on accessibility of the lesion and the potential for CNS damage. In most cases, stereotaxic biopsies can be performed without complications. However, in the presence of multiple lesions, it is likely that the therapeutic response to a variety of malignancies will be similar, regardless of diagnosis, and if a biopsy is not easily obtained, one might justifiably begin treatment with steroids and palliative radiotherapy.

In the event of a single, isolated intracranial lesion, neurosurgical consultation is warranted. Patients who undergo resection for a single intracranial metastasis appear to do considerably better than patients who receive cranial irradiation with or without additional treatments. This outcome is logical since surgical debulking may achieve better local control. The ability of radiation therapy to control disease is related to the size of the mass. The dose of radiation therapy needed to sterilize the field rises exponentially with the diameter of the mass. Thus, surgically debulking this lesion would produce a greater probability of achieving durable CNS control.

The assessment for surgical resectability generally rests on the anatomical location of the metastatic lesion. If the lesion is superficial or if removing the lesion is likely to produce little sensory or motor deficit, then surgical excision is clearly warranted (in the absence of medical contraindications to anesthesia and surgery). If, however, the excision of the lesion is likely to leave the patient with significant impairment, one must then balance the magnitude of the impairment and the quality of life achieved by removing the lesion versus the improvement of CNS control. Since brain metastases still define stage IV disease, if the surgery is likely to destroy functionality, one would not likely recommend this approach.

For the patient who develops brain metastases from breast cancer, the standard approach is whole-brain irradiation with boosts to areas of involvement and/or surgical excision (depending on the presence of a resectable, single lesion) followed by whole-brain irradiation. Initially, patients are given steroids to reduce edema and reduce the chance of neuronal loss from progressive intracranial pressure. The steroids are continued through the beginning of radiation therapy and then slowly tapered while carefully monitoring the neurological status to assess changes. Whole-brain irradiation is generally delivered in 10–15 fractions (300–240 cGy per fraction). Subsequent evaluation with MRI or CT contrast studies, 4–6 weeks after completion of radiotherapy, can sometimes define the level of CNS control. Few small residual lesions can sometimes undergo further therapy with radiosurgery techniques.

In recent years some investigators noted that chemotherapy occasionally produced regression of metastatic brain lesions. While the blood-brain barrier will not permit most agents that are useful for breast cancer to enter the CNS, overt metastases generally disturb the blood-brain barrier, and thus some of these agents can enter into the tumor. Therefore, it is not surprising that highly responsive tumors may show response when located in the CNS. However, the probability of producing an antitumor response with chemotherapy in the brain is considerably lower than the probability of achieving response with radiotherapy. Thus, chemotherapy should not be used as a substitute for radiotherapy, unless the patient has previously received cranial irradiation. In this setting, some of the newer agents, such as topotecan, may prove to be useful since it appears to penetrate the blood-brain barrier. However, in a theoretical concept, debulking the intracranial metastases may allow the subsequent brain irradiation to achieve better local control. Thus, in some instances in which the patient appears to be stable and can be carefully observed, one might start with chemotherapy, observe the course of the neurological signs and symptoms, and be prepared to intervene with immediate brain irradiation.

In the unusual instance in which a patient develops (or presents with) a single (isolated) CNS metastasis that has been resected and then irradiated, such patients are considered to be stage IV with no evidence of disease (NED). Since patients with stage IV disease will eventually develop metastases in other sites, one might justifiably ask whether adding chemotherapy is likely to change survival. There are only scanty data on this approach. In a series of abstracts presented from the M.D. Anderson Cancer Center, the investigators followed a group of patients with single metastases and administered FAC chemotherapy after the patients have been rendered "disease free." When this heterogeneous population was compared to historical controls, the investigators felt that the addition of early chemotherapy improved survival. While this work has been presented in abstract form, it has yet to be published in a final manuscript, and there is, as yet, no prospective evaluation of whether this approach can change outcome. Whether one can justify using chemotherapy and generating side effects when the patient is otherwise disease free must be given serious consideration with respect to the toxicity of chemotherapy and potential benefit that might be gained. As there is little evidence that this approach will cure patients, it is not recommended outside a study setting.

BIBLIOGRAPHY

Boogerd W, Dalesio O, Bais E, et al. Response of brain metastases from breast cancer to systemic chemotherapy. Cancer 1992; 69:972–980.

Borgelt B, Gelber R, Kramer S, et al. Ultra-rapid high dose irradiation schedules for the palliation of brain metastases: final results of the first two studies by the Radiation Therapy Oncology Group. Int J Radiat Oncol Biol Phys 1981; 7: 1633–1638.

Ferrara M, Bizzozzero F, Talamonti G, et al: Surgical treatment of 100 single brain metastases. J Neurolog Sci 1990; 34:303.

Holmes FA, Buzdar AU, Kau S-W, et al. Combined modality approach for patients with isolated recurrences of breast cancer (IV-NED). Breast Dis 1994; 7:7.

Patchell RA, Tibbs PA, Walsh JW, et al. A randomized trial of surgery in the treatment of single metastases to the brain. N Engl J Med 1990; 322:494.

Sunderaresan N, Galicich J. Surgical treatment of brain metastases: clinical and computerized tomography evaluation of the results of treatment. Cancer 1985; 55:1382.

H.7.   MENINGEAL CARCINOMATOSIS

Case #H.7.1
Goal: To discuss the management of meningeal carcinomatosis

THOMAS N. BYRNE

A 65-year-old woman, 7 years after adjuvant treatment for a stage II, hormone-receptor-positive breast cancer with tamoxifen, presents with diplopia. Examination reveals right 6th and 4th cranial nerve palsies. A CT scan of the head is negative for metastatic disease. The remainder of the metastatic workup is negative. She denies fever, chills, stiff neck, recent travel, or history of Lyme disease.

The neurological evaluation of the patient with a history of breast cancer and diplopia with no history of metastases presents a broad differ-

ential diagnosis; while this neurological abnormality may be the first manifestation of metastatic disease, one must not overlook an unrelated disorder.
In this case, diplopia may be due to disease in the brainstem (e.g., metastasis,
stroke, or less likely, given her age and lack of neurological history, de-
myelinating disease); or cranial nerves as they pass through the subarachnoid
space or epidural space of the cavernous sinus, superior orbital fissure, or
orbit (e.g., metastases or temporal arteritis); or neuromuscular junction disease (i.e., myasthenia gravis); muscle disease; or eye disease (e.g., retinal
metastases). Approaching the differential diagnosis in this fashion helps with
the localization as well as narrowing the differential diagnosis. From the
history, I would want to know whether the diplopia is associated with pain,
either headache or eye pain. Metastases to the cavernous sinus, superior
orbital fissure, and orbit are often painful and because of their small size
are often missed on routine computed-tomography (CT) scanning unless the
region of interest is specifically scanned looking for a metastatic deposit.
Patients with leptomeningeal metastases often have symptoms and/or signs
at multiple levels of the neuraxis; among these are headache or back pain.
Patients with temporal arteritis usually complain of headache and/or jaw
claudication.

  To further pursue a diagnosis of leptomeningeal metastases, I would
look for symptoms of cortical dysfunction (e.g., memory loss, dysphasia,
inattention), other cranial nerve symptoms (e.g., dysarthria, hearing loss),
and spinal cord or root disease (e.g., radiculopathic pain such as ''sciatica''
and sphincter disturbance). Again, symptoms of involvement at multiple
levels of the neuraxis, cerebral cortex, brainstem, spinal cord, and roots or
cauda equina suggest leptomeningeal disease. I would want to know the
duration of the diplopia and whether it was present in the morning upon
awakening or it occurred later in the day. The hallmark of myasthenia gravis
is weakness that develops after use of the muscle and, furthermore, is painless. I would query whether the patient had any other neurological symptoms
to suggest other cranial neuropathies, e.g., dysarthria, hearing loss, or sphincter disturbance. In considering disease of the brainstem itself, tailor the neurological examination to search for long tract signs.

  The workup of diplopia requires a detailed image of the posterior fossa
including brainstem, subarachnoid space, cavernous sinus, skull base, and
orbits. Magnetic resonance imaging (MRI) is significantly more sensitive
than CT scanning, but when metastases are being sought contrast enhancement is necessary to identify small parenchymal metastases or leptomeningeal metastases. MRI scanning may reveal several abnormalities in patients
with leptomeningeal metastases including leptomeningeal, subependymal,
dural, or cranial nerve enhancement; superficial cerebral metastases; intra-
medullary or leptomeningeal spinal metastases; and dilated ventricles due to

communicating hydrocephalus. In a study of 128 patients suspected of harboring leptomeningeal metastases, Freilich and colleagues found abnormal neuroimaging results in 70 patients (55%). If a diagnosis is not established, a lumbar puncture may be necessary to identify leptomeningeal metastases and look for other inflammatory diseases such as Lyme disease, other infection, or inflammatory disease. It is recognized that the yield of positive cytologies increases with greater volumes of CSF with each lumbar puncture. Many physicians send a minimum of 5 cc for cytological evaluation with each tap. If the first tap shows a negative cytology, then two or three repeat lumbar punctures may increase the yield. Despite multiple lumbar punctures, the cytology may remain negative. In the study by Freilich et al. cited above, cytology was positive in only 53 of 115 patients (46%).

Wasserstrom and colleagues reported the CSF results from 90 patients with leptomeningeal metastases from solid tumors. The most sensitive, albeit nonspecific, finding was elevated protein. These authors found an abnormal protein (>50 mg/dl) in 80% of patients undergoing multiple taps. Furthermore, they found CSF pleocytosis (>5/mm^3) in 65% but a low sugar (<40 mg/dl) in only 37%. Elevated CSF pressure was found in 64%. In their study, at least one abnormality was found on the initial CSF analysis in 97%; among patients undergoing multiple taps at least one abnormality was seen in 99%. Thus, while a positive CSF cytology may prove elusive, almost all patients with leptomeningeal metastases have some abnormality in their CSF. In patients in whom there is no evidence for metastatic disease elsewhere and who have negative CSF cytologies, it is important to exclude infectious and inflammatory causes of neurological dysfunction.

The treatment of leptomeningeal metastases from breast cancer is palliative. Since the diagnosis of leptomeningeal metastases is a diagnosis of malignant cells throughout the craniospinal axis, therapy must be directed at the entire neuraxis. Since total neuraxis irradiation compromises a large volume of bone marrow, treatment usually consists of irradiation of symptomatic sites and administration of intrathecal chemotherapy. The most commonly used agents for intrathecal chemotherapy are methotrexate, cytosine arabinoside, and thiotepa.

In a recent retrospective study of outcomes of patients with leptomeningeal metastases from breast cancer, Fizazi et al. compared patients treated before 1988 with intrathecal methotrexate, 15 mg once per week, with patients treated from 1989 to 1994 with high-dose methotrexate (MTX) (15 mg daily $\times$ 5 days repeated every 2 weeks and intrathecal hydrocortisone acetate, 125 mg on day 1, and folinic acid, 10 mg intramuscularly after each methotrexate injection). Most patients also received systemic treatment and radiation therapy. Median survival was 14 weeks for patients receiving the high-dose MTX regimen compared to 7 weeks for patients receiving the conventional regimen. The improved survival, however, carried a greater risk of hematological toxicity; grade 3 or 4 neutropenia occurred in 39% of patients treated with high-dose MTX compared to 33% treated with conventional MTX doses. In a univariate analysis, the authors found three prognostic factors that predicted response to therapy: controlled systemic disease at diagnosis; low initial CSF protein (<500 mg/dl); and systemic chemotherapy during intrathecal chemotherapy.

BIBLIOGRAPHY

Bleyer WA, Byrne TN. Leptomeningeal cancer in leukemia and solid tumors. Curr Probl Cancer 1988; 12:185–238.
Fizazi K, Asselain B, Vincent-Salomon A, et al. Meningeal carcinomatosis in patients with breast carcinoma. Clinical features, prognostic factors, and results of a high-dose intrathecal methotrexate regimen. Cancer 1996; 77:1315–1323.
Freilich R, Krol G, DeAngelis L. Neuroimaging and cerebrospinal fluid cytology in the diagnosis of leptomeningeal metastasis. Ann Neurol 1995; 38:51–57.
Wasserstrom WR, Glass JP, Posner JB. Diagnosis and treatment of leptomeningeal metastases from solid tumors: experience with 90 patients. Cancer 1982; 49: 759–772.

Case #H.7.2. Metastatic Epidural Spinal Cord Compression
Goal: To discuss the recognition and management of spinal cord compression

THOMAS N. BYRNE

A 55-year-old woman with a history of breast cancer metastatic to the lung presents with a history of progressive back and leg pain for 6 weeks. She reports that she had low back pain and sciatica periodically when she was in her 20s and 30s. The present pain is also in the low back but radiates into her anterior thigh and is not relieved by recumbency.

This patient with metastatic breast cancer and a new pain syndrome is at high risk for metastasis as the source of pain. In this case the patient thought the pain was her old "sciatica" returning. The features that distinguish sciatica from disc disease or lumbar spondylosis in this case are the location of the pain in the anterior thigh (L2 or L3) rather than in the posterior thigh and calf (L4, L5, or S1 distribution), the latter being the far more common location for lumbar spondylotic radiculopathy. Of course, there is no reason that a metastatic deposit cannot lodge in the lower lumbar spine causing a pain distribution identical to lumbar spondylotic radiculopathy. The other feature, which is consistent with metastatic disease, is that the pain is not relieved by bed rest. Unlike the pain of spondylotic disease, which is usually relieved by bed rest, pain from epidural metastatic disease to the spine may be unrelieved or even aggravated by bed rest.

Being concerned that this pain syndrome may be more than just "sciatica from arthritis," I would ask the patient to determine whether there are symptoms of metastatic disease elsewhere causing pain. I would consider leptomeningeal metastases in my differential diagnosis and seek to determine if there were symptoms of neurological dysfunction elsewhere along the neuraxis. I would be concerned as to cauda equina compression and determine whether there are bowel or bladder complaints, numbness of the sacral areas or legs, or leg weakness or gait difficulty. I would also consider whether the pain is related to a metastatic deposit in the hip, pelvis, or femur.

On examination of the patient I would survey the cerebral cortical functions, cranial nerves, and upper extremity neurological function to identify evidence for leptomeningeal metastases. In the lower extremities, I would carefully look for loss of reflexes, such as a dropped knee reflex, which might indicate an L2, L3, or L4 radiculopathy, weakness of the lower extremities, and sensory loss as well as loss of sphincter function. Mechanical signs may be helpful if present, but their absence does not rule out metastatic disease. For example, percussion tenderness of the spine is frequently absent in metastatic epidural spinal cord compression. If neck flexion, straight-leg raising or crossed-straight-leg raising causes radicular pain, the spine is often the source. Internal and external rotation of the hip (Patrick's maneuver) stresses the hip and femur without stretching the nerve root in the spine and, accordingly, is helpful in differentiating leg pain due to hip/leg disease from that arising from root compression.

Plain radiography and radionuclide bone scanning are readily available and often used in the evaluation of patients with breast cancer and pain thought to be due to spine metastases. While plain radiographs were found to be abnormal in approximately 85% of patients with epidural metastases, normal plain radiographs do not exclude the presence of vertebral metastases. In patients considered at high risk for metastatic disease, as in this case, normal plain radiographs have been reported to miss 67% of vertebral metastases without epidural extension. Radionuclide bone scanning is usually more sensitive but less specific than plain films. Spinal computed-tomography scan is sensitive and specific but the entire spinal axis cannot be readily surveyed. Magnetic resonance imaging (MRI) has become the imaging test of choice in evaluating the spine in patients suspected of spine metastases. MRI offers the ability to readily survey the entire spinal axis and usually distinguishes between metastatic disease and spondylosis.

What, then, is the diagnostic approach to the patient suspected of harboring a spine metastasis? Patients may be usually assigned to one of four different clinical presentations: (1) axial pain, normal neurological examination, and abnormal radiographs; (2) pain, normal neurological examination, and normal radiographs; (3) radiculopathy; (4) clinical manifestations of metastatic epidural compression. The diagnostic imaging approach to group 1 is controversial. Some authors suggest MRI of the symptomatic region to define radiotherapy ports while others irradiate symptomatic vertebral metastases using the plain film results without further imaging. The advantages and disadvantages of these two approaches have been discussed elsewhere. Among patients in group 2 who have unexplained pain and are at high risk for metastases, further imaging such as MRI is generally suggested to distinguish between metastatic and benign disease. In patients in group 3 with clinical manifestations of radiculopathy, there is a high incidence of metastatic epidural disease. Among those with cancer and abnormal plain radiographs, 88% have been found to harbor epidural tumor. Among those with normal radiographs, the frequency is 25%. Accordingly, in patients in group 3, MRI is ideally suited for identifying the rostrocaudal extent of epidural disease and planning radiotherapy ports. In patients in group 4 with clinical manifestations of metastatic epidural compression, imaging of the entire spinal axis is necessary to identify epidural tumor at sites remote from those already suspected.

The treatment for metastatic epidural compression includes corticosteroids, radiotherapy, and, in selected cases, surgery. Dexamethasone is administered as 10–100 mg intravenously followed by 4–24 mg four times per day and then tapered. The higher doses are reserved for patients with profound or rapidly progressing neurological deterioration. Most patients then proceed to radiotherapy. Laminectomy plus radiotherapy has not been found superior to radiotherapy alone. Alternatively, vertebral body resection and stabilization has been advocated by some authors in selected cases.

BIBLIOGRAPHY

Byrne TN. Spinal cord compression from epidural metastases. N Engl J Med 1992; 327:614–619.

Rodichok LD, Harper GR, Ruckdeschel JC, et al. Early diagnosis of spinal epidural metastases. Am J Med 1981; 70:1181–1188.

Siegal T, Siegal TZ. Current considerations in the management of neoplastic spinal cord compression. Spine 1989; 14:223–228.

H.8. PARANEOPLASTIC SYNDROMES

Case #H.8.1. Syndrome of Inappropriate Secretion of Antidiuretic Hormone (SIADH)
Goal: To discuss the incidence and management of SIADH in women with breast cancer

KEVIN R. FOX

A 43-year-old woman with metastatic breast cancer presents with seizures and confusion. Physical examination does not reveal any focal neurological deficits. The serum sodium is 103 meq/L.

This patient presents with profound hyponatremia and accompanying seizures. Although hyponatremia and the syndrome of inappropriate antidiuretic hormone production (SIADH) are not synonymous, SIADH must be considered the leading culprit in this patient or in any patient with cancer. Management of this patient requires immediate intervention for her life-threatening hyponatremia, combined with a thoughtful approach to the differential diagnosis. At the bedside, a rapid assessment of the patient's volume status should be made, but we can assume, for the sake of discussion, that her volume status will be normal to slightly decreased, consistent with the diagnosis of SIADH. One should not forget, however, that edematous disorders such as liver, cardiac, or renal failure may produce significant hyponatremia, although rarely to this degree.

Samples of blood and urine for measurement of osmolality should be obtained immediately. If one's suspicions are correct, then she will have a low serum osmolality and an inappropriately elevated urine osmolality. Intervention should begin immediately to correct the sodium and osmolality while awaiting these test results. The occurrence of seizures with this degree of hyponatremia is an indication for the administration of hypertonic (3%) NaCl. Guidelines recommend raising the serum sodium concentration by no more than 10 mEq/L in the first 24 hr, although, in urgent circumstances such as these, raising the concentration by as much as 1 mEq/L/phr is permissible for the first few hours. Overzealous correction of the sodium level may result in irreversible myelinolysis syndromes. The rate of hypertonic NaCl infusion can be estimated by calculating the patient's sodium deficit, or by calculating the patient's total body water in liters as 60% of body weight in kilograms. If she weighs 60 kg, her total body water will be 36 L, and thus raising her serum concentration by a total of 10 mEq/L will require the administration of 360 mEq of sodium in 24 hr. As 3% NaCl contains 513 mEq of Na/L, a volume of 700 cc will be required during the first 24 hr. Frequent measurements of the serum sodium are mandatory during this critical phase. The coadministration of a loop diuretic with strict attention to volume status may aid considerably in the safe recovery of this patient.

After the patient is stabilized and the first phase of correction is underway, the workup for causes of SIADH should continue. Fortunately, the differential diagnosis is relatively narrow. Given this patient's history of metastatic breast cancer, the diagnostic workup should begin with prompt evaluation of the central nervous system for the presence of metastatic disease. Although SIADH is an uncommon manifestation of metastatic breast cancer, the relatively high incidence of brain metastases and/or carcinomatous meningitis in breast cancer, and the ability of either of these conditions to cause SIADH, mandates emergent evaluation with contrast-enhanced brain magnetic resonance imaging (MRI). If the MRI is negative, lumbar puncture for cytological evaluation should be performed. Urgent consultation with radiation oncology should be obtained if evidence of CNS disease is diagnosed so that prompt palliative therapy can be initiated.

Even in the presence of documented CNS disease and its presumed causal association with SIADH, one must not forget other causes of this syndrome. Both hypothyroidism and hypoadrenalism may precipitate SIADH. Serum measurements of thyroxine, TSH, and cortisol may be obtained. A detailed treatment history must be obtained, because cyclophosphamide and vincristine are known precipitants of SIADH. (The author has a patient who developed seizures and a serum sodium level of 115 mEq/L within 12 hr of her first dose of intravenous cyclophosphamide. It was determined that the patient had taken the posttreatment recommendation to drink "liberal amounts of fluid" quite seriously and had consumed 2 gallons of free water in 8 hr following chemotherapy administration, thus compounding the SIADH-inducing effects of cyclophosphamide with water intoxication.)

After the initial hyponatremic crisis is treated, the diagnostic workup completed, and appropriate therapy is undertaken to correct the underlying cause, efforts must be maintained to allow the serum sodium level to drift toward normal. Modest fluid restriction (0.5–1.0 L/day) and infusions of isotonic intravenous fluids, with strict attention to maintaining normal volume status, are important. Care must be taken not to elevate the serum sodium level more than 10 mEq/day. Demeclocycline, at a dose of 600 mEq/day, should be reserved for stable, but symptomatic patients who fail to elevate their serum sodium levels above 130 mEq/L despite the above measures.

BIBLIOGRAPHY

Cerrill D, State R, Birge J, et al. Demeclocycline treatment in the syndrome of inappropriate anti-diuretic hormone secretion. Ann Intern Med 1975; 83:654.

Glover D, Glick J. Oncologic emergencies and special complications. In: Calabresi P, Schein P, Rosenberg S. Medical Oncology: Basic Principles and Clinical Management of Cancer. New York: Macmillan, 1985:1261.

Weisberg L, Cox M. Approach to the patient with hyponatremia. In: Kelley W. Textbook of Medicine. Philadelphia: Lippincott-Raven, 1997:950.

Case #H.8.2. Diabetes Insipidus
Goal: To recognize and manage diabetes insipidus (DI) in the breast cancer patient

WILLIAM N. HAIT

An 80-year-old woman presents with a 3-day history of polyuria, increasing thirst, and progressive weakness. She lives at home with her daughter, who noted an increased desire for cold beverages over the last few days. She denies fever or chills. She is on tamoxifen for the treatment of metastatic breast cancer. Evaluation reveals the presence of an enlarged, firm liver palpable 3 cm below the right costal margin. There is no jaundice. The serum sodium is 170 meq/L.

An elevated serum sodium in an elderly patient is secondary to free water depletion due to either inadequate water intake in the face of ongoing water loss or renal loss due to diabetes insipidus. In an elderly patient, one must be concerned about lack of access to water due to a senile or bedridden state, and the increased insensible loss of water due to fever or overheating from high ambient temperature. Essential hypernatremia, a rare condition at any age, is unlikely in this patient.

The most likely cause of the elevated serum sodium in elderly patients with breast cancer is decreased intake of free water due to frailty, fever, or lack of an air-conditioned environment. This can be readily confirmed by the history, urine electrolytes, and osmolality, which will show the UNa <10 and the Uosm markedly elevated. In that case the patient should be treated with gentle rehydration with hypotonic fluid (1/2 normal saline) aiming to correct the deficit over 2–3 days. In the case of severe volume depletion, one should begin with normal saline, realizing that it will still be hypotonic relative to the patient's serum.

In this case, the patient appears to be experiencing a rare complication of breast cancer, diabetes insipidus. It occurs most often in the setting of diffuse metastatic disease to the brain. The diagnosis can readily be confirmed by measuring urine and serum electrolytes and osmolality. The urine will show the failure of the kidney to concentrate urine in the presence of increased serum osmolality, and a relatively electrolyte-free urine. The abnormality is due to an inadequate production of or an inability of the kidney to respond to vasopressin. The development of severe hypernatremia implies an impairment of thirst or a lack of access to water. The cause is likely to be central in nature as a result of a metastases to the pituitary gland, a rare but reported event. This can be diagnosed best with magnetic resonance imaging.

Treatment requires calculation of the magnitude of the pure water deficit, which is estimated by the formula: (normal TBW) × (normal Sosm) = (current TBW) × (current Sosm). In a 60-kg woman with a serum Na of 170 mEq/L, the calculation is: TBW = (0.6 × 60) × (140/170), or 29.5 L. Therefore, the total water deficit is (36 − 29.5) = 6.5 L.

One must also be aware that repletion of the free water deficit carries significant risks, particularly cerebral edema when large amounts of new brain solutes have been produced. Approximately one-half of the water deficit should be replaced in the first 12 hr with careful monitoring of neurological status. The remainder can be replaced orally.

The long-term treatment of this patient requires control of the metastatic lesion to the pituitary with radiation. Any additional treatment would be controversial, since she progressed on tamoxifen and enters the clinical pathway at the point of recurrent disease with visceral crisis. Given the patient's age, I would recommend second-line hormonal therapy, with a drug such as anastrazole with close monitoring of her urine and serum osmalalities. Failure to control the disease would require vasopressin replacement with intranasal dDAVP (5–20 μg). If carcinomatous meningitis was present, intrathecal therapy with methotrexate could produce palliation.

BIBLIOGRAPHY

Arieff AI, DeFronzo RA, eds. Fluid Electrolyte and Acid-Base Disorders. New York: Churchill Livingstone Inc., 1985:203–204.

Yap HY, Tashima CK, Blumenschein GR, et al. Diabetes insipidus and breast cancer. Arch Intern Med 1979; 139:1009.

Case #H.8.3. Hypercalcemia
Goal: To discuss the diagnosis and management of hypercalcemia in breast cancer patients

MICHAEL REISS

A 65-year-old woman with hormone-receptor-positive breast cancer metastatic to bone presents with lethargy and back pain. She had recently been started on hydrochlorthiazide for hypertension. Physical examination reveals dehydration, mild confusion, and bony tenderness of the lumbo-sacral spine. Laboratory values include a serum calcium of 14 mg/dl, with normal serum proteins. Her electrolytes include a sodium of 148 meq/L, Cl 115 meq/L, potassium 4.6 meq/L, and bicarbonate 32 meq/L. The BUN is 40 mg/dl and the creatinine 1.2 mg/dl. The serum phosphate is low. Urine electrolytes are consistent with dehydration.

Based on the laboratory data provided, we can make a diagnosis of hypercalcemia. On the other hand, although hypercalcemia commonly causes confusion and lethargy, a change in mental status in combination with increasing back pain in a patient known to have extensive skeletal metastases should raise the concern that she may have developed lepto-meningeal carcinomatosis. In this case, the absence of focal neurological deficits referable to peripheral nerve root or cranial nerve involvement speaks against this possibility. However, should the patient's mental status fail to improve with aggressive hydration and prompt correction of the hypercalcemia, the presence of leptomeningeal carcinomatosis needs to be excluded.

Hypercalcemia of malignancy most commonly presents insidiously with fatigue, nausea, constipation, polyuria and dehydration, and progresses to increasing lethargy, confusion, and somnolence. Although the syndrome is usually a manifestation of disease progression, increasing bone pain and hypercalcemia can occur transiently in patients with metastatic breast cancer shortly after the introduction of endocrine therapy, the so-called "flare" phenomenon.

In the past, it was believed that hypercalcemia was caused by the direct osteoclastic activity of breast cancer metastases on bone. However, a significant proportion of patients develop hypercalcemia in the absence of skeletal metastases. In recent years, it has become clear that the hypercalcemia is caused by tumor-derived peptides that stimulate the activity of normal osteoclasts. The most important one of these peptides, parathormone-related peptide (PTH-RP), can be detected in the serum of the majority of patients with breast cancer who develop hypercalcemia. PTH-RP causes hypercalcemia both by activating osteoclast activity and by inhibiting tubular reabsorption of calcium. Thus, these patients typically display the same constellation of signs as found in primary hyperparathyroidism, including a metabolic alkalosis with hypophosphatemia, hyperchloremia, hyperphosphaturia, and an elevation of urinary cyclic AMP. Radioimmunoassays specific for native PTH and PTH-RP allow the clinician to definitively distinguish hypercalcemia caused by tumor-derived PTH-RP from primary hyperparathyroidism. Elevations of serum calcium in patients without obvious metastases and normal PTH and PTH-RP levels can be caused by excessive consumption of calcium and/or vitamin D, the use of thiazide diuretics, granulomatous diseases such as sarcoidosis, or hyperthyroidism.

Once the diagnosis of hypercalcemia is made, the clinician needs to assess whether hospitalization is required. Cases in which the serum calcium level does not exceed 12 mg/dl and the patient is alert, able to ingest fluids, has normal renal function, and has access to emergency care from home can be managed in the ambulatory setting. In contrast, patients with severe elevations of their serum calcium associated with dehydration, renal failure, and inability to ingest fluids because of mental impairment or nausea should be treated aggressively in a hospital setting. In the acute phase, the primary treatment goal is to stimulate calciuresis by correcting the dehydration and renal failure using intravenous and oral fluids. Furosemide can be added to improve calciuresis, but only after a normal hydration status has been achieved. Serum phosphate, potassium, and magnesium levels should be repleted intravenously as needed. Once the intravascular fluid volume has been replenished and adequate urine output has been restored, specific hypocalcemic drug treatment can be instituted.

In emergent situations, calcitonin can be used to rapidly decrease serum calcium levels within hours, although its duration of action is short. Biphosphonates, such as pamidronate and alendronate, effectively inhibit bone resorbtion, presumably by a direct toxic effect on osteoclasts. A single dose of pamidronate or alendronate will induce normocalcemia in the majority of patients, and this effect will last approximately 2–3 weeks. Alternatively, gallium nitrate can be used to block osteoclast activity while promoting bone deposition. Gallium nitrate is effective in 80–90% of unselected patients and may become the agent of choice to treat moderate to severe hypercalcemia depending on the outcome of comparative clinical studies of gallium nitrate and biphosphonates. Mild chronic hypercalcemia that is not associated with central nervous system impairment, nausea, or renal failure can safely be managed in an outpatient setting by encouraging oral hydration, reducing dietary calcium intake, and using biphosphonates or gallium nitrate to achieve normocalcemia.

Because hypercalcemia of malignancy is caused by tumor-cell-derived peptides, long-term correction of hypercalcemia will only be achieved if one can institute effective anticancer therapy. In most cases of advanced breast cancer, such treatment will be available. However, in a setting of far-advanced metastatic breast cancer that is refractory to therapy, one should seriously question the wisdom of correcting hypercalcemia if it arises.

Case #H.8.4. Dermato/polymyositis
Goal: To discuss the diagnosis and management of dermato/polymyositis

JEAN L. BOLOGNIA

A 58-year-old woman with metastatic carcinoma of the breast on megestrol acetate presents with increasing weakness. History reveals that this has been slowly progressive over the last 3–6 months. She now has difficulty climbing stairs or getting off the toilet seat without assistance. Examination reveals discoloration of the skin over the knuckles.

Dermatomyositis (DM) is generally classified, along with lupus erythematosus and scleroderma, as a connective tissue disease. However, in a significant portion of patients (up to a third in one case-control study), DM represents a paraneoplastic disorder, reflecting the presence of an internal malignancy or heralding its recurrence. Although the majority of patients with DM have cutaneous lesions as well as proximal muscle weakness, some individuals have only skin findings, a condition referred to as amyopathic DM or DM siné myositis (Table 1). In women with the paraneoplastic form of DM, the most common underlying malignancy is breast carcinoma, fol-

Table 1 Classification of Idiopathic Inflammatory Myopathies

Dermatomyositis
  Adult-onset dermatomyositis
  Dermatomyositis with malignancy
  Juvenile dermatomyositis
  Dermatomyositis as part of an overlap connective tissue disorder
  Amyopathic dermatomyositis
    Confirmed
      Biopsy-confirmed classic cutaneous manifestations of dermatomyositis
        without muscle weakness and with normal muscle enzyme levels for 2
        years or longer
    Provisional
      Biopsy-confirmed classic cutaneous manifestations of dermatomyositis
        without muscle weakness and with normal muscle enzyme levels for
        less than 2 years
Polymyositis
Inclusion-body myositis

Source: Adapted from Euwer RL, Sontheimer RD. Dermatologic aspects of myositis. Curr Opin Rheumatol 1994; 6:583–589, with permission of the publisher.

lowed by cancer of the lung, colon, and reproductive organs (endometrium and ovary). Clearly, clinicians who care for patients with a history of breast cancer or individuals at risk for its development must be able to recognize the cutaneous signs of DM.

The classic cutaneous eruption of DM is described as erythema of the face, a violet discoloration of the upper eyelids (heliotrope), and flat-topped papules on the distal interphalangeal (DIP), proximal interphalangeal (PIP), and metacarpophalangeal (MCP) joints (Gottron's papules) (Fig. 1). As is the case with any constellation of "classic" clinical findings, it often fails to appear in every patient or it may appear later in the course of the disease. However, several additional cutaneous clues can aid in the diagnosis of DM including erythema in a photodistribution, pink to pink-violet patches on the elbows and knees (Fig. 2), pruritus and scaling of the scalp, and swelling of the eyelids (Fig. 3). It may be easier to remember these clinical findings by recalling the misdiagnoses that patients with DM often carry: photosensitivity (e.g., photodrug eruption), new-onset psoriasis, and allergic contact dermatitis.

The nail fold changes that develop in patients with DM deserve special mention. Periungual telangiectasias are observed in three connective tissue diseases: systemic lupus, scleroderma, and DM. The telangiectasias in lupus resemble "glomeruli" while the telangiectasias in scleroderma and DM are simple dilated loops that alternate with avascular "skip" areas. These vascular changes are usually visible to the naked eye, but 10× magnification can aid in their detection. In addition to the periungual telangiectasias, the

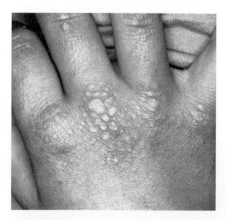

Figure 1 Gottron's papules over the MCP and PIP joints. (Courtesy Yale Resident's Slide Collection.)

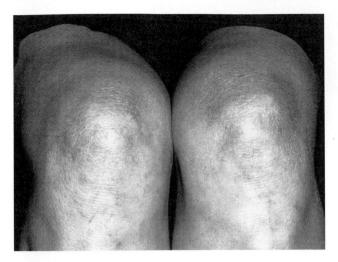

Figure 2 Pink to pink-violet patches on the knees. (Courtesy Yale Resident's Slide Collection.)

cuticles are often ragged in patients with DM (Fig. 4) and the nail fold changes may be accompanied by tenderness of the fingertips.

When the diagnosis of DM is suspected, a skin biopsy should be performed as well as measurement of serum levels of creatine phosphokinase (CPK) and aldolase. Histological findings include vacuolar degeneration of the basal cell layer, a superficial perivascular and lichenoid lymphocytic infiltrate, and sometimes, hemorrhage. There is, however, significant overlap between the histological features of DM and those of cutaneous lupus. The

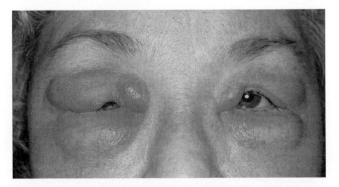

Figure 3 Periorbital swelling as the initial manifestation of DM.

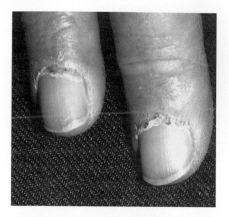

Figure 4 Prominent periungual teleangiectasias and ragged cuticles. The patient had an underlying ovarian carcinoma. (Courtesy Yale Resident's Slide Collection.)

majority of patients with DM have circulating antinuclear antibodies, but less than 20% have DM-specific anti-Mi-2 antibodies.

The classic criteria used to establish the diagnosis of DM are outlined in Table 2. However, these criteria were proposed before amyopathic DM was clearly defined as a clinical entity. Another recent advance is the use of magnetic resonance imaging (MRI) in the evaluation of patients suspected of having DM. The characteristic MRI findings are increased signal intensity on T_2-weighted images of proximal muscles (especially thigh and pelvic girdle), fat replacement of muscle groups, and atrophy. Such changes have even been observed in patients with normal CPK levels. MRI is also useful in determining the best site for a muscle biopsy and assessing disease activity.

Table 2 The Classic Diagnostic Criteria for Dermatomyositis

---

1. Typical skin rash of dermatomyositis
2. Proximal symmetrical muscle weakness
3. Elevation of serum muscle enzymes
4. Electromyographic features of myopathy
5. Muscle biopsy evidence of an inflammatory myopathy
Definite dermatomyositis—three or four criteria plus rash
Probable dermatomyositis—two criteria plus rash
Possible dermatomyositis—one criterion plus rash

Source: Bohan A, Peter JB. Polymyositis and dermatomyositis. N Engl J Med 1975; 292:345–347, 403–407.

In any patient with a history of breast cancer, the development of DM requires a search for recurrent disease. In retrospect, elevation of serum levels of AST and LDH may provide a clue to the diagnosis. Improvement in symptoms usually accompanies eradication of the tumor, but the cutaneous lesions may not resolve as quickly as the muscle weakness. Systemic corticosteroids should be instituted early in patients with evidence of muscle disease, especially in those where a complete response to chemotherapy or radiation therapy is rather unlikely. If side effects from the corticosteroids develop or the dosage cannot be tapered, an immunosuppressive agent such as azathioprine, methotrexate, cyclophosphamide, or cyclosporine can be added or high-dose intravenous immune globulin can be administered on a monthly basis. Antimalarials such as hydroxychloroquine are used to treat the cutaneous eruption in conjunction with topical sunscreens and potent topical corticosteroids. Persistent or severe cutaneous disease may require more aggressive therapy as outlined above.

BIBLIOGRAPHY

Bohan A, Peter JB. Polymyositis and dermatomyositis. N Engl J Med 1975; 292: 344–347, 403–407.

Callen JP. The value of malignancy evaluation in patients with dermatomyositis. J Am Acad Dermatol 1982; 6:253–259.

Euwer RL, Sontheimer RD. Dermatologic aspects of myositis. Cur Opin Rheum 1994; 6:583–589.

Manchul LA, Jin A, Pritchard KI, et al. The frequency of malignant neoplasms in patients with polymyositis-dermatomyositis. Arch Int Med 1985; 145:1835–1839.

Stonecipher MR, Jorizzo JL, Monu J, Walker F, Sutej PG. Dermatomyositis with normal muscle enzyme concentrations. Arch Dermatol 1994; 130;1294–1299.

H.9.   BRACHIAL PLEXUS RECURRENCE

Case #H.9.1
Goal: To discuss the differential diagnosis and management of breast cancer metastatic to the brachial plexus

MICHAEL H. TOROSIAN

A 57-year-old woman presents for evaluation. Six years ago she underwent right lumpectomy; axillary node dissection; breast, axillary, and supraclavicular nodal irradiation; and CAF chemotherapy for a 1.9-cm, 6/17 node-positive breast cancer. Recently she developed new right arm lymphedema. Physical examination reveals radiation changes persisting in the right breast and decreased flexor and extensor strength in the right forearm and wrist.

Ipsilateral upper extremity lymphedema can occur immediately or its appearance can be delayed following axillary dissection or radiation therapy to the axilla. The incidence of lymphedema has declined in recent years since standard axillary dissection techniques have evolved to include removal of only level I and II lymph nodes (preserving level III lymph nodes if uninvolved) without transection or removal of the pectoralis minor muscle. Attention to these surgical details and limitation of surgical dissection to the inferior aspect of the axillary vein allow preservation of collateral lymphatics, which minimizes the risk of lymphedema. Factors that predispose to the development of lymphedema include complete removal of all axillary lymphatics, transection or removal of the pectoralis minor muscle, radiation therapy to the axilla, and metastatic carcinoma to the lymphatics. Delayed development of lymphedema can occur following infection, trauma (blunt, penetrating, or thermal), or axillary recurrence of cancer.

New-onset lymphedema accompanied by ipsilateral neurological deficits in this patient with high-risk breast carcinoma is an ominous sign of recurrence. Despite the absence of palpable adenopathy, axillary recurrence of carcinoma is strongly suspected. Magnetic resonance imaging (MRI) is the recommended diagnostic test to evaluate the axilla. MRI- or computed-tomography-guided needle biopsy can be performed in the absence of a palpable mass to establish the diagnosis of recurrent malignancy. If a diagnosis of recurrence cannot be confirmed in this manner, open surgical biopsy is indicated.

Brachial plexus recurrence is not amenable to surgical therapy—in contrast to isolated axillary recurrence inferior to the brachial plexus for which surgical resection is clearly indicated. Since this patient has had prior radiation therapy to the axilla, chemotherapy with or without tamoxifen is recommended at this time. In patients who have not received radiation therapy and who present with isolated brachial plexus recurrence, radiation therapy to the ipsilateral axilla and supraclavicular regions is indicated.

Editors' comment: Another item in the differential diagnosis of lymphedema with associated neurological deficits following radiation therapy for breast cancer is radiation neuritis. This may be hard to differentiate radiographically. We therefore wholeheartedly concur with the recommendation for biopsy in this clinical setting.

BIBLIOGRAPHY

Bonnerot V, Dao T, Campana F, et al. Evaluation of MR imaging for detecting recurrent tumor within irradiated brachial plexus. Radiology 1993; 189:151.

Halverson KJ, Perez CA, Kuske RR, et al. Isolated local-regional recurrence of breast cancer following mastectomy: radiotherapeutic management. Int J Radiat Oncol Biol Phys 1990; 19:851.

Recht A, Pierce SM, Abner A, et al. Regional nodal failure after conservative surgery and radiotherapy for early-stage breast carcinoma. J Clin Oncol 1991; 9:988.

Tennvall-Nittby L, Tenegrup I, Landberg T. The total incidence of loco-regional recurrence in a randomized trail of breast cancer TNM stage II: the South Sweden Breast Cancer Trial. Acta Oncol 1993; 32:641.

H.10. BREAST CANCER DURING PREGNANCY

Case #H.10.1
Goal: To discuss the management of breast cancer in a pregnant patient

ROBERT S. DIPAOLA

A gravida 6, para 1, 33-year-old woman seeks an opinion following excisional biopsy of a 2.3-cm left breast mass that reveals high-grade invasive ductal carcinoma. The margins are negative. She is 16 weeks' pregnant, states that she has had five first-trimester miscarriages while trying to have a desperately desired second child. The patient wishes to do everything possible to carry the baby to term and to maximize her chances of living to see her 7-year-old child grow up.

This is a case of a 33-year-old woman with a second-trimester pregnancy and a 2.3-cm, high-grade, invasive ductal cancer. The prognosis of breast cancer in pregnant patients is thought to be worse than in nonpregnant patients. However, breast cancer is diagnosed in more advanced stages in pregnant than in nonpregnant patients; survival is similar to that of nonpregnant patients at similar stages. The later stage at presentation may be secondary to delayed diagnosis during pregnancy.

The benefit of therapeutic abortion has not been demonstrated. Therefore, the overall prognosis of breast cancer in the pregnant patient should not be different from that of nonpregnant patients. Maintaining pregnancy once a diagnosis of breast cancer is made does not appear to affect prognosis.

The management of breast cancer in pregnancy must include the known benefits of surgery and chemotherapy in breast cancer without pregnancy and the potential risk of these modalities to the fetus. The risks of surgery and general anesthesia in pregnancy are minimal and surgery should be performed with curative intent. As radiation therapy is contraindicated in pregnancy, a modified radical mastectomy should be performed. The lymph node dissection may add information to future management after delivery. Adjuvant chemotherapy would be expected to reduce the risk of recurrence by 30–40%, as for nonpregnant patients.

Fortunately, the risk of adjuvant chemotherapy to the fetus in the second trimester is low. A review of all known toxicity from chemotherapy agents used to treat breast cancer supports the contention that the risk is low enough to treat patients with standard agents. The risk of fetal malformations from alkylating agents, antimetabolites, antitumor antibiotics, and plant alkaloids in 150 patients in the second or third trimester was 1.3%. The use of doxorubicin and cyclophosphamide for four cycles following mastectomy would be reasonable in this case. If this patient were in the first trimester of pregnancy, the risk of chemotherapy would be high; either abortion or waiting to treat in the second trimester should be considered. With all of these agents, however, the potential for neoplastic disease in later life may be increased in an individual who has been exposed in utero.

BIBLIOGRAPHY

DiPaola RS, Goodin S, Ratzell M, Florczyk, M, Karp G, Ravikumar TS. Chemotherapy for metastatic melanoma during pregnancy. Gynecol Oncol 1997 (in press).
Early Breast Cancer Trialists' Collaborative Group. Systemic treatment of early breast cancer by hormonal, cytotoxic, or immune therapy. Lancet 1992; 339: 1–71.
Petrek JA, Dukoff R, Rogatko A. Prognosis of pregnancy-associated breast cancer. Cancer 1991; 67:869.

H.11.   LYMPHEDEMA

Case #H.11.1
Goal: To discuss the management of upper extremity lymphedema following axillary lymph node dissection for breast cancer

JAY K. HARNESS

A 53-year-old woman develops bothersome right arm lymphedema 3 years after right lumpectomy and axillary lymph node dissection (0/36 nodes) for an 8-mm tubular cancer. The axilla was not irradiated.

Upper extremity lymphedema is one of the most distressing complications following operations for breast cancer. In the days of the Halsted
radical mastectomy, clinically significant lymphedema was reported to occur
in as many as 60% of patients. The incidence of lymphedema has decreased
to 5–20% with more conservative (less radical) breast cancer operations,
depending on the means of assessment.

Several independent risk factors contribute to the development of lymphedema. They include: (a) extensive axillary lymphadenectomy; (b) axillary
radiotherapy; (c) presence of nodal metastases; (d) postoperative wound
complications; and (e) recurrent episodes of arm cellulitis. In the current era
of more conservative breast cancer operations, extensive axillary lymph node
dissection followed by axillary radiotherapy has the highest incidence
(nearly 40%) of patients developing postoperative lymphedema. Limiting
axillary dissection to the removal of the level I and II lymph nodes *below*
the axillary vein preserves lymphatic channels around and above this important structure. This type of dissection should also prevent trauma to the
vein, which in turn could result in axillary vein thrombosis (another cause
of upper extremity edema).

The wide variation in the reported incidence of lymphedema is the
result of a lack of uniform diagnostic criteria. Subjective criteria include
size, appearance, heaviness, and functional activity. Circumferential or vol-
umetric measurements are objective ways of characterizing lymphedema.

Evaluation of the new onset of lymphedema should include a careful
history and physical examination. It is important to rule out axillary or in-
breast recurrences as possible causes through the judicious use of mammography, computed tomography (CT), and/or magnetic resonance imaging
(MRI). Recurrent episodes of upper extremity cellulitis could also cause late
onset of lymphedema.

Noninvasive imaging modalities currently used to evaluate patients
with lymphedema include lymphoscintigraphy, CT, and MRI. A duplex examination of the axillary vein can be used to rule out axillary vein thrombosis as a cause of the edema. I would personally recommend ruling out
axillary and/or in-breast recurrence, axillary vein thrombosis, and other
causes of late-onset lymphedema. Once this has been accomplished, focusing
on management of the problem is the next step.

Management of upper extremity lymphedema is almost exclusively
nonoperative. Mechanical therapy is the main component of nonoperative
management. Reducing the size of the arm and preventing cellulitis are the
primary goals of therapy. Early in the course of the disease, when the tissues
are still soft, it may be possible to return the arm to its original size. After
fibrosis develops, the brawny tissue typically cannot be restored to normal.

Elevation is a simple and effective method for reducing lymphedema.
Simple massage of the affected arm, performed on a regular basis, can help

to promote lymphatic drainage and keep the tissue soft and decompressed. This method has been popular in Europe. Weight reduction, range-of-motion, and upper extremity muscle exercises can be used as adjuncts in the treatment of lymphedema.

Sequential pneumatic compression devices are utilized in more advanced cases. They produce a distal-to-proximal milking action on the arm with pressures of 100 mmHg or more in cycles ranging from 20 sec to 1 or 2 min. Protocols for these devices often include an initial 2–3-day hospitalization and daily 6–8-hr treatment sessions. Once maximum volume reduction has taken place, maintenance of limb volume is achieved by a custom-made, two-way, stretch elastic compression sleeve.

The latest compression device on the market is a nonpneumatic sleeve (Fig. 1). The Reid sleeve (Peninsula Medical, Stanford, CA) is made from a soft foam core and is designed to provide consistent pressures in the range of 40–50 mmHg. Pressures are controlled by series of Velco straps adjusted using a pressure gauge. The device is worn at night. Initial trials indicate that the device is as effective as sequential pneumatic devices.

For this patient, I would recommend an initial program of meticulous upper extremity hygiene, range-of-motion exercises, and muscle activities (e.g., repetitive squeezing of a rubber ball in the hand), plus simple elevation. If that fails to provide significant relief, I would recommend a nonpneumatic sleeve as the next step. Depending on the success of these efforts, a pneumatic sequential compression device may or may not be needed. Also, a static compression stocking may be necessary to maintain the reduced arm volume.

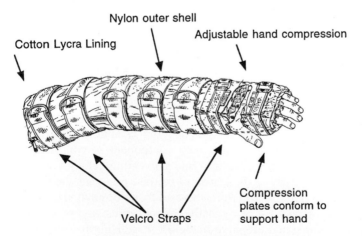

Figure 1 Reid sleeve. (Courtesy of Peninsula Medical, Stanford, CA.)

Editors' comment: The perplexing issue is why this woman with a small tubular carcinoma developed lymphedema. The removal of 36 lymph nodes may have contributed to the problem. Generally, one must consider undertaking a workup for recurrent disease when: the lymphedema is extensive; lymphedema develops more than 2 years after surgery; the original primary was "high risk"; or history and physical examination suggest recurrent tumor. Evaluation with mammography is almost always indicated. CT and/or MRI scans to evaluate high axillary and brachial plexus recurrences should be considered.

BIBLIOGRAPHY

Hayward JL, Winter PJ, Tong D, et al. A new approach to the conservative treatment of early breast cancer. Surgery 1984; 95:270.

Kissin MW, della Rovere GQ, Easton D, Wetbury G. Risk of lymphoedema following the treatment of breast cancer. Br J Surg 1986; 73:580.

Leis HP. Selective moderate surgical approach for potentially curable breast cancer. In: Gallagher HS, Leis HP, Snyderman RK, Urban JA, eds. The Breast. St Louis: CV Mosby, 1978:232–247.

Lobb AW, Harkins HN. Postmastectomy swelling of the arm with note on effect of segmental resection of axillary vein at time of radical mastectomy. West J Surg 1949; 57:550.

H.12. HORMONE REPLACEMENT THERAPY

Case #H.12.1
Goal: To discuss the use of hormone replacement therapy in a woman at high risk for breast cancer

TERESA GILEWSKI and LARRY NORTON

A 51-year-old, perimenopausal woman seeks an opinion regarding the advisability of hormone replacement therapy. She experiences occasional hot flashes. She has had three prior breast biopsies, the most recent of which 4 years ago showed multiple foci of atypical lobular hyperplasia. Her mother had breast cancer at age 61 and died from a heart attack at age 64; her younger sister had breast cancer at age 38 and is currently alive and well.

This perimenopausal women presents with four concerns: vasomotor instability (hot flashes), the potential for osteoporosis, coronary heart disease, and risk factors for breast cancer. She has a family history of premenopausal and postmenopausal breast cancer and myocardial infarction. She herself has atypical lobular hyperplasia of the breast. We do not know if she is osteoporotic or if she has a family history of osteoporosis. We do not know if she is hyperlipidemic. It is presumed, probably correctly, that her vasomotor symptoms are associated with spontaneous estrogen withdrawal secondary to age-related ovarian failure.

What would the oral administration of estrogen and progesterone do for her? Estrogen alone or in combination with progestogens can ameliorate symptoms due to vasomotor instability and urogenital atrophy, improve bone mineralization, increase high-density-lipoprotein cholesterol, and decrease low-density-lipoprotein serum cholesterol. A reduction in the risk of major coronary heart disease has also been documented. A recent analysis of the Nurses' Health Study found a reduction in overall mortality for current users of postmenopausal hormones compared to those who had never used them. The most significant decrease in mortality was from that attributed to coronary heart disease. However, this benefit was offset by an increased risk of death after long-term ($\geq$10 years) current use primarily due to an increased risk of breast cancer. Although the data in other studies concerning the potential risk of breast cancer and hormone replacement therapy are conflicting, there appears to be a small increased risk in certain groups (i.e., long-term users).

There is minimal information available regarding the use of hormone replacement therapy (HRT) in those with a history of prior benign breast disease. Several studies indicate no significant increased risk of breast cancer in women who use HRT. However, this patient is already at an increased risk for breast cancer based on the presence of atypical lobular hyperplasia without HRT. A family history of breast cancer may augment the risk of breast cancer from HRT, although again the data are conflicting. Whether HRT can be safely used in women with known *BRCA1* or *BRCA2* mutations who do not have breast cancer is unknown.

A variety of hormone replacement therapy regimens are available. Owing to the higher incidence of endometrial carcinoma with unopposed estrogens, most current regimens add a progestin to estrogen. However, the combination of estrogen and progestin does not decrease the risk of breast cancer in studies thus far. Some earlier data suggested there may be an increased risk of breast cancer with the combination, but this remains unclear.

Men with *BRCA1* mutations do not have a higher-than-expected incidence of breast cancer, so physiological estrogen clearly plays a role in women with these germline mutations. The safety of hormone replacement therapy in women who have a history of breast cancer is unclear at this time.

Are there any alternatives for this patient? Hot flashes may be greatly improved by the use of 20–40 mg/day of megestrol acetate, which is a drug that has anti-breast-cancer activity when used at 160 mg/day. Vitamins, clonidine, and antidepressants have also been of benefit in anecdotal situations. She may not have or be predisposed to the development of osteoporosis, but if she has objective reason to be treated for this condition, calcium supplements or a variety of bisphosphonates are available (i.e., risedronate, clodronate, alendronate). If her serum lipids are unfavorable for cardiovascular health, then diet, exercise, and cholesterol-lowering drugs are effective and do not increase her risk of developing breast cancer. Exercise may actually decrease breast cancer risk.

Hence, the use of estrogens in such a postmenopausal woman should not be an automatic response. When the risks and benefits are weighed, alternatives may be superior in certain situations. This is especially so since raloxifene has just been approved by the Food and Drug Administration for the indication of preventing osteoporosis in postmenopausal women. This drug may well impact beneficially on cardiovascular lipid profiles and is not clearly associated with higher-than-expected rates of either breast or endometrial cancer. In fact, the possibility that long-term use in postmenopausal women may decrease incidence rates for breast cancer is now being explored.

BIBLIOGRAPHY

Armstrong BK. Oestrogen therapy after the menopause—boon or bane? Med J Aust 1988; 148:213–214.

Belchetz PA. Hormonal treatment of postmenopausal women. N Engl J Med 1994; 330;1062–1071.

Col NF, Eckman MH, Karas RH, et al. Patient-specific decision about hormone replacement therapy in postmenopausal women. JAMA 1997; 277:1140–1147.

Colditz GA, Egan KM, Stampfer JM. Hormone replacement therapy and risk of breast cancer: results from epidemiologic studies. Obstet Gynecol 1993; 168: 1473–1480.

Colditz GA, Hankinson SE, Hunter DJ, et al. The use of estrogens and progestins and the risk of breast cancer in postmenopausal women. N Engl J Med 1995; 332:1589–1593.

Darling GM, Johns JA, McCloud PI, et al. Estrogen and progestin compared with simvastatin for hypercholesterolemia in postmenopausal women. N Engl J Med 1997; 337:595–601.

Delmas PD, Balena R, Confravreux E, et al. Bisphosphonate risedronate prevents bone loss in women with artificial menopause due to chemotherapy of breast cancer: a double-blind, placebo-controlled study. J Clin Oncol 1997; 15:955–962.

Delmas PD, Bjarnason NH, Mitlak BH, et al. Effects of raloxifene on bone mineral density, serum cholesterol concentration, and uterine endometrium in post menopausal women. N Engl J Med 1997; 337:1641–1647.

Dupont WD, Page DL. Menopausal estrogen replacement therapy and breast cancer. Arch Intern Med 1991; 151:67–72.

Friedman LS, Gayther SA, Kurosaki T, et al. Mutation analysis of *BRCA1* and *BRCA2* in a male breast cancer population. Am J Hum Genet 1997; 60:313–319.

Grady D, Ernster V. Invited commentary: does postmenopausal hormone therapy cause breast cancer? Am J Epidemiol 1991; 134:1396–1400.

Grodstein F, Stampfer MJ, Manson JE, et al. Postmenopausal estrogen and progestin use and the risk of cardiovascular disease. N Engl J Med 1996; 335:453–461.

Grodstein F, Stampfer MJ, Colditz GA, et al. Postmenopausal hormone therapy and mortality. N Engl J Med 1997; 336:1769–1775.

Liberman UA, Weiss SR, Broll J, et al. Effect of oral alendronate on bone mineral density and the incidence of fractures in postmenopausal osteoporosis. N Engl J Med 1995; 333:1437–1443.

Loprinzi CL, Michalak JC, Quella SK, et al. Megestrol acetate for the prevention of hot flashes. N Engl J Med 1994; 331:347–352.

Newcomb PA, Longnecker MP, Storer BE, et al. Long-term hormone replacement therapy and risk of breast cancer in postmenopausal women. Am J Epidemiol 1995; 142:788–795.

Roy JA, Sawka CA, Pritchard KI. Hormone replacement therapy in women with breast cancer: do the risks outweigh the benefits? J Clin Oncol 1996; 14:997–1006.

Saarto T, Blomqvist C, Valimaki M, et al. Chemical castration induced by adjuvant cyclophosphamide, methotrexate, and fluorouracil chemotherapy causes rapid bone loss that is reduced by clodronate: a randomized study in premenopausal breast cancer patients. J Clin Oncol 1997; 15:1341–1347.

Sillcro-Arenas M, Delgado-Rodriguez M, Rodigues-Canteras R, et al. Menopausal hormone replacement therapy and breast cancer: a meta-analysis. Obstet Gynecol 1992; 79:286–294.

Steinberg KK, Thacker SB, Smith SJ, et al. A meta-analysis of the effect of estrogen replacement therapy on the risk of breast cancer. JAMA 1991; 265:1985–1990.

Thune I, Brenn T, Lund E, et al. Physical activity and the risk of breast cancer. N Engl J Med 1997; 336:1269–1275.

Case #H.12.2
Goal: To discuss the use of hormone replacement therapy in women with a past history of breast cancer

SANDRA F. SCHNALL

A 52-year-old woman, 8 years post right lumpectomy, axillary lymph node dissection, and radiation therapy for a node-positive (1/12), estrogen-receptor-positive, 1.3-cm, infiltrating ductal carcinoma (treated adjuvantly with CMF), is now experiencing increasing difficulty with hot flashes, mood swings, insomnia, and dyspareunia. She wishes to initiate hormone replacement therapy.

As the number of breast cancer survivors increase, their nononcological health problems occupy a growing concern. The menopausal symptoms of hot flashes, dyspareunia, atrophic vaginitis, sleep disorders, mood swings, coronary vascular disease, and osteoporosis can be at the very least annoying and often debilitating. The reluctance to use hormone replacement therapy (HRT) in breast cancer survivors may diminish their quality of life and possibly diminish their overall survival (i.e., from coronary vascular disease).

The role of HRT after treatment of an invasive breast carcinoma is controversial. Several reports on the role of HRT in breast cancer survivors have now been reported. None demonstrate a strikingly adverse effect. However, these are small and anecdotal and do not represent formal, randomized clinical trials.

The theoretical risk of HRT in breast cancer survivors includes the concern that: (a) estrogen may stimulate growth of residual malignant cells, (b) hormone replacement therapy/estrogens may increase the risk of a new primary breast cancer, and (c) HRT may increase breast density making detection of abnormalities on subsequent mammograms difficult.

The benefits of HRT in the treatment of osteoporosis are well known. Osteoporosis can cause substantial morbidity. More than 1.5 million osteoporotic-related bone fractures are reported in the United States annually. HRT has also been associated with reduction in the risk of coronary vascular disease in postmenopausal women.

There are alternatives to hormone intervention for the treatment of menopausal related symptoms. In one study, low-dose megestrol acetate was used for the treatment of hot flashes in women with breast cancer and was well tolerated. Vaginal dryness can also be treated with lubricants. However, in some women the role of a low-dose estrogen vaginal cream may well be worth the theoretical small risk of breast cancer stimulation.

Tamoxifen, which is commonly used for the treatment of breast cancer in postmenopausal women, has been shown to maintain bone mass and density and decrease the risk of coronary vascular disease. Theoretically, tamoxifen may improve or prevent certain postmenopausal symptoms in breast cancer survivors without the risks of standard estrogen replacement. These results will be clarified upon completion of an ongoing trial of tamoxifen in the prevention of breast cancer in women at high risk.

Therefore, which breast cancer patients would most benefit from hormone replacement therapy is not clear. Most medical oncologists in the United States have been reluctant to prescribe hormone replacement therapy. Obstetricians/gynecologists seem to be less hesitant. Nonetheless, prescribing hormone replacement therapy in a breast cancer survivor requires careful evaluation of the risks and benefits for each individual patient and a detailed discussion with the patient. If symptoms cannot be controlled with nonhormone replacement, a brief trial of HRT may be warranted.

A recent study from Australia supports the role of HRT in some patients surviving breast cancer. They treated women with debilitating symptoms beginning at a median survival of 3 years from diagnosis with low-dose estrogen replacement. Once symptoms were controlled, they often reduced the dose of the hormone and commonly stopped all treatment within 1–2 years. In this study, symptoms were well controlled and no greater-than-expected increase of tumor recurrences occurred.

However, until randomized, large-scale clinical trials are complete, the answer to the question of HRT in breast cancer survivors is still open. A physician must individualize the severity of the symptoms and the risk. In my patients who fail nonhormonal modalities, I weigh the severity of their symptoms, the quality of life, and the overall prognosis from their tumor. If a patient is greater than 5 years since diagnosis, I offer low-dose hormone therapy for a brief trial. However, the patient must understand that the risks, toxicity, and safety of this treatment are not fully known.

BIBLIOGRAPHY

Creasman WT. Estrogen replacement therapy; is previously treated cancer a contraindication? Obstet Gynecol 1991; 77:308–312.
Ethan JA. A case controlled study of combined continuous estrogen-progesterone replacement therapy among women with a personal history of breast cancer. J Menopause 1995; 2:67–72.
Loprinzi CL, Michalak JC, Quella SK. Megestrol acetate for the prevention of hot flashes. N Engl J Med 1994; 331:347–352.
Marchant DJ. Estrogen replacement after breast cancer. Risk versus benefits. Cancer 1993; 71:2169–2176.

H.13.   BREAST RECONSTRUCTION

Case #H.13.1
Goal: To discuss surgical options for immediate breast reconstruction in older women

MIHYE CHOI

An otherwise healthy, 68-year-old woman is diagnosed with a 1.4-cm, invasive lobular carcinoma with clinically negative axillary nodes. She chooses to undergo modified radical mastectomy and wishes to have an immediate reconstruction. She will not consider use of a prosthetic implant and requests information concerning "that tummy tuck operation that makes a breast from the extra fat on my stomach."

One of the interesting issues to be addressed in this case is the patient's age. Currently fewer women over the age of 68 choose to undergo breast reconstruction compared to younger women. A survey of female mastectomy patients reported that advanced age was one of the main factors influencing them in their decision against breast reconstruction. It is not clear how much the decision is influenced by reluctance of the oncological and reconstructive surgeons to offering reconstruction to elderly women and how much by elderly women's lack of interest. As a greater number of older people enjoy improved health and maintain active life-styles, it is probable that interest in breast reconstruction in the elderly will rise. The risks involved in breast reconstruction in the elderly population appear comparable to those in younger women. Indeed, a study by August et al. reported lower complication rates of both immediate and delayed breast reconstruction in the elderly population as compared with the younger population. General health and risk factors of an individual patient are of greater importance in choosing a reconstructive procedure than strictly chronological age. The psychological and physical benefits of breast reconstruction should be readily available to the elderly population.

While patients often present to the plastic surgeon's office with a specific type of reconstruction in mind, the various options of reconstruction should be discussed with the patient to ensure that she is sufficiently informed about alternatives. During the consultation with this particular patient, the plastic surgeon should gently explore her reason for disinterest in prosthetic breast reconstruction. Although many patients are aware of the silicone implant controversy, patients' data fund is frequently inaccurate and may lead to misinformed decisions.

Breast reconstruction can be classified as autogenous or prosthetic. The advantages of *prosthetic breast reconstruction* include shorter initial operating time and recovery period and lack of donor site morbidity. The disadvantages include periprosthetic capsular contracture (approximately 10%), implant failure, need for additional procedures such as capsulectomy and revisions (as high as 30%), and less-natural-appearing breast. The current standard in prosthetic breast reconstruction is to use an anatomically designed expander to preferentially inflate the inferior pole of the breast to give a more natural appearance. Most plastic surgeons prefer to place the prosthesis under the pectoralis and serratus muscles and to use a textured, saline-filled implant to minimize the risks of implant exposure and periprosthetic capsular contracture. The silicone-gel prosthesis is no longer available in the United States, although there is little scientific evidence that silicone gel implants cause or contribute to autoimmune disease.

Autogenous reconstruction can be achieved with a pedicled myocutaneous flap or with a free flap. The general advantages of autogenous reconstruction are the appearance of the reconstructed breast, the lack of foreign material, and the secondary abdominoplasty effect in the case of the transverse rectus abdominis myocutaneous (TRAM) flap. The disadvantages include prolonged operative time with greater blood loss, longer recovery period, and donor site morbidity. A pedicled flap such as the latissimus dorsi flap can be used alone for a small-sized breast reconstruction or in conjunction with an implant for larger breast reconstruction. This flap has the advantage of autogenous reconstruction when used alone; however, it has the disadvantage of donor site morbidity including seroma formation and wound dehiscence. When this flap is used in conjunction with an implant, a 30% capsular contracture rate is reported. The current gold standard in autogenous breast reconstruction is the TRAM flap owing to its versatility, natural appearance, and the additional benefit of abdominoplasty. A TRAM flap is contraindicated when there has been a previous injury to the vascular pedicle (superior epigastric artery) such as from a subcostal incision. The other factors that increase the complication rate associated with this flap include obesity, smoking, diabetes, autoimmune disease, and pulmonary and cardiac diseases. One of the disadvantages of the pedicled TRAM flap is the relatively precarious blood supply; flap ischemia may result in fat necrosis or partial flap loss. The donor site morbidity includes abdominal wall weakness and ventral hernia. Owing to these limitations, the free TRAM with the more direct blood supply from the inferior epigastric artery has been advocated. The apparent advantages include a lower incidence of partial flap loss and fat necrosis, and less abdominal wall morbidity. Disadvantages include longer operative time with greater blood loss. Furthermore, failure of this flap (2–5%) may result in substantial soft-tissue loss and a devastating cosmetic result. The flap of choice by most reconstructive surgeons currently remains the pedicled TRAM. However, the free TRAM flap may be preferred for reconstruction of a large breast.

Coordination between the oncological and reconstructive surgeons is critical in achieving the best reconstructive result. The reconstructive surgeon should be involved in designing the mastectomy incision with the oncological surgeon so that the reconstruction can be planned accordingly. Viability of the mastectomy skin flap is crucial to avoid implant exposure and infection, particularly with the prosthetic reconstruction. With autogenous reconstruction, the breast skin incision can be copied directly onto the flap using a template to match the skin deficit precisely. A team approach with the oncological and reconstructive surgeons working simultaneously is an attractive option to shorten the operating time with TRAM reconstruction. This is valuable especially with a free-flap reconstruction so that the reconstructive surgeon can start to dissect out the recipient vessels in the axilla immediately after the flap is raised and the mastectomy is completed.

BIBLIOGRAPHY

August DA, Wilkins E, Rea T. Breast reconstruction in older women. Surgery 1994; 115:663–668.

Baldwin BJ, Schustermann MA, Miller MJ, Kroll SS, Wang BG. Bilateral breast reconstruction: conventional versus free TRAM. Plast Reconstr Surg 1994; 93:1410–1416.

Council on Scientific Affairs, American Medical Association. Silicone gel breast implants. JAMA 1993; 270(21):2602.

Grotting JC. Immediate breast reconstruction using free TRAM flap. Clin Plast Surg 1994; 21:207.

Handel N, Silverstein MJ, Waisman E, Weisman JR. Reasons why mastectomy patients do not have breast reconstruction. Plast Reconstr Surg 1990; 86:118–122.

Moore TS, Farrell LD. Latissimus dorsi myocutaneous flap for breast reconstruction: long term results. Plast Reconstr Surg 1992; 89:666.

Shusterman MA: The free transverse rectus abdominis musculocutaneous flap for breast reconstruction. Ann Plast Surg 1994; 32:234.

Winer EP, Fee-Fulkerson K, Fulkerson CC, Georgiade G, Catoe KE, Conway M, Brunatti C, Holmes V, Rimer BK. Silicone controversy: a survey of women with breast cancer and silicone implants. J Natl Cancer Inst 1993; 85:1407–1411.

Case #H.13.2
Goal: To discuss factors relevant to decision making for breast reconstruction

PHILIP D. WEY

A 43-year-old woman is found on breast biopsy to have a 3.8-cm, high-grade, subareolar, invasive ductal carcinoma with 2 palpable, 1.5-cm, hard, mobile axillary lymph nodes. Mastectomy is recommended because the biopsy margins are positive. The patient is reluctant to undergo reexcision because of distortion after removal of the nipple-areolar complex. An active cross-country skier and tennis player, she is 85% of her ideal body weight and wishes to consider immediate breast reconstruction.

Reconstructive breast surgery offers a chance to "restore wholeness" after mastectomy. The ability to focus on quality-of-life issues is due to the substantial improvement in treatment of primary as well as recurrent breast cancer using a multidisciplinary approach involving oncologists, surgeons, radiation therapists, and other caregivers. Plastic surgery of the breast has advanced beyond merely restoring a breast mound. Current approaches often result in a natural-appearing, reconstructed breast and nipple that match the opposite side. The outcome is a symmetrical, harmonious, and proportionate reconstruction.

Although the prospects for reconstruction may ease the emotional distress women encounter when facing loss of the breast, the decision for mastectomy should be made independent of the decision for reconstruction. In the unlikely event of complications resulting in loss of the reconstruction, one does not wish for the event to simulate another mastectomy, and it would be an unfortunate situation for a woman to regret her decision for mastectomy (vs. conservation surgery) because of the inability to complete the reconstruction process.

Decision making regarding breast reconstruction follows a logical progression once the decision for mastectomy has been made. Is an immediate or delayed reconstruction desired? What type of reconstruction is desired? Is surgery to the opposite breast for reasons of symmetry acceptable? Reasons for immediate reconstruction include: (a) reducing the number of operations required; (b) technical ease; and (c) reducing body image distortion from the mastectomy defect. Reasons to delay the procedure include: (a) patient's preference to handle ablative surgery issues separately from reconstruction issues; (b) indecision regarding method of reconstruction; and (c) planned postoperative chest wall radiation. The few absolute contraindications to breast reconstruction include comorbid illness making additional surgical and anesthetic risks for elective reconstructive surgery unacceptable. Advanced stage (i.e., locally advanced) cancer is also of concern when coordinating multimodality therapy.

The patient presented has palpable axillary adenopathy. It is advised to prepare her for the potential need for adjuvant radiation therapy if four or more lymph nodes are found to contain metastatic cancer. The presence of a breast implant or tissue expander does not interfere with effective administration of radiation therapy. Unfortunately, the converse is not true, as chest wall irradiation has deleterious effects on breast reconstruction. Radiation delivered to a tissue expander or breast implant often results in capsular contracture. Therefore, most plastic surgeons favor the use of autogenous tissue methods (such as the TRAM flap), which have a better ability to tolerate the effects of radiation on normal tissues. Autogenous tissue reconstruction, when exposed to radiation, may develop some tissue fibrosis, although it is impossible to predict to what extent. In the individual who has already undergone radiation therapy and is considering a delayed reconstruction procedure, tissue expansion is not routinely recommended owing to the unacceptably high risk of complications such as capsular contracture, wound healing problems, and exposure or extrusion of the device (expander or implant).

If this patient does not undergo radiation therapy and is otherwise healthy, she could consider any of the available reconstruction options, including expanders, implants, autogenous tissue, and combinations thereof. Currently, silicone gel implants are available for use in breast reconstruction only in clinical study protocols, and a saline implant may be chosen as an acceptable substitute. In women of childbearing age, the use of an abdominal donor site (TRAM) in autogenous tissue reconstruction may be undesirable, and a saline breast implant would be a good option. The durability of the device is not known, and follow-up examination for leakage or rupture is recommended.

Autogenous tissue would be an excellent treatment option and has the advantages of: (a) avoiding medical and mechanical devices; (b) a softer, more natural feel; and (c) better aesthetic match to a greater variety of breast shapes and contours. As this patient would presumably like to maintain a high level of physical activity postoperatively, a single muscle pedicle TRAM flap as opposed to the recruitment of both muscles would be preferred. The use of microvascular TRAM free-tissue transfer can substantially reduce abdominal muscle requirements and, thus, donor site morbidity. In the motivated patient, distant microvascular donor sites (such as the gluteus free flap) would also preserve the abdominal donor site for heavy activity.

BIBLIOGRAPHY

Evans GR, Schusterman MA, Kroll SS, Miller MJ, Reece GP, Robb GL, et al. Reconstruction and the radiated breast: is there a role for implants? Plast Reconstr Surg 1995; 96:1111.

King GM, Rademaker AW, Mustoe TA. Abdominal-wall recovery following TRAM flap: a functional outcome study. Plast Reconstr Surg 1997; 99:417.

Nemecek JR, Young VL. Postmastectomy reconstruction. In: Marsh JL, ed. Decision Making in Plastic Surgery. St Louis: Mosby–Year Book, 1993.

Paletta CE, Bostwick J, Nahai F. The inferior gluteal free flap in breast reconstruction. Plast Reconstr Surg 1989; 84:875.

Shaw WW. Breast reconstruction by superior gluteal microvascular free flaps without silicone implants. Plast Reconstr Surg 1983; 72:490.

Sultan MR, Smith ML, Esatbrook A, Schnabel F, Singh D. Immediate breast reconstruction in patients with locally advanced disease. Ann Plast Surg 1997; 38: 345.

Williams JK, Carlson GW, Bostwick J, Bried JT, Mackay G. The effects of radiation treatment after TRAM flap breast reconstruction. Plast Reconstr Surg 1997; 100:1153.

Case #H.13.3
Goal: To discuss factors relevant to decision making for breast reconstruction

MIHYE CHOI

A 44-year-old, small-breasted woman is evaluated for a 4-cm, invasive ductal carcinoma. There is extensive angiolymphatic invasion. The biopsy margins are positive. Her mammograms reveal microcalcifications extending over much of the breast. Examination reveals palpable axillary lymph nodes. She is 85% of ideal body weight. You recommend a modified radical mastectomy. The patient desires breast reconstruction.

This case raises the potential problems encountered in breast reconstruction in a patient requiring adjuvant chemotherapy and radiation. For example, adriamycin is known to adversely affect wound healing. Radiation therapy is a significant problem for all types of breast reconstruction, causing fat necrosis in the autogenous flaps and periprosthetic capsular contracture in the implant-reconstructed breast. In addition, any complication involving the reconstructed breast, such as partial flap loss or implant exposure, may delay the adjuvant treatment. Owing to these concerns, some reconstructive surgeons would not recommend immediate breast reconstruction, especially for the patient who needs to undergo postoperative radiotherapy. These concerns regarding immediate breast reconstruction should be carefully weighed against the psychological benefit of immediate breast reconstruction. Schain reported that the earlier reconstruction is performed, the less severe the postmastectomy depression. The psychological benefits should not be overlooked in patients undergoing immunosupressive and cytotoxic treatments. A well-healed, reconstructed breast does not interfere with the effectiveness of chemotherapy and radiation therapy. Neither does it affect the detection of local recurrences. Locoregional recurrences develop in the native skin and subcutaneous tissue adjacent to the mastectomy site, not in the subpectoral region. In summary, although delayed breast reconstruction may be preferable in this patient, there is no absolute contraindication to immediate breast reconstruction. If the patient reaches a well-informed decision to proceed with immediate reconstruction with the understanding that the result may be suboptimal and necessitate subsequent revisions, this option can be approached with a careful plan to coordinate the postoperative care and the adjuvant treatment schedule.

This patient, who is 85% of ideal body weight, is unlikely to have sufficient abdominal or back adipose tissue to create an adequate breast mound with a TRAM or latissimus dorsi flap alone. Unfortunately, immediate reconstruction using a tissue expander after adjuvant radiotherapy is associated with discomfort and difficulty expanding the irradiated tissues. The result is often an inadequate breast mound with minimal ptosis. One way to deal with this problem is to complete the skin expansion before the radiotherapy, while the patient is receiving chemotherapy. The capsulectomy for the inevitable pericapsular contracture that will follow radiation therapy can be performed during the second-stage operation for the placement of a permanent implant. The breast expander should be placed under the pectoralis and serratus muscles to completely cover the prosthesis. This will minimize prosthesis exposure resulting from possible skin complications following the radiation therapy. At the time of mastectomy, skin flaps should be carefully inspected. The placement of the prosthesis should not be undertaken if the vascularity of the skin flap is compromised. Another option in this patient is to use the latissimus dorsi flap with a prosthesis for either the immediate or delayed reconstruction. This flap provides well-vascularized tissue to cover the prosthetic reconstruction, mitigating the effects of the radiation therapy on wound healing.

In conclusion, there are few reasons to delay breast reconstruction in a patient who meets the criteria for mastectomy. Relative contraindications for immediate breast reconstructions include medical conditions precluding an extensive or prolonged operation, locally advanced breast cancer, and probable need for adjuvant irradiation. Adjuvant radiotherapy more so than chemotherapy hinders the aesthetic result of immediate breast reconstruction regardless of the type of reconstruction used. It raises the likelihood of additional surgeries for capsulectomy or excision of fat necrosis. These disadvantages should be carefully weighed against the psychological benefit of immediate reconstruction.

BIBLIOGRAPHY

Bland KL. Experimental and clinical observations of the effects of cytotoxic chemotherapeutic drugs on wound healing. Ann Surg 1984; 199:782.

Dowden RV. Selection criteria for successful immediate breast reconstruction following mastectomy. Br J Plast Surg 1984; 37:369.

McGinley PH, Powell WR, Bostwick J III. Dosimetry of a silicone breast prosthesis. Radiology 1980; 135:223.

Schain WS. The sooner the better: a study of psychological factors in women undergoing immediate versus delayed breast reconstruction. Am J Psychiatry 1985; 142:40.

Slavin SA. Improving the latissimus dorsi myocutaneous flap with tissue expansion. Plast Reconstr Surg 1994; 93:811.

Slavin SA, Love SM, Golwyn RM. Recurrent breast cancer following immediate
    reconstruction with myocutaneous flaps. Plast Reconstr Surg 1994; 93:1191.
von Smitten K, Sundell B. The impact of adjunctive radiotherapy and cytotoxic
    chemotherapy on the outcome of immediate breast reconstruction by tissue
    expansion after mastectomy for breast cancer. Eur J Surg Oncol 1992; 18:
    119–123.

Case #H.13.4
Goal: To discuss breast reconstruction in a poor-prognosis patient

PHILIP D. WEY

*A 43-year-old woman has recently been diagnosed with a T2N1M0 (22
positive lymph nodes) breast cancer and is about to embark on high-dose
chemotherapy with stem cell rescue. She would like to have breast
reconstruction and is referred for discussion regarding "timing" of the
procedure.*

Immediate breast reconstruction following mastectomy for early-stage
breast cancer is well established. Administration of conventional chemotherapy on schedule and without an increased frequency of wound complications is well documented. Studies have shown that in the routine setting,
the patient undergoing immediate breast reconstruction faces no significant
additional risk when exposed to standard adjuvant chemotherapy.

Morbidity and mortality among patients receiving more aggressive adjuvant chemotherapy regimens, including high-dose chemotherapy with colony-stimulating factor support or stem cell support, can be more problematic
and presents new challenges to the reconstructive breast surgeon. Concerns
arise whether immediate breast reconstruction can and should be offered to
high-risk patients, and if so, what precautions are needed. It is acknowledged
that the reconstructive choices are continually evolving. In immediate breast
reconstruction, patients are encouraged to consider a single-stage reconstructive approach of autogenous tissue donor sites, or in multistaged procedures
be prepared for significant delays in completion of reconstruction due to
immunosuppression.

In the case presented for consideration of delayed breast reconstruction, the patient should be encouraged to complete high-dose chemotherapy
and stem cell transplantation with or without radiation therapy as indicated.
Recovery from such a protocol could last 3–6 months. Tissue expansion is
actively discouraged postradiation owing to the high risk of skin and wound
complications requiring device removal, as well as predictably high rates of

capsular contracture. The preferred option for breast reconstruction in this patient would utilize autogenous tissue with or without an implant.

Successful treatment of the high-risk breast cancer patient requires open communication among interdisciplinary personnel. It is to be hoped that as survival among women with advanced-stage primary breast cancer increases, the opportunity for immediate breast reconstruction can be routinely offered.

BIBLIOGRAPHY

Ahles TA, Tope DM, Furstenberg C, et al. Psychologic and neuropsychologic impact of autologous bone marrow transplantation. J Clin Oncol 1996; 14:1457.

Ayash LJ, Elias A, Wheeler C, Tepler I, Schwartz G, Schnipper L, et al. High dose chemotherapy with autologous stem cell support for breast cancer: a review of the Dana-Farber Cancer Institute/Beth Israel Hospital experience. J Hematother 1993; 2:507.

Ayash LJ, Wheeler C, Fairclough D, Schwartz G, Reich E, Warren D, et al. Prognostic factors for prolonged progression-free survival with high-dose chemotherapy with autologous stem-cell support for advanced breast cancer. J Clin Oncol 1995; 13:2043.

Furey PC, Macgillivray DC, Castiglione CL, Allen L. Wound complications in patients receiving adjuvant chemotherapy after mastectomy and immediate breast reconstruction for breast cancer. J Surg Oncol 1994; 55:194.

Holland HK, Dix SP, Geller RB, Devine, SM, Heffner LT, et al. Minimal toxicity and mortality in high-risk breast cancer patients receiving high-dose cyclophosphamide, thiotepa, and carboplatin plus autologous marrow/stem-cell transplantation and comprehensive supportive care. J Clin Oncol 1996; 14: 1156.

Myers SE, Williams SF. Role of high-dose chemotherapy and autologous stem cell support in treatment of breast cancer. Hematol Oncol Clin North Am 1993; 7:631.

Peters WP, Ross M, Vredenburgh JJ, Meisenberg B, Marks LB, Winer E, et al. High-dose chemotherapy and autologous bone marrow support as consolidation after standard-dose adjuvant therapy for high-risk primary breast cancer. J Clin Oncol 1993; 11:1132.

Sultan MR, Smith ML, Esatbrook A, Schnabel F, Singh D. Immediate breast reconstruction in patients with locally advanced disease. Ann Plast Surg 1997; 38: 345.

Wey PD, Highstein JB, Borah GL. Immediate breast reconstruction in the high-risk adjuvant setting. Ann Plast Surg 1997; 38:342.

Yule GJ, Concannon MJ, Croll G, Puckett CL. Is there liability with chemotherapy following immediate breast reconstruction? Plast Reconstr Surg 1996; 97:969.

H.14.   MANAGEMENT OF MEDICAL COMPLICATIONS

Case #H.14.1
Goal: To discuss the use of doxorubicin chemotherapy in the presence of Gilbert's disease

JOSEPH AISNER

A 42-year-old woman is set to begin adjuvant chemotherapy with CAF. Laboratory studies reveal a bilirubin of 2.5, 50% indirect. A hemolysis workup is negative. CT of the liver is normal. She states that jaundice runs in the family.

This is an interesting situation that tests the dosing algorithms for anthracyclines in the presence of abnormal bilirubin levels. Elevated bilirubin may indicate the presence of liver disease, which can significantly alter doxorubicin (or other anthracycline) metabolism resulting in increased area under the curve (AUC) and thus increased toxicity. This does not necessarily apply to the situation of hereditary bilirubin metabolism.

Assuming that this patient has an inherited disease causing *unconjugated* hyperbilirubinemia (Gilbert's disease) rather than hemolysis, which is readily ruled out, and assuming further the patient has no other disturbances of hepatic function, I would proceed with the first course of CA chemotherapy without dose modification. Subsequent dose modifications would then be based on the toxicities encountered with the first course.

There are several inherited disorders in bilirubin metabolism, including, an abnormality in glucuronide formation (Gilbert's disease) and abnormal transport of bilirubin (Dubin-Johnson syndrome); both can lead to episodic hyperbilirubinemia that is often associated with fevers or during periods of fasting or illness. However, these patients can and often do have increased bilirubin levels without underlying exacerbations. There is no indication from the literature that patients with these inherited diseases have any greater incidence of mucositis or myelosuppression with anthracycline therapy than the normal population without bilirubin disturbances. One might therefore infer that there is little change in the area under the curve for conventional doses of doxorubicin. Furthermore, the dose-reduction algorithms for elevated bilirubin that are included in the package insert for doxorubicin were derived from retrospective data, and these algorithms have not been prospectively validated. Thus, in the absence of other liver function abnormalities, these dosing guidelines probably represent an overestimate of the need to modify (reduce) the dose of doxorubicin. Dose modification for Gilbert's disease, however, may need specific validation for other drugs known to have hepatic clearance. Given the mechanism of abnormal glucuronide formation, it is likely that Gilbert's disease may generate toxicity problems associated with other drugs such as the camptothecin derivatives. The entire field of drug dosing, exposure, and pharmacodynamics in the presence of altered organ function is an important research activity and defining these kinetics for each new drug is clearly warranted.

BIBLIOGRAPHY

Brenner DE, Wiernik PH, Wesley M, Bachur NR. Acute doxorubicin toxicity. Relationship to pre-treatment liver function, response, and pharmacokinetics in patients with acute non-lymphocytic leukemia. Cancer 1984; 53:1042–1048.

Johnson PJ, Dobbs N, Kalayci C, et al. Clinical efficacy and toxicity of standard dose adriamycin in hyperbilirubinaemic patients with hepatocellular carcinoma: relation to liver tests and pharmacokinetic parameters. Br J Cancer 1992; 65:751.

Robert J, Gianni L. Pharmacokinetics and metabolism of anthracyclines. Cancer Surv 1993; 17:219.

Scharschmidt BF. Bilirubin metabolism and hyperbilirubinemia. In: Wyngaarden JG, Smith LH, eds. Cecil's Textbook of Medicine, 18th ed. Philadelphia: WB Saunders, 1988.

Sulkes A, Collins JM. Re-appraisal of some dosage adjustment guidelines. Cancer Treat Rep 1987; 71:229–233.

Case #H.14.2
Goal: To discuss the management of malignant pericardial effusion

WILLIAM N. HAIT

A 45-year-old woman presents with chest discomfort and shortness of breath. Physical examination reveals a woman in no acute distress, a blood pressure of 90/70, heart rate 120, and respiratory rate 18. Workup reveals a large pericardial effusion with signs of tamponade. She is 3 years post treatment with lumpectomy followed by radiation therapy and adjuvant CAF for a hormone-receptor-positive, stage II, invasive lobular cancer of the left breast. She has been on tamoxifen since the completion of chemotherapy. She has a negative past medical history. There is a strong family history of atherosclerotic cardiovascular disease.

The differential diagnosis of chest discomfort and shortness of breath in a 45-year-old woman with a history of breast cancer and a family history of coronary artery disease can be divided anatomically into disorders of the heart (arteries, valves, and cardiac muscle), lungs (parenchyma and vasculature), pleura, and chest wall (musculature and ribs). Despite the broad differential, we are told that a workup revealed a large pericardial effusion with signs of tamponade. Therefore, the differential narrows to the various causes of pericardial tamponade, which may be traumatic, infectious, granulomatous, inflammatory (e.g., secondary to radiation), or malignant. Given the history of stage II lobular invasive carcinoma and the approximate risk of recurrence of 50% within the first 5 years, this is an example of malignant pericarditis until proven otherwise. The possibility of radiation-induced pericarditis should also be considered.

Cardiac mortality is increased in patients receiving radiation for breast cancer. In older series, the risk appeared to be due to an increase in ischemic heart disease, attributable perhaps to increased exposure of the left anterior descending coronary artery. Pericarditis is a common complication of radiation therapy to the mediastinum but an uncommon complication of radiation to the breast following lumpectomy. Its onset peaks within the first year following treatment and is uncommon thereafter.

Malignant pericarditis is present in 25% of patients with metastatic breast cancer by the time of death, but is responsible for death in <5% of patients. The median survival of patients with malignant pericarditis from breast cancer ranges from 12 to 20 months.

Pericardial tamponade is a medical emergency that can lead to sudden death. The initial approach is both diagnostic and therapeutic. Following a chest X-ray, which may show the classic globular enlargement of the heart, clear lung fields, and small left>right pleural effusions, a more definitive approach is taken. A two-dimensional cardiac echo should be obtained to confirm the presence of pericardial fluid and or thickening, as well as the presence of collapse of the right atrium and right ventricle during diastole, the former being an earlier finding than the later. These findings are highly sensitive (92%) and specific (100%) predictors of cardiac tamponade. I would recommend immediate evaluation by a cardiologist, who should place a Swan-Ganz catheter to measure ventricular and atrial filling pressures. Next, a pigtail catheter should be inserted into the pericardial space and pericardial pressure measured. Equalization of all pressure measurements, ventricular, atrial, and pericardial, would suggest a hemodynamically more significant problem. Next, 50 cc of fluid should be removed from the pericardial space and one red-top tube should be filled to observe for clotting. Clotting of the fluid indicates that it comes from the ventricle rather than the pericardium, since any blood in the pericardial fluid would be post-clot and lysis. The cardiac pressures should be immediately repeated to evaluate whether removal of a small amount of fluid decreased intraventricular pressures. If so, the underlying pathophysiological process is likely to favor pericardial tamponade rather than pericardial constriction. Next, the remainder of the fluid should be drained and the pigtail catheter left in place attached to suction. As much fluid as possible should be sent immediately, unpreserved, for cytology. At this point, the intraventricular and intrapericardial pressures should be normal. Failure of the intracardiac pressures to return to normal despite complete drainage of the pericardium and the expected decrease in pericardial pressure suggests the presence of occult constriction. In this case, the diagnosis of subacute, effusive, constrictive pericarditis should be considered, and depending on the course over the next 24–48 hr, an operative procedure should be entertained.

If, at any point, the hemodynamic situation begins to deteriorate and there is no strong evidence for constriction, a pericardial window via the subxiphoid approach should be undertaken. A useful alternative is a thorascopic pericardiectomy, which can now be done safely at many institutions. A decision should be made early on as to whether surgical intervention is indicated, since use of a thorascopic approach is simpler before the pericardium is drained. In the presence of tamponade, the long-term results are somewhat better following surgical intervention.

Once the clinical situation is stable, definitive treatment must be considered. If a diagnosis of malignant pericarditis is confirmed by cytology, the patient would enter the clinical pathways as a stage IV patient experiencing a first recurrence. In most cases, I would recommend that this patient be enrolled on a clinical research protocol, but given the urgency of the situation, such a protocol would have to contain at least one of the known active drugs, such as a taxane, or vinca alkaloid. Methotrexate must be avoided because of the risk of serious side effects secondary to third spacing of the drug.

BIBLIOGRAPHY

Buck M, Ingle JN, Guilani ER, et al. Pericardial effusion in women with breast cancer. Cancer 1987; 60:263.

Cuzick J, Stewart H, Rutqvist L, et al. Cause-specific mortality in long-term survivors of breast cancer who participated in trials of radiotherapy. J Clin Oncol 1994; 12:447.

Fuller S, Haybittle J, Sith R, et al. Cardiac doses in post-operative breast irradiation. Radiother Oncol 1992; 25:19.

Gillam LD, Guyer DE, Gibson TC, et al. Hydrodynamic compression of the right atrium: a new echocardiographic sign of cardiac tamponade. Circulation 1983; 68:294.

Hagemeister FB, Buzdar AU, Luna MA, et al. Causes of death in breast cancer. Cancer 1980; 46:162.

Mack MJ, Landreneau, RJ, Hazelrigg SR, et al. Video thorascopic management of benign and malignant pericardial effusions. Chest 1993; 103:390S.

Mann T, Brodie BR, Grossman W, McLaurin L. Effusive-constrictive hemodynamic pattern due to neoplastic involvement of the pericardium. Am J Cardiol 1978; 41:781–786.

Singh S, Wann S, Schuchard GH, et al. Right ventricular and right atrial collapse in patients with cardiac tamponade: a combined echocardiographic and hemodynamic study. Circulation 1984; 70:966.

Case #H.14.3
Goal: To discuss the management of malignant pleural effusions

KEVIN R. FOX

A 42-year-old woman presents with shortness of breath. She is 3 years post treatment with CAF for a stage II, infiltrating ductal carcinoma. Chest X-ray reveals a large left pleural effusion.

Malignant pleural effusions occur commonly in patients with breast cancer. In fact, breast cancer is the most common cause of malignant pleural effusion in women. Because this patient is symptomatic, treatment should produce rapid, short-term relief of symptoms while ensuring the greatest degree of long-term stabilization. Although the institution of systemic chemotherapy may provide resolution of the effusion, such a response may take weeks to months, too slow for immediate consideration here, if proper palliation is to be effected.

Proper management, therefore, requires some means of mechanical drainage of the pleural effusion. Bedside percutaneous thoracentesis will produce immediate symptom relief, but should only be relied upon if the concurrent administration of systemic therapy is expected to produce a high likelihood of response. While this approach might be appropriate in a patient with a small, minimally symptomatic effusion in the setting of known hormone-receptor-positive breast cancer with little or no prior exposure to hormonal therapy, it is not advisable in our patient, who has a large effusion, is receptor-negative, and has a likelihood of response to systemic therapy below 50%. In our patient, simple thoracentesis virtually guarantees that reaccumulation of the effusion will occur within a few days.

Instead, a definitive surgical procedure should be performed for purposes of long-term clearance of the effusion. Placement of a chest tube at the bedside, or clearance of the pleural space by direct videothoracoscopy with intraoperative pleurodesis, are two viable options. Before either procedure is undertaken, a decubitus film should be obtained to ensure that the effusion is free-flowing. A free-flowing effusion can be managed with bedside placement of a chest tube with minimal morbidity. The success of this intervention requires the near-complete drainage of the pleural space, thus allowing direct apposition of the visceral and parietal pleura. The process usually takes several days to reach a daily output of the chest tube below 200 cc/day under conditions of low suction. At this point, a sclerosing agent is instilled directly into the drained pleural space. Many experts maintain that talc is the most effective agent for this purpose, and thus talc instillation has become the standard pleurodesis agent at our hospital. The direct instillation of a talc slurry into the pleural tube should initiate the intense pleural reaction required to obliterate the pleural space and prevent subsequent reaccumulation of fluid.

If the decubitus film demonstrates fluid loculations or unsuspected pleural masses, then bedside placement of a chest tube may be ineffective, and consideration should be given to operative intervention with thoracoscopy, direct visualization of the pleural space, and the intraoperative instillation of a sclerosing agent, again preferably talc. A preoperative computed-tomography scan of the chest is advised before this procedure is undertaken. Much of the experience with talc has not been by instillation via chest tube, but by direct instillation during more extensive surgical procedures such as thoracoscopy or thoracotomy. Whether thoracoscopic intervention is superior to simple chest tube placement in uncomplicated patients remains controversial, and the choice of procedure may be guided largely by the preferences of one's institution and thoracic surgical team. The success rate of properly executed talc pleurodesis may be as high as 90%, as compared to a success rate of approximately 75% with tetracycline.

Following the optimal local treatment of the pleural effusion, this patient should be considered a candidate for systemic therapy. Given the 3-year interval since adjuvant treatment with CAF, this patient may not be truly "doxorubicin-resistant," and she might respond to reinstitution of the same regimen. However, because most adjuvant CAF regimens administer from 360 to 400 mg/m^2 of doxorubicin, this patient would reach a reasonable limit of doxorubicin exposure within a short period of time, making doxorubicin-based therapy of little practical value in this case.

The highest response rates in patients with metastatic breast cancer and prior doxorubicin exposure have been achieved with the taxanes. Whether docetaxel (Taxotere) or paclitaxel (Taxol) is the superior agent in this setting is arguable and is the subject of an ongoing randomized clinical trial. Data from phase II and cross-comparisons from phase III trials suggest that taxotere may produce somewhat higher response rates. Therefore, the use of a taxane constitutes the most appropriate chemotherapeutic intervention at this point. There is no evidence that the combination of a taxane with another nonanthracycline chemotherapeutic agent will necessarily provide any advantage to this particular patient.

There exist many controversial questions regarding the management of this patient. If her pleural effusion, after a proper metastatic evaluation, is her only site of disease, and if it has been managed appropriately by local means, is chemotherapy necessary at all? Furthermore, would high-dose chemotherapy provide any long-term advantage? This author remains skeptical as to the true benefit of high-dose approaches to metastatic breast cancer, but would favor a course of taxane-based therapy as a temporary hedge against further disease progression and dissemination.

BIBLIOGRAPHY

Fentiman I, Rubens R, Hayward J. A comparison of intracavitary talc and tetracycline for the control of pleural effusions secondary to breast cancer. Eur J Can Clin Oncol 1986; 22:1079.

Hansheer F, Yarbro J. Diagnosis and treatment of malignant pleural effusion. Semin Oncol 1985; 12:54.

Hartman D, Gaither J, Kesler K, et al. Comparison of insufflated talc under thoracoscopic guidance with standard tetracycline and bleomycin pleurodesis for control of malignant pleural effusions. J Thorac Cardiovasc Surg 1993; 105: 743.

Case #H.14.4
Goal: To discuss the role of surgery and radiation therapy in the management of metastases to weight-bearing bones

KEVIN R. FOX

A 58-year-old woman presents with pain in the anterior thigh. Your astute fellow makes the diagnosis of bony metastases to the hip. A bone scan is consistent with metastases to the femoral neck. A plain film reveals erosion of the cortex.

The development of bone metastases is a common problem in breast cancer and will be the first manifestation of metastatic disease in up to 40% of patients. The goals of therapy are palliation of pain, prevention of pathological fracture, and restoration of full ambulatory function. The management of this patient is driven by the location of this particular lesion, and by the fact that it is symptomatic. Although radiation therapy might provide excellent relief of pain, this treatment modality alone may not be considered adequate. The risk of pathological fracture may remain and healing and restoration of normal bone may be delayed by external-beam radiation. Therefore, urgent orthopedic consultation should be sought.

Immediate management prior to orthopedic consultation should include strict limitation of activity to essential functional necessities, thus minimizing weight bearing. Strict bed rest is probably not required, but use of a walker or crutches is prudent until orthopedic evaluation can be arranged. In this patient, a bone scan has been completed and should always be considered as a first diagnostic step (in conjunction with plain films of symptomatic areas) to rule out coexisting lesions in other long bones.

The fundamental question is whether orthopedic fixation is required. General guidelines have traditionally included (a) destruction of more than 50% of cortical width and (b) lesions more than 2.5 cm in diameter. However, such criteria may not be accurate predictors of fracture risk in breast cancer patients, and a "scoring system" as proposed by Mirels (see Table 1) may better predict this particular patient's risk. If one notes that "functional pain" in this instance is defined as pain with weight bearing, then her score will be at least eight by this method, and her risk of fracture in the next 6 months, if the condition is untreated, will be unacceptably high. I would favor orthopedic intervention without delay.

The choice of the orthopedic procedure should be deferred to the orthopedic surgeon. As this lesion is located in the femoral neck, an intermedullary compression screw and side plate device could be considered, but total hip replacement may be a better long-term option. Many orthopedic

Table 1   A Predictive Model for Fracture Risk

	Score		
	1	2	3
Site	Upper limb	Lower limb	Peritrochanteric
Pain	Mild	Moderate	Functional
Lesion size (fraction of bone diam.)	Blastic <1/3	Mixed 1/3–2/3	Lytic >2/3

Fracture risk by score	
Score	Risk (%)
0–7	5
8	15
>9	33

surgeons expert in the management of bone metastases will now obtain magnetic resonance imaging (MRI) scanning of the hip to better assess the full extent of the lesion and thus make the best surgical decision on the patient's behalf. In borderline cases, one should favor orthopedic intervention, as plain films may underestimate the patient's risk for injury without fixation. MRI scanning should be considered in all cases where the need for surgery is unclear.

After appropriate orthopedic management, the value of adjunctive radiation therapy must be considered. Because this patient's lesion was symptomatic at diagnosis, and the use of a compression screw will not likely palliate her pain, radiation therapy is indicated. However, if a total hip replacement is chosen, and the lesion thus surgically extirpated, the need for adjunctive radiation therapy will be obviated.

Following appropriate local treatment, systemic therapy considerations will be relatively straightforward and should follow general oncological algorithms. The ultimate choices will depend on the patient's prior systemic therapy, whether her original tumor was hormone-receptor-positive, and whether she has other sites of metastatic disease. If this femoral lesion is the only site of disease in this patient and has been surgically extirpated, then "adjuvant" hormonal therapy can be considered if she was receptor-positive and has relatively little prior exposure to hormonal intervention. The inevitable appearance of other systemic metastases may be delayed by hormonal therapy. If she had been receptor-negative, then the use of adjunctive combination chemotherapy should be considered for an arbitrary period of 3–6 months. The use of bisphosphonate compounds such as pamidronate has not been studied in patients with solitary, surgically treated metastases and is probably best reserved until additional lytic lesions appear.

Editors' comment: The importance of adjunctive radiation therapy following orthopedic intervention is important. Retrospective studies have shown that the risk of refracture and functional outcome are improved with radiation.

BIBLIOGRAPHY

Harrington K. Orthopedic Management of Metastatic Bone Disease. St Louis: Mosby, 1988.

Mirels H. Metastatic disease in long bones. Clin Orthop 1988; 249:256.

Tong D, Gillick L, Hendrickson F. The palliation of symptomatic osseous metastases: final results of the Radiation Therapy Oncology Group. Cancer 1982; 50:893.

Case #H.14.5
Goal: To discuss the use of hematopoietic growth factors in the management of patients receiving adjuvant chemotherapy

I. CRAIG HENDERSON

A 34-year-old woman is being treated for high-risk, stage I disease with dose-intensified CA. You have obtained weekly blood counts during her first cycle, which revealed a nadir at day 14 of 400 total neutrophils. Other than feeling tired, she had no symptoms during this cycle.

This patient has invasive, operable breast cancer and adjuvant chemotherapy has been selected. Although she is on "dose-intensified" adjuvant chemotherapy, it is not clear precisely what doses she has received. She has afebrile neutropenia after cycle 1. I would repeat cycle 2 at the same doses.

Although higher doses of cyclophosphamide and doxorubicin (CA) are associated with a deeper white cell nadir, there is little prolongation of the nadir as a result of higher doses. Most patients will have recovered to "safe levels" within 2–3 days after the nadir and will be able to receive their next course of treatment on time even if the white cell count at day 21 (assuming the usual 3-week cycle of CA) is somewhat below that at the beginning of treatment. Unlike CMF, there is rarely cumulative myelosuppression. Thus, patients on CA rarely have febrile neutropenia or serious infectious complications. This was shown elegantly in the early 1970s. The first preparative regimen used for autologous bone marrow transplant was CA. Since the nadirs were consistently short regardless of dose, it is was difficult to demonstrate that the autologous marrow was engrafting.

It might be argued that dose reduction would be appropriate for this patient, but this would depend somewhat on what doses she received on cycle 1. It has been shown in a large, randomized trial that reduction of CAF doses from $600/60/600$ mg/m^2 of cyclophosphamide, doxorubicin, and 5-fluorouracil, respectively, to $300/30/300$ mg/m^2 decreased (or possibly eliminated) the survival benefit from adjuvant chemotherapy. However, a more modest decrease in dose from $600/60/600$ mg/m^2 to $450/45/450$ had no effect. (It should be noted that only four cycles of therapy at either $600/60/660$ mg/m^2 or $300/30/300$ mg/m^2 were given while patients randomized to receive $450/45/450$ mg/m^2 received six cycles.) A subsequent study that randomized patients to higher doses of cyclophosphamide (1200 mg/m^2 at 3-weekly intervals) did not demonstrate either a disease-free or overall survival advantage for the higher dose. Studies evaluating cyclophosphamide doses of 2400 mg/m^2 and doxorubicin doses of up to 90 mg/m^2 have completed enrollment by the NSABP and the CALGB, but no results have yet been reported. Until all of the data are available, it is wise to be cautious about reducing chemotherapy doses, but at the same time doses much higher than those in the conventional range (e.g., cyclophosphamide 600 mg/m^2 and doxorubicin 60 mg/m^2) cannot be justified in the face of life-threatening toxicities.

If this patient develops febrile neutropenia on a subsequent course of therapy, I would be inclined to continue the same dose but add G-CSF in subsequent courses. This is the indication approved by the Food and Drug Administration (FDA) and recommended by the American Society of Clinical Oncology, since the doses of CA that might reasonably be used outside of a protocol should not result in febrile neutropenia in more than 40% of courses. The choice of G-CSF over GM-CSF is largely historical; G-CSF was originally evaluated and approved by the FDA for support of conventional chemotherapy while GM-CSF was originally developed in studies of very-high-dose chemotherapy and autologous bone marrow transplantation. G-CSF may be associated with a more rapid recovery of neutrophils while GM-CSF may have a greater benefit in the prevention of thrombocytopenia. The NSABP evaluated each cytokine in the pilot studies for their randomized trials in which cyclophosphamide doses of 1200 mg/m^2 and 2400 mg/m^2 were compared to lower doses. They concluded that the two cytokines were probably equally efficacious but that G-CSF caused more rapid recovery of neutrophils, was associated with marginally fewer hospitalizations, and was slightly less toxic. Based on studies performed to date, either G-CSF or GM-CSF can reasonably be used to prevent febrile neutropenia.

BIBLIOGRAPHY

American Society of Clinical Oncology. Recommendations for the use of hematopoietic colony-stimulating factors: evidence-based, clinical practice guidelines. J Clin Oncol 1994; 12:2471–2508.

Bregni M, Siena S, Di Nicola M, Dodero A, Peccatori F, Ravagnani F, Danesini G, Laffranchi A, Bonadonna G, Gianni AM. Comparative effects of granulocyte-macrophage colony-stimulating factor and granulocyte colony-stimulating factor after high-dose cyclophosphamide cancer therapy. J Clin Oncol 1996; 14: 628–635.

Domine M, Estevez L, Andrade J, Robles L, Casimiro C, Paniagua C, Barbolla L, Vicente L, Lobo F. Randomized trial of granulocyte-macrophage colony-stimulating factor (GM-CSF) versus granulocyte colony-stimulating factor (G-CSF) after high-dose chemotherapy with peripheral blood progenitor cell (PBPC) rescue. Proc Annu Meet Am Soc Clin Oncol 1997; 16:A419 (abstract).

Fisher B, Anderson S, Wickerham DL, DeCillis A, Dimitrov N, Mamounas E, Wolmark N, Pugh R, Atkins JN, Meyers FJ, Abramson N, Wolter J, Bornstein RS,

Levy L, Romond EH, et al. Increased intensification and total dose of cyclo-phosphamide in a doxorubicin-cyclophosphamide regimen for the treatment of primary breast cancer: findings from National Surgical Adjuvant Breast and Bowel Project B-22. J Clin Oncol 1997; 15:1858–1869.

Tobias JS, Weiner RS, Griffiths CT, Richman CM, Parker LM, Yankee RA. Expe-rience with cryopreserved autologous marrow infusion following high dose chemotherapy. Eur J Cancer 1977; 13:269–277.

Wood WC, Budman DR, Korzun AH, Cooper MR, Younger J, Hart RD, Moore A, Ellerton JA, Norton L, Ferree CR, Ballow AC, Frei I, Emil, Henderson IC. Dose and dose intensity of adjuvant chemotherapy for stage II, node-positive breast carcinoma. N Engl J Med 1994; 330:1253–1259.

Case #H.14.6
Goal: To discuss the management of intractable nausea and vomiting

SUSAN GOODIN

A 39-year-old woman is being treated on a randomized clinical trial for high-risk, stage II breast cancer, and is receiving CA, with an escalated dose of cyclophosphamide ($1g/m^2$ every 21 days). Her pretreatment antiemetics included ondansetron, compazine, and dexamethasone. She started vomiting 12 hr after completion of her cytoxan, and despite increased use of ativan and dexamethasone, she remained ill for over 1 week.

Nausea and vomiting may have several causes in patients with cancer. These can include physical complications of the disease, brain metastases, metabolic complications such as hypercalcemia, or bowel obstruction. In the absence of underlying causes, nausea and vomiting occurring soon after the administration of antineoplastics can be assumed to be induced by chemo-therapy. Many factors can influence the incidence of chemotherapy-induced nausea and vomiting. The most important treatment-related factor is the intrinsic emetogenicity of the chemotherapy regimen. The incidence and severity of nausea and vomiting are related to the emetogenic potential of the drug, dose, route of administration, schedule, infusion rate, and drug combination administered. The emetogenic potential of individual antineo-plastic agents has been categorized from high to low based on induction of emesis when administered as single agents with no antiemetics (Table 1). Since few antineoplastics are administered as single agents, a recently pub-lished algorithm helps determine the emetogenicity of combination regimens (Table 2).

There is a high degree of interindividual variability in the magnitude of nausea and vomiting experienced by patients, and a number of factors

Table 1 Emetogenic Potential of Single-Agent Chemotherapy

Level	Frequency of emesis (%)	Agent
5	>90	Carmustine > 250 mg/m^2
		Cisplatin $\geq$ 50 mg/m^2
		Cyclophosphamide > 1500 mg/m^2
		Dacarbazine
		Mechlorethamine
		Streptozocin
4	60–90	Carboplatin
		Carmustine < 250 mg/m^2
		Cisplatin $\leq$ 50 mg/m^2
		Cyclophosphamide > 750 mg/m^2 $\leq$ 1500 mg/m^2
		Cytarabine > 1 g/m^2
		Doxorubicin > 60 mg/m^2
		Methotrexate > 1 g/m^2
		Procarbazine (oral)
3	30–60	Cyclophosphamide < 750 mg/m^2
		Cyclophosphamide (oral)
		Doxorubicin 20–60 mg/m^2
		Epirubicin < 90 mg/m^2
		Hexamethylmelamine (oral)
		Idarubicin
		Ifosfamide
		Methotrexate 250–1000 mg/m^2
		Mitoxantrone < 15 mg/m^2
2	10–30	Docetaxel
		Etoposide
		5-Fluorouracil < 1000 mg/m^2
		Gemcitabine
		Methotrexate > 50 mg/m^2 < 250 mg/m^2
		Mitomycin
		Paclitaxel
1	<10	Bleomycin
		Busulfan
		Chlorambucil (oral)
		2-Chlorodeoxyadenosine
		Fludarabine
		Hydroxyurea
		Methotrexate $\leq$ 50 mg/m^2
		L-Phenylalanine mustard (oral)
		Thioguanine (oral)
		Vinblastine
		Vincristine
		Vinorelbine

Table 2 Algorithm for Defining the Emetogenicity of Combination
Chemotherapy

1. Identify the most emetogenic agent in the combination.
2. Assess the relative contribution of other agents to the emetogenicity of the
   combination. When considering other agents, the following rules apply:
   a. Level 1 agents do not contribute to the emetogenicity of a given regimen.
   b. Adding one or more level 2 agents increases the emetogenicity of the
      combination by one level greater than the most emetogenic agent in the
      combination (e.g., 2 + 2 = 3; 2 + 2 + 2 = 3)
   c. Adding level 3 or 4 agents increases the emetogenicity of the combination
      by one level per agent. (e.g., 3 + 2 = 4; 3 + 2 + 2 = 4; 3 + 3 + 3 = 5)

have been identified that influence a patient's risk. Beyond the emetogenicity
of the chemotherapy regimen, other factors that influence a patient's risk
include gender (females are at a much higher risk for nausea and vomiting),
age (decreased risk with increasing age), alcohol intake (decreased risk with
history of alcohol abuse), and prior experience with chemotherapy. In addition, patients with a previous history of motion sickness, emesis during
pregnancy, and patients with anxiety are at higher risk to experience nausea
and vomiting.

Antineoplastics are associated with three types of nausea and vomiting:
acute, delayed, and anticipatory. The acute syndrome is most common and
is associated with high frequency and severity occurring within the first 24
hr after administration of the antineoplastic agent. Delayed nausea and vomiting is often less severe than the acute syndrome and occurs 1–5 days after
chemotherapy administration, with a peak frequency between 48 and 72 hr.
Anticipatory nausea and vomiting is a conditioned response that occurs before or very soon after chemotherapy administration and can be triggered
by psychological factors.

A wide range of antiemetic agents have been used to control nausea
and vomiting. These agents target neurotransmitters that have been identified
as having a role in chemotherapy-induced nausea and vomiting. Dopamine
receptors within the chemoreceptor trigger zone (CTZ) and the upper gastrointestinal tract are the target of the dopamine antagonists phenothiazines,
butyrophenones, and the substituted benzamides. These agents are effective
in the acute setting for low, moderate, and highly emetogenic regimens.
Although the pathophysiology of delayed emesis is not well understood, the
dopamine antagonists also appear to be effective in this setting.

Serotonin (5-HT) is the target of the serotonin antagonists ondansetron,
granisetron, and dolasetron. These agents inhibit serotonin from binding to
5-HT3 receptors located in the gastrointestinal tract and the CTZ, preventing

acute emesis from low, moderate, and highly emetogenic chemotherapy regimens. Although studies are lacking in the delayed setting, serotonin antagonists currently do not appear to play a significant role in the prevention of emesis that begins greater than 24 hr following emetogenic chemotherapy.

The corticosteroids dexamethasone and methylprednisolone do not target a specific neurotransmitter. It is currently believed that inhibition of prostaglandin synthesis and changes in cellular permeability are responsible for their effectiveness as antiemetics. Regardless of their mechanism, corticosteroids are potent antiemetics in the acute and delayed setting. When combined with the serotonin antagonists or metoclopramide, corticosteroids significantly enhance effectiveness. Finally, the benzodiazepines are most effective as an adjuvant to more well-established antiemetic agents. Their major contribution to the antiemetic regimen appears to be their anxiolytic, amnestic, and sedative properties. This makes the use of lorazepam attractive in the prevention and treatment of anticipatory nausea and vomiting.

The aggressiveness of antiemetic therapy should be determined by both the antiemetic potential of the treatment regimen and patient characteristics that would help predict the risk of acute, delayed, or anticipatory nausea and vomiting. The CA regimen, utilizing 1 g/m^2 of cyclophosphamide, would be classified as a level 5, or highly emetogenic, regimen. Adding to the risk of emesis, this patient's gender also increases her susceptibility to emesis. A cyclophosphamide-based regimen, which is associated with both acute and delayed emesis, would typically be pretreated with a regimen similar to what this patient received: a 5-HT3 antagonist and a steroid. Since her breakthrough emesis occurred 12 hr after completion of the chemotherapy, a number of factors could explain the failure of the regimen and therefore provide alternatives for future cycles. Assuming that she received adequate doses of antiemetics, additional doses of the serotonin antagonist with a steroid could be administered at 12 hr after the chemotherapy on her next cycle. However, recent data have shown that repeated dosing of the serotonin antagonist within the first 24 hr does not improve control in the acute setting. The patient also suffered from a week of delayed emesis, which was ineffectively treated with lorazepam and dexamethasone. Repeated antiemetic dosing at 12 hr may help control delayed emesis, but the doses must be administered on a scheduled basis and continued for 4–5 days after the chemotherapy. In addition, the use of a dopamine D2 antagonist with dexamethasone has been shown to be beneficial in preventing delayed emesis.

For the next cycle of therapy, the patient should be given a scheduled dose of lorazepam the evening before and 30 min prior to chemotherapy, as well as a serotonin antagonist, dexamethasone, and metoclopramide for prevention of the acute phase of emesis. Prophylaxis for delayed emesis should be started 12 hr after chemotherapy and continued until day 4 with scheduled doses of Compazine Spansules, 15 mg twice a day, dexamethasone 8 mg twice a day, and lorazepam at bedtime.

BIBLIOGRAPHY

Hesketh PJ, Gandara DR, Hainsworth J, et al. Addition of dopamine D2 antagonist prochlorperazine to granisetron/dexamethasone: improved control of acute emesis from high-dose cisplatin. Proc Am Soc Clin Oncol 1996; 15:540.

Hesketh PJ, Kris MG, Grungerg SM, Beck T, Hainsworth JD, Harker G, Aapro MS, Gandara D, Lindley C. Proposal for classifying the acute emetogenicity of cancer chemotherapy. J Clin Oncol 1997; 15(1):103–109.

Kris M, Pendergrass KB, Navari RM, et al. Prevention of acute emesis in cancer patients following high-dose cisplatin with the combination of oral dolasetron and dexamethasone. J Clin Oncol 1997; 15(5):2135–2138.

Marty M, Pouillart P, Scholl S, et al. Comparison of the 5-hydroxytryptamine 3 antagonist ondansetron with high-dose metoclopramide in the control of cisplatin-induced emesis. N Engl J Med 1990; 322:816–821.

Rittenberg CN, Gralla RJ, Lettow LA, et al. Combination antiemetic trials for delayed emesis. Proc Am Soc Clin Oncol 1994; 13:452.

H.15.   PALLIATION AND SUPPORTIVE CARE

Case #H.15.1
Goal: Management of intractable pain

SUSAN GOODIN

A 59-year-old woman presents with intractable bone pain. She has a 4-year history of metastatic breast cancer, hormone receptor positive, which is no longer responsive to therapy. She has received radiation therapy to multiple bony sites and both she and her radiation therapist are unwilling to radiate previously radiated areas that remain painful. She is on 240 mg twice daily of a slow-release morphine preparation, a nonsteroidal anti-inflammatory drug, and morphine sulfate for breakthrough pain.

Bone metastases are a major cause of morbidity in advanced breast cancer. Although bone metastases are associated with a poor prognosis, many patients survive for years after diagnosis of these lesions.

Pain is one complication of cancer that has metastasized to the bone. The mechanism causing pain in skeletal malignancy is not known, although it may result from direct tumor involvement of bone with activation of local nociceptors or compression of adjacent nerves, vascular structures, and soft tissue. The mechanisms of pain relief are also poorly understood. The goal of pain therapy in patients with advanced disease is to provide sufficient relief to allow function at a level they choose and to eventually die relatively pain free.

Strategies for controlling metastatic bone pain include the use of several modalities alone or in combination. These include antineoplastic drugs, hormonal agents, radiation therapy, opioids, nonsteroidal anti-inflammatory agents, radiopharmaceuticals, and more recently, the bisphosphonates. Before additional therapies are added, however, the assessment of the patient's pain and the efficacy of the current regimen must be determined.

Bone pain is usually described as dull and aching, localized to the area of metastasis, and is increased by movement. In addition to the pain assessment, the breakthrough drug regimen must be monitored closely to assure that the patient is receiving adequate doses of breakthrough opioid medication as well as scheduled medications. The treatment of persistent or moderate to severe pain should initially be an increase of the dosage of the opioid.

As prostaglandins are frequently associated with painful bone metastases because of their involvement in bone resorption, the non-steroidal anti-inflammatory drugs (NSAIDs) are thought to be essential in the treatment of bone pain. Their analgesic effect is based on inhibition of the mediators of the inflammatory process. Tumor growth produces inflammation and mechanical effects in adjacent tissues that can trigger the release of prostaglandins, bradykinin, and serotonin, which may precipitate or exacerbate pain in the surrounding tissue. By virtue of their mechanism of action, i.e., targeting the chemical mediators of the inflammatory process, the NSAIDs work well as adjunct therapy in the treatment of metastatic bone pain. However, unlike the opioid analgesics, the NSAIDs have a ceiling effect and increasing doses above the maximum daily dose will only increase toxicities without improving analgesia. Switching to a different class of NSAID has proven beneficial when maximum doses have been reached, rather than discontinuing the use of NSAIDs completely. In addition, corticosteroids can be utilized in refractory cases for the same mechanistic reason that NSAIDs are effective in the treatment of painful bone metastases.

Several radiopharmaceuticals have been used to treat pain from metastatic disease to bone. The beta-emitting radionuclides work by localizing in the area of increased osteoblastic activity causing local tissue damage, reducing pain-producing enzymes, and suppressing tumor growth by irradiation. Phosphorus-32-orthophosphate produces partial or complete relief of pain in about 80% of patients with bone metastases from breast cancer and prostate cancer. However, its use is limited by severe hematological toxicity in over 30% of patients. Although the majority of the data are for prostate cancer, strontium 89 is also effective in breast cancer, with 89% of patients achieving significant palliation. Regular monitoring of hematological status is essential, as there may be a 30% drop in blood counts from baseline. Onset to pain relief is approximately 10–20 days with a duration of pain relief from 4 to 15 months.

Activation of osteoclasts, the normal bone-resorbing cells, may represent the fundamental process underlying the development and progression of bone metastases. Bisphosphonates are inhibitors of osteoclastic bone resorption. Pamidronate has been shown to reduce skeletal morbidity, including pain, in breast cancer patients. In addition, pamidronate has also been shown to prevent skeletal complications in women with metastatic breast cancer who have osteolytic bone metastases.

Treatment of chronic cancer pain is often difficult and frustrating because there is no specific formula for success. As the patient under discussion is not a candidate for additional radiation or hormonal therapy, the current treatment regimen should be optimized after an assessment of the pain and the adequate use of breakthrough medications. If the upper limit of the recommended dose of the NSAID is reached (for example, 3200 mg/day of ibuprofen) and pain relief is not achieved, that drug should be discontinued and another NSAID from a different chemical class should be tried (e.g., choline magnesium trisalicylate 3000 mg/day).

The patient could receive pamidronate for the treatment of the pain in addition to the potential prevention of future skeletal complications. If the pain persists or increases, the addition of a radiopharmaceutical would be an appropriate choice for palliation of the painful bone lesions.

BIBLIOGRAPHY

Hortobagyi GN, Theriault RL, Porter L, et al. Efficacy of pamidronate in reducing skeletal complications in patients with breast cancer and lytic bone metastases. N Engl J Med 1996; 335:1785–1791.

Jacox AK, Carr DB, Payne R, et al. Management of Cancer Pain. Clinical Practice Guideline no. 9. Rockville, MD: Agency for Health Care Policy and Research, 1994. AHCPR publication no. 94-0592.

Robinson RG, Spicer JA, Preston DF, et al. Tratment of metastatic bone pain with strontium-89. Nucl Med Biol 1987; 14:219–222.

Silberstein EB. The treatment of painful osseous metastases with phosphorus-32-labeled phosphates. Semin Oncol 1993; 20(Suppl 2):10–21.

Tyrrell CT, Bruning PF, May-Levin F, et al. Pamidronate infusions as single-agent therapy for bone metastases: a phase II trial in patients with breast cancer. Eur J Cancer 1995; 31A(12):1976–1980.

H.16. PSYCHOSOCIAL SUPPORT

Case #H.16.1
Goal: To discuss the management of high-risk psychosocial patients and the use of alternative therapies

ALAN AXELROD

A 42-year-old woman presents for a fifth medical opinion regarding treatment of a biopsy-proven, 3.4-cm, invasive breast cancer with palpable axillary lymph nodes. She started a macrobiotic diet soon after the breast cancer was diagnosed. She is reluctant to undergo "standard therapy" because of the effect she anticipates the resulting recuperation, disfigurement, and fatigue will have on her 7-year-old daughter.

The diagnosis and treatment of cancer routinely raises so many psychosocial issues that it is sometimes difficult to determine what lies within the range of "normal" adjustment to this stress and what constitutes "abnormal" adjustment. Vulnerable/high-psychosocial-risk patients tend to be those with long-standing premorbid personality and or social/family problems. The additional stress related to illness and its treatment will frequently exacerbate these preexisting problems.

The first indication that a patient may be at high psychosocial risk may be difficulties maneuvering within the prescribed limits necessary to effect successful implementation of a mutually agreed upon treatment plan. In this case example, the fact that the patient presents for a fifth medical opinion indicates an inability to even begin treatment because of problems related to accepting a treatment plan suggested by four previous physicians. Although patient autonomy must always be respected and successful treatment must enlist the cooperation of the patient and family, decision making that seems to jeopardize the patient's health, such as an inability to agree to suggested treatment options, or an inability, once agreed upon, to carry through, is an indicator that something more than "normal" adjustment is happening, and that the patient's ability to problem-solve is ineffective in the current situation.

An initial history and physical will net pertinent psychosocial information as will the routine demographics collected at the time of intake. Is the person married, employed, covered by medical insurance? Are there young children in the family who may be affected by the disruptions caused by cancer? What is the patient's history of tobacco and alcohol use? Is there a history of physical and/or emotional illness or difficulties? All of the answers to these and other routine questions provide insight into the patient's social situation and emotional stressors. In the illustrative case example, the patient has a 7-year-old daughter and she states that she is concerned about the effect that "standard therapy" will have on her. This information should prompt exploration into the patient's marital status and general social support system. Is the patient a single mother and is her concern really with her ability to care for herself and her child? Is the child a vehicle for the projection of her own worries and fears concerning "disfigurement and fatigue"?

Many patients, as does the one in the case example, integrate "alternative therapies" into their treatment plans. Many are hesitant to speak about this with their physicians for fear of alienating them. Medical personnel must always impress upon the patient that information about "alternative therapies" must be provided to their treating physicians because of contraindications that may arise in combination with "traditional" medical treatment. Many physicians have become accustomed to their patients' inclusion of "other" forms of treatment into their self-care. "Complementary therapies," not to be confused with "alternative therapies," are gaining acceptance in the lay and medical communities. These therapies, which often include cognitive/behavioral interventions, have shown effectiveness in symptom reduction and improvement in quality of life. They enable the patient to feel a sense of empowerment and control. There are currently studies that are investigating the possibility that these interventions can influence disease progression and mortality.

The psychosocial resources available to cancer patients and their families vary widely from institution to institution and from locality to locality. Social work staff is available in many hospital and outpatient settings to assess, treat, and/or refer patients for psychotherapy/counseling. Social service agencies such as Cancer Care and local branches of the American Cancer Society provide support for patients and families. Support groups are numerous, especially self-help groups such as Us-Too for prostate cancer patients. The consultation and liaison service of hospital-based psychiatry departments is availble for consultation with hospitalized patients and can frequently call upon the expertise of psychiatry, psychology, and psychiatric nursing. Referral for follow-up is made to hospital-based mental health clinics or community mental health centers.

Identifying patients who are vulnerable and at high psychosocial risk is important to insure that the patient and family can avail themselves of appropriate medical care. Those psychosocial problems that interfere with this specific area of functioning must be addressed before treatment can proceed. It is not the role of the mental health professional to try to effect major characterological change in patients and families who present with psychosocial problems, although this may certainly be an outgrowth of effective intervention. Long-standing, premorbid psychiatric problems are to be referred out to appropriate resources in the community, with close communication between the treating physician and the psychotherapist in the community to maximize the patient's efforts of successfully completing the recommended and mutually agreed upon treatment plan.

PSYCHOSOCIAL HIGH-RISK CRITERIA FOR ONCOLOGY PATIENTS

1. Patient who is experiencing emotional difficulties that interfere with his/her ability to receive prescribed care.
2. Family member who is experiencing emotional difficulties that interfere with his/her ability to provide prescribed care to patient.
3. Patient whose life situation has become functionally altered (inability to work, care for family, etc.) because of diagnosis and/or disease progression.
4. Patient identified as having inadequate social support (single parent, elderly and living alone, etc.).
5. Patient experiencing difficulty making treatment decisions, or in conflict with family members concerning treatment decisions (including advance directives).
6. Patient not complying with treatment schedules.
7. Patient who has experienced "life events" impacting on current functioning (death of spouse, unemployment, illness of family member).
8. Patient whose change in functional status requires home care or institutional care planning.
9. Patient without adequate resources to obtain ongoing medical care (medical insurance, housing, transportation).
10. Patient who requests social work intervention.

Case #H.16.2
Goal: Management of cancer-phobic patients
SUSAN A. MCMANUS

A 38-year-old woman requests evaluation for prophylactic mastectomies. She has had two mammograms (both negative) and two breast biopsies (performed for palpable masses and revealing fibrocystic changes without atypia) in the past 2 years. Her mother died of breast cancer at age 71; there is no other family history of breast cancer.

This patient is so fearful of developing breast cancer that she seeks prophylactic mastectomy. Her actual risk for developing cancer, based on her family history and pathology reports, is not much higher than that of the normal population (relative risk 1.5, with postmenopausal first-degree relative, and no increased risk with a biopsy that shows no proliferative or atypical changes). However, cancerphobic patients are likely to perceive their risk as much higher than their actual risk.

Cancerphobia was identified as a growing problem in 1975 by Ingelfinger. It appears to parallel medical preoccupation with the disease. Cancerphobia can be sparked by intense media coverage, interaction with friends and co-workers who have the disease, or watching a family member suffer with cancer. It has been subdivided into transient and fixed chronic types. The transient type is frequently seen in individuals who are exposed to cancer patients and sometimes requires clinical examination and laboratory testing for reassurance. Transient cancerphobia may develop in anyone who has had personal contact with a cancer patient, especially one who has not survived.

The fixed chronic type of cancerphobia may develop in individuals who are at enhanced risk of developing cancer, such as those with a positive family history of breast cancer, in siblings of a child who dies of cancer, and in hypochondriacal patients. A careful medical workup should be done to provide reassurance. Reassurance is also obtained by regular follow-up examinations, but is characteristically short-lived.

Classification of the type of cancerphobia guides further workup. The transient type is more amenable to management with careful follow-up and reassurance. The chronic-type patient may continue the search for a surgeon who will perform the mastectomies.

Management of this patient should begin with a careful history and clinical examination, including review of the mammograms and pathology reports with the patient. A careful discussion of risk factors together with printed materials is helpful reinforcement. The patient may also benefit from genetic counseling. Next, a surveillance program should be developed. Frequent examinations by a physician and yearly mammograms may be reassuring. Life-style adjustments, such as increasing physical activity, maintaining ideal body weight, and limiting alcohol consumption, should be recommended. Breast self-examination should be taught and performed regularly.

Leventhal points out that a certain level of fear can spur action toward preventive behaviors, but he and others have found that levels of fear that are too high or too low may result in a patient being less adherent to breast self-examination and mammography.

Hopefully, the plan outlined above would allow the patient a degree of comfort and assurance to put off her search for prophylactic mastectomies. The Society of Surgical Oncology has established guidelines regarding this procedure. Through development of a volunteer registry of patients who underwent prophylactic mastectomy, Borgen and colleagues have found that patients who requested bilateral mastectomies were less likely to be dissatisfied with their decision than patients who had the operation recommended by a physician. Despite this, I believe that efforts should be made to convince this patient to postpone her decision, to comply with the surveillance program, and to seek the benefits of an improved life-style.

BIBLIOGRAPHY

Holland JC, Rowan JH. Handbook of Psycho:oncology: Care of the Patient with Cancer. New York: Oxford University Press, 1989.
Leventhal H. Fear communication in the acceptance of preventive health practices. Bull NY Acad Med 1965; 41:1144–1168.
Lopez MJ, Porter KA. Current role of prophylactic mastectomy. Surg Clin North Am 1996; 76:231–242.
Smith BL, Gadd MA, Lawler C, et al. Perception of breast cancer risk among women in breast center and primary care settings: correlation with age and family history of breast cancer. Surgery 1996; 120:297–303.
Stefanek ME, Helzlsouer KJ, Wilcox PM, Houn F. Predictors of and satisfaction with bilateral prophylactic mastectomy. Prev Med 1995; 24(4):412–419.

H.17. PROPHYLACTIC MASTECTOMY

Case #H.17.1
Goal: To discuss the role of prophylactic mastectomy
MONICA MORROW

A 43-year-old woman presents for counseling. Her mother died of bilateral breast cancer at age 51 (first cancer diagnosed at age 44) and her grandmother died of breast cancer at age 56. Her 38-year-old sister is alive and well. The patient has had three breast biopsies over the past 30 months, two of which demonstrated atypical ductal hyperplasia and one of which revealed a single, 1-mm focus of ductal carcinoma in situ.

This patient has several risk factors for breast cancer development. Her family history of breast cancer could carry a lifetime breast cancer risk between 30% and 85%, depending on whether a mutation of a breast cancer predisposition gene (*BRCA1, BRCA2*) is present. Additional information on the number of unaffected relatives (maternal aunts, cousins) and the presence or absence of family history of ovarian carcinoma would aid in determining the risk of a genetic mutation. Genetic mutation is present in only about 10% of breast cancer cases, and this pedigree is not clearly indicative of genetic disease. Genetic testing could help to clarify this patient's level of risk. Unfortunately, neither of her affected relatives is alive to undergo testing to determine if a *BRCA1* or *BRCA2* mutation is present in an affected relative. Thus, a positive test in this patient will provide useful information, but a negative test does not exclude the possibility of a mutation in another, as-yet-unidentified, breast cancer predisposition gene. Since the risks and benefits of genetic testing are a complex subject, I would refer this patient to a genetic counselor for a detailed discussion of this subject.

In addition to a family history of breast cancer, this patient has atypical hyperplasia (AH) and ductal carcinoma in situ (DCIS), two lesions associated with an increased risk of breast cancer development. AH in a patient with a family history of breast cancer increases the relative risk of breast cancer development by a factor of 9, so approximately 20% of patients with this combination of risk factors will develop breast cancer in a 15-year period. The natural history of very small amounts of DCIS is less well understood as these lesions were rarely identified prior to the use of screening mammography, and the impact of a family history of breast cancer on the risk of invasive cancer in the patient with DCIS is unclear. I would estimate the risk of invasive cancer after a diagnosis of a 1-mm focus of DCIS to be approximately 1% per year.

The indication for prophylactic mastectomy is an increase in breast cancer risk that is unacceptable to the patient. This patient, whose lifetime risk of breast cancer exceeds 20%, is clearly at increased risk. Whether a woman opts for prophylactic mastectomy in part depends on what aspect of breast cancer causes her most concern: fear of death or fear of disfigurement. In this era of breast-conserving therapy for established carcinoma, many women regard prophylactic removal of both breasts as unacceptably radical, particularly since it is not 100% protective against breast cancer development. Psychological assessment is an important part of the counseling process for the woman considering prophylactic surgery.

If prophylactic mastectomy is undertaken, the procedure should be a total (simple) mastectomy with the same anatomical boundaries as a therapeutic mastectomy. Care should be taken to remove the axillary tail of the breast and to create thin skin flaps, since residual breast tissue is a potential source of future breast carcinoma. Subcutaneous mastectomy with preservation of the nipple does not provide optimal removal of breast tissue, leaving behind the major ducts at the nipple, and should not be done. Prophylactic mastectomy is usually done with immediate reconstruction. The use of a skin-sparing mastectomy, with removal of only the nipple areolar complex and preservation of the breast skin, minimizes scarring and improves the cosmetic result of the procedure. Additional exposure to ensure maximal removal of breast tissue is gained by incising the skin as needed. Consultation with a reconstructive surgeon is part of the decision-making process for patients considering prophylactic surgery.

The efficacy of prophylactic mastectomy in the high-risk woman is uncertain. Although risk is clearly reduced, carcinoma can develop even after a well-performed prophylactic mastectomy, and risk reduction is not proportional to the amount of breast tissue removed. The literature on prophylactic mastectomy is not particularly helpful since many women undergoing the procedure in the past would not be classified as high risk today, and careful follow-up was not usually performed. In the woman with a *BRCA1* mutation the risk of ovarian carcinoma must also be considered when prophylactic mastectomy is undertaken.

BIBLIOGRAPHY

Bilimoria M, Morrow M. The woman at increased risk for breast cancer: evaluation and management strategies. Ca Cancer J Clin 1995; 45:263–278.

Hoskins KF, Stopfer JE, Calzone KA, et al. Assessment and counseling for women with a family history of breast cancer. A guide for clinicians. JAMA 1995; 273:577–585.

Morrow M. Identification and management of the woman at increased risk for breast cancer development. Breast Cancer Res Treat 1994; 31:53–60.

Case #H.17.2
Goal: To discuss management options for an in-breast recurrence following lumpectomy and radiation therapy for breast cancer

ROSEMARY B. DUDA

A 36-year-old woman presents for a second opinion regarding an in-breast recurrence. Two years prior to this she underwent lumpectomy and radiation therapy for a 2.5-cm lesion located in the extreme tail of the breast. She received six cycles of CMF. Two weeks ago she noted a lump "under her arm." Workup revealed a recurrence in the most lateral aspect of the remaining breast tissue. An excisional biopsy left positive margins. Her surgeon feels that she can be managed with a reexcision, since no greater margin will be achieved by a mastectomy. After multiple opinions, the patient has expressed a strong preference for a mastectomy of the involved breast and a prophylactic mastectomy of the uninvolved breast. She is a fashion model, recently divorced, without children. She is an avid exercise enthusiast, who enjoys running, biking, and playing tennis. Physical examination is unremarkable. Metastatic workup is negative.

The overall survival rates for women who undergo breast-conserving therapy are equivalent to those for women who are treated with a modified radical mastectomy. The local recurrence rate following lumpectomy and axillary dissection ranges from 8% to 20% with 10 years of observation. A higher rate of local failure may be associated with histologically positive margins of resection, associated intraductal carcinoma, an inadequate radiation dose, and a delay in beginning radiation treatment.

Local recurrences can be difficult to detect. Mammography alone may detect approximately 30–50% of local recurrences while the clinical examination with or without mammography will detect the remainder of the lesions.

The management of a local recurrence following breast conservation is salvage mastectomy or wide local excision with or without brachytherapy. Salvage mastectomy is the standard of care, although clinical investigations continue to evaluate the roles of conservative surgery and radiation implants. Systemic therapy as the only treatment for a local recurrence is not effective.

A local recurrence after breast-conserving surgery and radiation therapy has a better prognosis than a local recurrence after a mastectomy. In most series, the longer the time to treatment failure, the better the prognosis. The 5-year relapse-free survival with salvage mastectomy is 60–75% and the overall or cause-specific disease-free survival is 80–85%. Local/regional control with salvage mastectomy is reported to be 88–95%. Patients with skin involvement may have a rapid recurrence on the chest wall following mastectomy.

There is far less information on the use of breast-conserving surgery to treat a local recurrence compared to that of salvage mastectomy. In a series of 50 patients treated with a wide excision for an in-breast recurrence, 16 (32%) developed subsequent local failures. The 5-year local control in this study was 92% for recurrences occurring more than 5 years after the initial treatment. The local control was only 49% if the recurrence was less than 5 years from the time of the initial conservative therapy. In addition, the local control was 73% if histologically negative margins could be achieved compared to 36% for positive or indeterminate margins.

There are only small reported series of women treated with wide excision and radiation with interstitial implants for patients with in-breast recurrences following lumpectomy and radiation. In these patients local treatment failure occurred 20–25% of the time. The role of systemic therapy in the treatment of in-breast recurrence is yet to be determined. Based on the available information, this patient's best treatment would be a salvage mastectomy.

As was expressed by this patient, the issue of prophylactic contralateral mastectomy is often raised. There is an approximate fivefold increased risk of developing a second primary breast cancer in the contralateral breast because of her history of breast cancer. This risk is inversely related to age at presentation of the first primary breast cancer. Approximately 0.5% of women with a previous history of unilateral breast cancer will develop a second primary breast cancer each year for at least the next 15 years. In a large series of breast cancer patients followed for 10 years by the NSABP, the incidence of contralateral breast cancer was 4.2%. This study suggested that the overall survival of women with breast cancer was not influenced by the development of a contralateral breast cancer as the second primary was at a comparable or earlier stage than the initial breast cancer.

This patient's risk of dying of breast cancer during the next 5 years on the basis of her local recurrence is 15–20%. It may be logical to think that a prophylactic mastectomy is superior to close and careful evaluation with mammography and clinical examinations, but this has yet to be proven. So a prophylactic mastectomy, for which no solid data exist for prevention of an occurrence of a cancer, will have little impact on her overall survival from the primary breast cancer. It may, however, provide a major psychological advantage to the patient.

The goal of reconstruction is to alleviate the deformities that are caused by a mastectomy. Reconstruction can be performed immediately following a mastectomy or as a delayed procedure. The advantages of immediate reconstruction are that the patient is not faced with the physical and psychological trauma of coping with the deformity of the mastectomy. An immediate procedure also spares the patient an additional procedure and its associated risks from anesthesia. Reconstruction should be made available to this patient, regardless of the previous radiation therapy. The options include a saline prosthesis or autogenous tissue, usually a latissimus dorsi or transverse rectus abdominis (TRAM) myocutaneous flap, and less commonly, a gluteus maximus flap. Autogenous tissue provides the best cosmetic result and, in light of the previous radiation therapy, offers the safest option. The most appropriate reconstructive procedure should be based on body habitus, personal preferences, realistic expectations of results, smoking history, and previous surgery at the operative sites. All types of reconstructive procedures can provide excellent cosmetic results when the choice of surgery is individualized.

Physical limitations following myocutaneous flaps are generally few in the motivated patient. A physical therapy program can be implemented to hasten recovery. The standard latissimus dorsi flap does not have enough bulk to create an acceptable cosmetic result for most woman and is frequently used with a saline implant. It does not cause a functional loss of the shoulder, although it does result in a large scar on the back.

The TRAM flap is a more complex surgical procedure and an adequate blood supply based on the inferior epigastric pedicle is critical to the survival of the flap. It offers the advantage of having enough bulk that an implant is not required, the incision is on the lower abdomen and in general is more cosmetically pleasing, and it does offer the advantage of removing sometimes pendulous tissue from the abdomen. A disadvantage of a TRAM flap is a longer hospitalization and recovery time, protrusion of the lower abdominal wall, and an abdominal wall hernia. The TRAM flap can be performed as a pedicled flap or as a microvascular tissue transfer flap.

The gluteus maximus myocutaneous flap is a good option for a free muscle transfer flap, based on the superior or inferior gluteal artery. The advantages of this flap are that there is usually sufficient tissue for use even in slender women, the scar is cosmetically hidden in the buttocks region, and the recovery time is less than that of the TRAM. This flap is technically more demanding than the TRAM flap, thereby limiting its use.

Saline implants offer the advantage of adding the least amount of time to the surgical procedure and offer an excellent cosmetic result in a slender woman, particularly when bilateral. However, following irradiation, the elasticity of the skin may be limited, and therefore limit the amount of expansion that can be performed. In addition, palpable folds are present, there is a high deflation rate, and capsular contracture may develop.

Appropriate psychological support for this patient may include a social worker, therapist, or counselor, a psychiatrist, and patient support groups for herself and her family members. The goals of a support system, which could include one or all of the listed resources, are to provide emotional support, provide education, maintain a social identity, provide a tangible environmental support, and provide social affiliation. The five needs identified from a patient survey are the need for hope, honesty, information, emotional expression, and to discuss issues related to death and dying. Every patient with breast cancer should have access to psychosocial resources.

BIBLIOGRAPHY

Cella DF, Telch MJ. Cancer support groups: the state of the art. Cancer Pract 1993; 1:56–61.

Chaudary MA, Millis RR, Hoskins EO, et al. Bilateral primary breast cancer: a prospective study of disease incidence. Br J Surg 1984; 71:711–714.

Clark R, Wilkinson R, Miceli P, et al. Breast cancer: experiences with conservation therapy. Am J Clin Oncol 1987; 49:461.

Clarke DH, Le MG, Sarrazin D, et al. Analysis of local-regional relapses in patients with early breast cancers treated by excision and radiotherapy: experience of the Institut Gustave-Roussy. Int J Radiat Oncol Biol Phys 1985; 11:137–145.

Fisher B, Bauer M, Margolese R, et al. Five year results of a randomized clinical trial comparing total mastectomy and segmental mastectomy with or without radiation in the treatment of breast cancer. N Engl J Med, 1985; 312:665–673.

Fisher ER, Fisher B, Sass R, et al. Pathologic findings from the National Surgical Adjuvant Breast Project (Protocol No. 4). XI. Bilateral breast cancer. Cancer 1984; 54:3002–3011.

Fowble B, Solin L, Schultz D, et al. Breast recurrence following conservative surgery and radiation: patterns of failure, prognosis, and pathologic findings from mastectomy specimens with implications for treatment. Int J Radiat Oncol Biol Phys 1990; 19:833.

Harris JR, Connolly JL, Schnitt SJ, et al. The use of pathologic features in selecting the extent of surgical resection necessary for breast cancer patients treated by primary radiation therapy. Ann Surg 1985; 201:164–169.

Hislop TG, Elwood JM, Coldman AJ, et al. Second primary cancers of the breast: incidence and risk factors. Br J Cancer 1984; 49:79–85.

Kurtz JM, Amalric R, Brandone H, et al. Local recurrence after breast-conserving surgery and radiotherapy. Cancer 1989; 63:1912–1917.

Kurtz KM, Jacquemier J, Amalric R, et al. Is breast conservation after local recurrence feasible? Eur J Cancer 1991; 27:240–244.

Mackay GJ, Bostwick III. Reconstructive breast surgery. In: Harris, Lippman, Morrow, Hellman, eds. Disease of the Breast. Philadelphia: Lippincott-Raven, 1996:601–619.

Recht A, Hayes DF, Eberlein TJ, Sadowsky NL. Local regional recurrence after mastectomy or breast-conserving therapy. In: Harris, Lippman, Morrow, Hellman, eds. Disease of the Breast. Philadelphia: Lippincott-Raven, 1996:649–667.

Sarrazin D, Monique LE, Rousse J, et al. Conservative treatment versus mastectomy in breast cancer tumors with macroscopic diameter of 20 millimeters or less: the experience of the Institut Gustave-Roussy. Cancer 1984; 53:1209–1213.

Schnitt SJ, Connolly JL, Harris JR, et al. Pathologic predictors of early local recurrence in stage I and II breast cancer treated by primary radiation therapy. Cancer 1984; 53:1049–1057.

Stomper PC, Recht A, Berenberg AL. Mammographic detection of recurrent cancer in the irradiated breast. AJR 1987; 148:39.

Veronesi U, Salvadori B, Luini A, et al. Conservative treatment of early breast cancer: long term results of 1232 cases treated with quadrantectomy, axillary dissection, and radiotherapy. Ann Surg 1990; 211:250.

Young-Brockopp D. Cancer patient's perceptions of five psychological needs. Oncol Nurs Forum 1982; 9:31–35.

H.18.   HIGH-RISK COUNSELING

Case #H.18.1
Goal: To discuss the appropriate use of genetic screening/ counseling

BARBARA L. WEBER

One of your patients with stage II breast cancer in remission comes to your office to discuss her 23-year-old daughter, who is in excellent health. The mother is terrified that she has passed on "the gene for breast cancer" and wants your advice regarding genetic testing and surveillance. The mother's breast cancer was diagnosed at age 47, she is of Irish descent, and there are no other known family members with breast or ovarian cancer.

As a result of the widespread media coverage of recent progress in understanding the molecular basis of some forms of inherited breast cancer, this is a common occurrence in clinical practice. In this clinical setting, the likelihood that the mother has a germline (heritable) mutation in *BRCA1* or *BRCA2* is low; thus the likelihood that the daughter has such a mutation is similarly quite low. To provide the best available information to the mother, several steps may be undertaken. First, one can provide the mother with an estimate of the likelihood that she carries a *BRCA1* or *BRCA2* mutation. The published literature suggests that in women with breast cancer diagnosed before age 40, *BRCA1* mutations are present in approximately 10%, and by extrapolation, *BRCA2* mutations are present in approximately 3%. These numbers decrease further as the age of breast-cancer diagnosis increases. While direct mutation studies are not available, an extrapolation suggests that, in the absence of a family history, in a non-Ashkenazi Jewish family, the likelihood that the mother carriers either a *BRCA1* or *BRCA2* alteration is in the range of 2%. Given that the daughter has a 50% chance of having inherited a mutation if present, the daughter's risk of being a carrier is approximately 1%. For comparison, the mutation carrier rate in the general population is estimated at 0.1%.

In families with a very low likelihood of finding a *BRCA1* or *BRCA2* mutation, testing is perhaps to be discouraged, as the difficulty in interpreting a negative test is a significant consideration. The problem with a negative test arises in the setting of a family where the molecular explanation for breast cancer has not been elucidated. In this setting, a negative result may indicate that no heritable cause for breast cancer is present in the family, or may simply indicate that whatever the cause may be has not been tested for.

In addition, it is estimated that at least 10% of *BRCA1* and *BRCA2* mutations are not detectable by currently available commercial testing—a feature common to all laboratories offering *BRCA1* and *BRCA2* mutation analysis. Thus, individuals should not be falsely reassured in the setting of a negative test. As a final consideration in this setting, the mother should be reminded that this information may best be relayed to her daughter by a health professional familiar with genetic susceptibility testing, and that the decision of whether to pursue testing ultimately needs to be made by her daughter without outside pressure.

As a final step in assisting the mother, one can estimate the daughter's lifetime risk for developing breast cancer using the Claus model. In this setting, the daughter has a current risk of 0.1%, reaches a risk of 0.5% at age 35 (and should begin having annual mammograms at this age, as this is the average risk of 40-year-old women in the United States), and has a lifetime breast-cancer risk of 13.2%. Additionally, the daughter should be encouraged to learn and practice monthly breast self-examination. This approach to evaluating the daughter's risk should provide reassurance to the mother as well as offer a sensible plan for surveillance for the daughter.

BIBLIOGRAPHY

Claus EB, Risch N, Thompson WD. Autosomal dominant inheritance of early-onset breast cancer. Cancer 1994; 73:643–651.

Fitzgerald MG, MacDonald DJ, Krainer M, et al. Germline *BRCA1* mutations in Jewish and non-Jewish women with early onset breast cancer. N Engl J Med 1996; 334:143.

Krainer M, Silva-Arrieta S, FitzGerald MG, et al. Differential contributions of *BRCA1* and *BRCA2* to early-onset breast cancer. N Engl J Med 1997; 336(20): 1448–1449.

Langston AA, Malone KE, Thompson JD, et al. *BRCA1* mutations in a population-based sample of young women with breast cancer. N Engl J Med 1996; 334:137.

Case #H.18.2
Goal: To discuss the appropriate use of genetic screening/ counseling

DEBORAH L. TOPPMEYER

A 26-year-old woman is seen by you in consultation following the recent diagnosis of metastatic breast cancer in her 34-year-old sister. Her mother died at age 50 of metastatic breast cancer. She has a 2-year-old daughter and two siblings, a younger sister and brother. What do you recommend for surveillance?

Genetic factors contribute to approximately 5–10% of all cases of breast cancer and 25% of cases diagnosed in women less than 30 years of age. Inherited predisposition to cancer or heritable cancer is thought to be the result of a mutation in a single, highly penetrant, autosomal dominant breast cancer susceptibility gene such as *BRCA1* and *BRCA2*.

Cancer risk assessment refers to the process of quantifying the statistical probability of an individual's developing cancer due to the presence of variables such as family history, environmental exposures, life-style, and chance. An estimate of cancer risk is often offered in comparison to the "baseline" risk of cancer for the general population. Family history is the most important factor used to determine a person's risk for the development of breast cancer. Maternal and paternal contribution must be considered. A pedigree must be constructed with affected and unaffected individuals over at least three generations recorded when taking a family history.

High- and moderate-risk families differ with respect to degree of risk for individual family members, the method one uses to quantitate an individual's risk, and the underlying molecular basis for cancer susceptibility. The high-risk family is characterized by the presence of multiple cases of breast cancer in close relatives (at least three), early age of onset (less than 45 years), higher incidence of bilateral breast cancer, and the presence of ovarian cancer. The moderate-risk family, in comparison, has a less striking family history, absence of ovarian cancer, and an older average age at the time of diagnosis. In addition, certain populations, in particular individuals of Ashkenazi Jewish decent, have a prevalence of select *BRCA1* and *BRCA2* mutations of approximately 2.5%. Thus, if there is a family history of ovarian cancer or early-onset breast cancer, those individuals may be considered as a part of the high-risk pool.

For women classified as being members of a moderate-risk family, one of two risk prediction models for breast cancer assessment is used. The more frequently used Claus model best predicts risk for women with a family history of breast cancer. Claus et al. analyzed data from the Cancer and Steroid Hormone (CASH) study of breast cancer incidence in a population with limited screening. Their focus was predicting breast cancer risk in women with positive family histories. As such, tables were constructed to permit estimation of risk on the basis of the number of relatives with breast cancer, their relationship to the proband, and the age of onset of breast cancer in affected relatives. For the patient classified as being at high risk, this model is not applicable. Such families have a high probability of carrying a mutation in a dominant breast cancer susceptibility gene. The inheritance of such a gene follows the classic Mendelian pattern of autosomal dominant transmission, with each child of mutation carriers having a 50% chance of inheriting such a gene alteration. Families meeting the criteria of high risk are counseled using the Mendelian model.

Relative to this case, analysis of the pedigree demonstrates a limited or uninformative family history. We are told of only two affected first-degree relatives, the patient's mother, who was likely diagnosed with breast cancer before the age of 50, and the patient's sister, who was diagnosed with metastatic breast cancer at age 34. In assessing the proband's risk, it would be helpful to have information regarding unaffected relatives. For example, the significance of the proband's mother's breast cancer would be viewed differently if she was an only child as opposed to being the only one of eight sibs affected. In the latter case, invoking Mendelian law, the probability of an autosomal dominant cancer susceptibility gene accounting for the breast cancer in this family would be low. Rather, the most appropriate model to use for counseling this patient would be the Claus model. Applying this model, the proband's lifetime risk for the development of breast cancer is calculated to be 39%, having two first-degree relatives aged 34 and 50 affected with breast cancer.

Counseling the moderate risk regarding DNA predictive testing poses some of the greatest challenges in this area. Ideally, DNA predictive testing should be performed as part of a comprehensive genetic testing and counseling program. Since *BRCA1* and *BRCA2* were cloned, commercial availability has resulted in less discriminating use of the genetic test. The question of when and to whom to offer predictive testing is complex and controversial with far-reaching consequences. Although the ability to identify a patient at risk holds potential promise regarding increased surveillance or prevention, it is also fraught with numerous pitfalls, including risk of insurance or employer discrimination; these issues need to be addressed through informed consent prior to performing predictive testing. Genetic testing should not be offered in a capricious manner. This family does not meet the criteria for a high-risk family and would typically not be considered for genetic testing. However, if the pedigree analysis did indeed show the family to be uninformative (i.e., mother was an only child and grandmother died at a very young age from pneumonia) and the family was strongly motivated to be screened, one could offer DNA predictive testing. Extensive pretest counseling should take place including a detailed discussion of the limitations of testing, the meaning of a positive and negative test result, and potential ramifications of genetic testing, as part of the informed consent process. The American Society of Clinical Oncology has outlined the basic elements for informed consent given the complexity of germline DNA testing. The following issues must be discussed with the patient prior to testing: (a) information on the specific test being done, (b) implications of a positive or negative test result, (c) the possibility that the test will be uninformative, (d) options for risk examination without genetic testing, (e) risk of "passing" a mutation to their children, (f) technical accuracy of the test, (g) fees involved in testing and counseling, (h) risk of psychological distress, (i) risk of employment and insurance discrimination, (j) need for confidentiality, and (k) options and limitations of medical surveillance and screening after testing.

It is essential to identify the highest-risk individual for testing. Given that greater than 800 mutations have been found for *BRCA1* and *BRCA2*, it is not possible to offer genetic testing in the absence of an affected living relative. In this case, as the proband's mother is deceased, the most informative individual to test would be her 34-year-old sister. Only if she was identified as having a mutation in *BRCA1* or *BRCA2* of functional significance would the proband and interested family members be offered testing for this specific mutation. If the proband tested negative for this specific mutation, her breast cancer risk would drop to that of the general population. If positive, she would have a lifetime risk approaching 87%. On the other hand, if the proband's sister tested negative, we would be unable to provide any further refinement of our original risk assessment.

The most important point to remember in genetic testing is that *failure to find a* BRCA1 *mutation in a high-risk but currently cancer-free family member is clinically useful only if a specific* BRCA1 *mutation has been identified in an affected first-degree relative.* A negative test result (that is, no *BRCA1* mutation was found) in a patient with breast cancer from a multiplex family in which a *BRCA1* mutation has not been previously proved has multiple possible explanations: (a) a *BRCA1* mutation is present but has been overlooked (that is, a false-negative result); (b) a different, highly penetrant gene is responsible for the family's inherited susceptibility; (c) multiple genes of lower penetrance are the basis for the familial aggregation; (d) the cluster is a chance event—that is, not an inherited problem; or (e) this is a genetic family, but the specific patient chosen for initial testing and screening represents a sporadic case.

The case highlights the many complex issues that are raised when counseling families with uninformative pedigrees whose actual risk may lie anywhere along the spectrum from moderate to high.

BIBLIOGRAPHY

American Association of Clinical Oncology Statement of the American Society of Clinical Oncology: genetic testing for cancer susceptibility. J Clin Oncol 1996; 14(5):1730–1736.

Claus EB, Risch N, Thompson WD. Autosomal dominant inheritance of early-onset
   breast cancer: implications for risk prediction. Cancer 1994; 73(3):643–651.

Case #H.18.3
Goal: To discuss the appropriate use of genetic screening/ counseling in the setting of Li-Fraumeni syndrome

BARBARA L. WEBER

*A 25-year-old woman is referred for evaluation of a new breast mass,
which on excisional biopsy is found to be an infiltrating ductal carcinoma.
Her mother died at age 43 from breast cancer, a younger brother died of
osteosarcoma at age 12, and a first cousin died of leukemia at age 4. She
seeks advice regarding her 18-year-old sister, who is in excellent health.*

This family fits the description of a family with Li-Fraumeni syndrome
(LFS), a rare genetic cancer-susceptibility syndrome. LFS was first identified
as a syndrome in 1969 in a description of four kindreds in which cousins
or siblings both had childhood soft tissue sarcomas, and other relatives had
excessive cancer occurrence. Subsequent studies have further elucidated the
major component cancers, which now include breast cancer, soft tissue and
osteosarcomas, brain tumors, leukemias, and adrenocortical carcinomas.
Like the cancer associated with mutations in *BRCA1* and *BRCA2*, cancer
susceptibility in Li-Fraumeni families follows an autosomal dominant pattern of transmission, with as many as 90% of carriers affected with at least
one cancer by age 70. Nearly 30% of tumors in reported families occur
before age 15 years.

   In 1990, germline mutations were identified in the p53 tumor suppressor gene in affected members of LFS families. Mutations were clustered
in the conserved sequences of the gene (exons 5–9), an observation that
was thought to increase the significance of these findings. To date, approximately 50% of carefully defined families with a clinical picture of LFS
have had detectable alterations in the p53 gene. While mutations are more
frequently identified in "hot spots" within the conserved sequences, they
have been seen throughout the gene. p53 genes, which are ostensibly normal
by sequencing, but with abnormal functional assays or expression, have also
been observed.

   The clinical issues involved with presymptomatic testing for LFS are
among the most difficult in genetics and have been compared to the problems associated with testing for Huntington disease. One of the major issues
is that many of the malignancies arise in childhood, raising concerns about
the genetic testing of minors, and the emotional impact on parents and chil-

dren alike of the very high cancer risks associated with a positive test. A complicating factor is that screening for most of the component tumors is not associated with improved survival—breast cancer is the one LFS-related tumor for which screening for early-stage disease would be expected to be beneficial. Experience in centers dealing with genetic testing for cancer susceptibility suggests that great care should be exercised in counseling these families. Some family members may prefer to remain ignorant of the fact that a cancer syndrome exists in their family, even by clinical description, when little can be done to alter the risk of dying from cancer associated with p53 germline alterations. Others may be interested in hearing that an explanation may exist, but shy away from testing for the same reasons, or because of concerns about privacy and insurability. Still others may desire p53 germline mutation analysis, with the recognition that identification as a noncarrier in a family with a known mutation offers significant relief of anxiety as well as the knowledge that identification as a carrier offers little other than increased breast cancer surveillance as a possible intervention. Because of the marked difficulties in counseling these families and providing testing in a supportive setting, it is recommended that these families be referred to centers with investigational protocols for such testing, or at least with extensive experience. Such centers may be identified by contacting the Institute for Human Genome Research at the National Institutes of Health.

BIBLIOGRAPHY

Li FP, Fraumeni JF Jr. Soft-tissue sarcomas, breast cancer, and other neoplasms: a familial syndrome? Ann Intern Med 1969; 71:747–752.

Li FP, Fraumeni JF Jr, Mulvihill JJ, et al. A cancer family syndrome in twenty-four kindreds. Cancer Res 1988; 48:5358–5362.

Li FP, Garber JE, Friend SH, et al. Recommendations on predictive testing for germ line p53 mutations among cancer-prone individuals. J Natl Cancer Inst 1992; 84:1156–1160.

Malkin D, Li FP, Strong LC, et al. Germline p53 mutations in a familial syndrome of breast cancer, sarcomas, and other neoplasms. Science 1990; 250(4985): 1233–1238.

Case #H.18.4
Goal: To discuss the appropriate use of genetic testing/counseling in the setting of a likely *BRCA1* mutation

BARBARA L. WEBER

A 32-year-old woman is referred for adjuvant treatment of a high-grade, infiltrating ductal carcinoma (T2N0M0). Her family history is remarkable

*for a father who died of colon cancer at age 50, a paternal aunt who is
alive and well after treatment of a stage I breast cancer at age 35, and a
paternal grandmother diagnosed with breast cancer at age 43 who died of
stage IV ovarian cancer at age 76. Her paternal grandparents were
Russian Jewish immigrants at the turn of the century; her maternal
grandparents were also Jewish, but no information is available from this
branch of the family as all but the patient's mother died in the Holocaust.
She has two younger sisters and an older brother who are in excellent
health.*

This family has many characteristics that suggest with high likelihood
that the pattern of cancer occurrence in this family is due to a germline
alteration in *BRCA1*. The strongest predictor of finding a *BRCA1* mutation
in this family is the presence of both breast and ovarian cancer in a single
individual (the patient's paternal grandmother). Other significant predictors
include Ashkenazi Jewish ancestry and the young average age of breast
cancer diagnosis in this family (average age 37). Using the tables generated
by Couch et al., the predicted probability that a *BRCA1* alteration explains
the pattern of cancer in this family is approximately 90%. As the patient
under consideration is herself affected with breast cancer, the probability
that she carries such a mutation is also 90%. The likelihood of finding a
BRCA2 mutation is comparatively lower, as the majority of breast and ovarian cancer in Jewish families are due to *BRCA1* mutations, predominantly
the two-base deletion in exon 2 called 185delAG.

If this patient wishes to pursue the option of testing for *BRCA1* and
BRCA2, she should give fully informed consent before proceeding. A detailed list of what constitutes informed consent for testing in this setting is
described in a position paper on genetic susceptibility testing prepared by
the American Society of Clinical Oncology and summarized in Table 1.
Specifically, she should be aware of the cancer risks associated with a
BRCA1 mutation, the problems in devising recommendations for surveillance and prevention strategies, and the potential risks to insurability.

The breast cancer risk associated with a *BRCA1* mutation is estimated
to be 60–80% by age 80, and such alterations are also associated with a
20–40% lifetime risk of ovarian cancer. *BRCA2* has a risk profile similar
but not identical to *BRCA1*, and lifetime breast cancer risk to *BRCA2* mutation carriers also is estimated to be 60–80%, with ovarian cancer risk in
the range of 10–20%. *BRCA2* mutations also are associated with a 6%
lifetime risk of male breast cancer. Although in absolute terms this represents
significantly less cancer risk to men than women, the relative risk represents
a similar 100-fold increase over the general population risk. Other cancer
risks are likely to be associated with *BRCA2* mutations, but remain poorly

Table 1 Basic Elements of Informed Consent for Germline DNA Testing

1. Information on the specific test being performed
2. Implications of a positive and negative result
3. Possibility that the test will not be informative
4. Options for risk estimation without genetic testing
5. Risk of passing a mutation to children
6. Technical accuracy of the test
7. Fees involved in testing and counseling
8. Risk of psychological distress
9. Risk of insurance or employer discrimination
10. Confidentiality
11. Options and limitations of medical surveillance and screening
    following testing

defined. Second breast cancers may occur in as many as 60% of women who carry a *BRCA1* or *BRCA2* mutation and survive a first breast cancer. Colon and prostate cancer may also be increased in *BRCA1* and *BRCA2* mutation carriers. Thus, while this patient has a breast cancer diagnosis, she should be apprised of the risk for other cancers. Hearing this information in the setting of a newly diagnosed cancer may be particularly difficult. Current recommendations for future management of this patient, based on the scanty data currently available, are provided in Table 2. When discussing these recommendations, this patient should be aware that there are few data available to estimate risk reduction associated with prophylactic mastectomy or oophorectomy (although they are likely to be significant), nor are there data to determine if any survival benefit is associated with frequent surveillance (although, again, this is likely to be the case). As studies examining various options are completed, it is hoped that in the future we will be able to offer

Table 2 Recommendations for Management of Known Carriers of *BRCA1* or *BRCA2* Mutations

Mammograms every 6–12 months beginning at age 25
or
Prophylactic mastectomy
and
Physical examination every 6 months
Prophylactic oophorectomy after childbearing with estrogen replacement therapy at
   least until age 50

more definitive information, and perhaps make recommendations, but at present such data do not exist.

As noted above, this woman also needs to be educated about the lack of information provided by a negative test—particularly in this setting, as the family history strongly suggests an inherited cancer susceptibility, which is not negated by a negative test result. She must also be advised about the potential risk for loss of health insurance associated with genetic testing. While this is, at present, a largely theoretically concern and legislative steps are being taken to protect individuals who opt to undergo genetic testing for *BRCA1* and *BRCA2* mutations, it remains a major source of concern for individuals undergoing testing and a primary reason that some patients are deferring testing.

In considering the approach to testing in this individual, it would be reasonable to advise that she proceed initially with a limited test looking only for the three mutations in *BRCA1* and *BRCA2* that occur with significantly increased frequency in Ashkenazi Jewish breast/ovarian cancer families. This approach will save money and is the most likely test to detect a mutation in this case. If this screen is negative, the patient should be advised that the most complete information available will be obtained by completing the full analysis of both *BRCA1* and *BRCA2*, as current evidence suggests that about 1 in 30 Ashkenazi breast cancer families with a *BRCA1* or *BRCA2* mutation have a mutation other than one of the three common mutations.

Finally, if a *BRCA1* or *BRCA2* mutation were to be identified in this woman, testing would be available for other adult family members should they choose to pursue this option. The cost of testing will be decreased significantly as compared to full-length screening, and the predictive value of the test will greatly increase. However, each family member should go through the process of pretest counseling to insure that they fully understand the implications of testing and agree to proceed. In considering testing for other family members, it is important to provide a genetic test that includes the mutation detected in the original family member, as well as the other mutations common in the Ashkenazi population. Several families have been described where two different mutations are segregating independently, and based on the population frequency of these mutations, it is expected that such families will continue to be identified. Particularly in this family, with the unfortunate but not uncommon circumstance of having no cancer history information from a branch of the family lost due to Nazi atrocities during World War II, this possibility cannot be excluded. Obviously, significant errors in risk evaluation exist if the assumption that there is a single mutation in the family is not correct. In contrast, it is generally recommended in non-Ashkenazi families to screen only for the known family mutation, as the population frequency is an order of magnitude lower, reducing likelihood of finding a family with more than one mutation. In addition, the testing would require full screening on every individual as there have not been identifiable common mutations that are useful for testing in an American population.

BIBLIOGRAPHY

Couch FJ, Blackwood MA, DeShano ML, et al. *BRCA1* mutations in women attending clinics that evaluate the risk of breast cancer. N Engl J Med 1997; 336(20):1409–1415.

Easton DF, Bishop DT, Ford D, Crockford GP, and the Breast Cancer Linkage Consortium. Genetic linkage analysis in familial breast and ovarian cancer—results from 214 families. Am J Hum Genet 1993; 52:678–701.

Hoskins KF, Stopfer JE, Calzone KA, et al. Assessment and counseling for familial cancer risk: a guide for clinicians. JAMA 1995; 273:577–585.

Statement of the American Society of Clinical Oncology: genetic testing for cancer susceptibility. J Clin Oncol 1996; 14(5):1730–1736.

Streuwing JP, Hartge P, Wacholder S, et al. Cancer risk with 185delAG and 5382insC mutations of *BRCA1* and the 6174delT mutation of *BRCA2* among Ashkenazi Jews. N Engl J Med 1997; 336(20):1401–1408.

Wooster R, Neuhausen S, Mangion J, Quirk Y, Ford D, Collins N, et al. Localization of a breast cancer susceptibility gene, *BRCA2*, to chromosome 13q12–13. Science 1994; 265:2088–2090.

Case #H.18.5
Goal: To recognize the familial syndrome of Cowden disease (multiple-hamartoma syndrome)

JEAN L. BOLOGNIA

A 31-year-old woman is referred for evaluation of a stage I, infiltrating ductal carcinoma of the breast. There is a strong family history of breast cancer, including a sister who had bilateral disease diagnosed in her early forties. On physical examination you are struck by the presence of small, wart-like lesions of the face.

In addition to the familial breast cancer syndromes associated with *BRCA1* and *BRCA2* gene mutations, there is the autosomal dominant disorder Cowden disease. It is also referred to as the multiple-hamartoma syndrome because benign tumors frequently develop in affected individuals, especially in the breast and thyroid gland. However, approximately 30–50% of women with Cowden disease also develop breast cancer.

The three most commonly affected organs in patients with Cowden disease are the breast, thyroid, and gastrointestinal (GI) tract. In the breast, both benign fibroadenomas and fibrocystic disease are seen in addition to ductal adenocarcinoma. Of the women who develop breast cancer, up to one-third will have bilateral primary tumors. Goiter and the formation of adenomas are the primary thyroid abnormalities with follicular carcinomas occurring less frequently (<10% of patients). At least one-third of affected individuals also have multiple, nonadenomatous polyps of the upper as well as the lower GI tract. Of note, patients with Cowden disease can develop brain tumors, in particular cerebellar gangliocytomatosis (the latter is also referred to as Lhermitte-Duclos disease).

Aside from a family history of hamartomas or carcinomas, the clinical suspicion of Cowden disease usually arises from a recognition of the mucocutaneous signs of this disorder (seen in 99–100% of patients). Although wart-like papules on the face, cobblestoning of the oral mucosa (Fig. 1), and palmoplantar and acral keratoses (Fig. 2) are the characteristic findings, one should exclude the diagnosis in any woman with breast cancer and a "bumpy" face or mouth. Biopsy specimens of the facial papules often show a form of benign appendageal tumor with follicular differentiation known as a trichilemmoma. (Trichilemmomas are uncommon enough that their presence should raise the possibility of Cowden disease and a reexamination of the patient to determine whether there are multiple lesions.) Additional pathological diagnoses include tumor of the follicular infundibulum, benign papillomas, and sclerotic fibromas.

Once the diagnosis of Cowden disease is highly suspected or clinically confirmed (e.g., multiple trichilemmomas in a patient with breast cancer; Table 1), genetic analysis of the *PTEN* gene can be considered. Based on

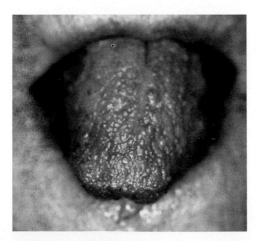

Figure 1 Multiple papillomas of the tongue in a patient with Cowden disease. (Courtesy Yale Residents' Slide Collection.)

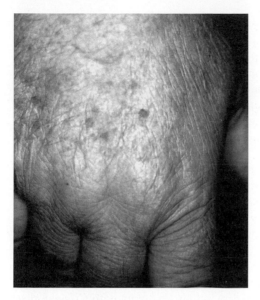

Figure 2 Multiple acral keratoses on the dorsum of the hand in a patient with Cowden disease. (Courtesy Yale Residents' Slide Collection.)

Table 1 International Cowden Consortium Cowden Disease Diagnostic Criteria

Pathognomonic criteria
  Six or more papules, of which three or more must be trichilemmomas
or
  Cutaneous facial papules plus oral mucosal papillomatosis
or
  Oral mucosal papillomatosis plus acral keratoses or palmoplantar keratoses ($\geq$6)

Major criteria	Minor criteria
Breast cancer	Thyroid lesions, e.g., goiter
Thyroid cancer	Mental retardation (IQ $\leq$ 75)
Macrocephaly ($\geq$97th percentile)	GI hamartomas
Lhermitte-Duclos disease	Fibrocystic disease of the breast
	Lipomas
	Fibromas
	Genitourinary tumors or
	malformations

Diagnosis of Cowden disease—2 major criteria where one is either macrocephaly or Lhermitte-Duclos disease; 1 major with 3 minor criteria; 4 minor criteria

Source: From Nelen MR, Padberg GW, Peeters EAJ, et al. Localization of the gene for Cowden disease to chromosome 10q22–23. Nature Genet 1996; 13:114–116.

linkage analyses performed in several families with Cowden disease, the putative susceptibility gene was localized to chromosome 10q22–23 in 1996. The next year, building on the observation that sporadic breast, brain, and prostate cancers contained somatic mutations in the *PTEN* tumor suppressor gene (it resides within the q22–23 region of chromosome 10), investigators described germline mutations in four of five families with Cowden disease. The protein product of this gene has regions that are homologous with both tyrosine phosphatases and tensin, a protein involved in focal cellular adhesions.

As is the case with familial cutaneous melanoma, mutations have not been found in all of the patients with Cowden disease. Therefore, a negative result remains inconclusive. A debate of the pros and cons of genetic screening for breast cancer susceptibility is clearly beyond the scope of this case discussion and is covered elsewhere in this book. However, it is important to remember that because the mucocutaneous findings of Cowden disease appear during the second decade of life, teenage daughters can be screened clinically, preferably in conjunction with a dermatologist. As with women with known *BRCA1* and *BRCA2* gene mutations, patients with Cowden disease face the dilemma of prophylactic bilateral mastectomy. In one review of the literature, the median age at which breast cancer was diagnosed was 41 years with a range of 20–62 years.

BIBLIOGRAPHY

Brownstein MH, Wolf M, Bikowski JB. Cowden's disease. A cutaneous marker of breast cancer. Cancer 1978; 41:2393–2398.

Liaw D, Marsh DJ, Li J, et al. Germline mutations of the *PTEN* gene in Cowden disease, an inherited breast and thyroid cancer syndrome. Nature Genet 1997; 16:64–67.

Starink TM. Cowden's disease: analysis of fourteen new cases. J Am Acad Dermatol 1984; 11:1127–1141.

Case #H.18.6
Goal: To discuss the use of screening mammography in high-risk patients

CAROL H. LEE

A 35-year-old woman, 14 years post chemotherapy plus mantle irradiation for stage III Hodgkin's disease, presents with microcalcifications on routine screening mammograms.

Young women who have undergone radiation therapy for Hodgkin's disease are at increased risk for the subsequent development of breast cancer, with the estimated incidence approaching 35% by age 40. Based on the results of two studies, the magnitude of the risk appears to vary significantly with the age of the patient at the time of treatment with the greatest risk occurring in those treated between the ages of 10 and 16. The relative risk, which was 136 for women treated before the age of 15, declined with increasing age at the time of treatment but remained elevated for women younger than 30 years at the time of irradiation. The relative risk for all women treated before the age of 30 was 19; for those over the age of 30, the relative risk was 0.7. For women treated with both chemotherapy and radiation therapy, the relative risk for developing breast cancer was not significantly increased above that of women receiving radiation alone but the latency period between the time of treatment and the diagnosis of breast cancer was shorter. The breast cancers occurred at intervals of 4.5–23 years after irradiation, with a mean of 15 years. The majority of the cancers occurred within or at the margins of the radiation field.

In addition to women who have been irradiated, other young women at increased risk for breast cancer include those with a mother or sister with premenopausal breast cancer (relative risk 3.1), with additional risk if the cancer in that premenopausal, first-degree relative was bilateral (relative risk 8.5–9). Another group at increased risk for breast cancer at a young age are women with the *BRCA1* or *BRCA2* genetic mutation. These women have an estimated breast cancer incidence of 50% before age 50.

While the efficacy of screening mammography for decreasing mortality from breast cancer among women over age 40 has been demonstrated by several large, randomized, controlled trials, the value of regular screening mammography for women younger than 40 who are at increased risk for developing breast cancer has not been evaluated. Mammography has a lower sensitivity for detecting breast cancer in younger women, perhaps owing to overall greater density of the breasts in younger women, which can obscure an underlying malignancy. It has been demonstrated, however, that a high proportion of cancers occurring in young women, including those who were radiated for Hodgkin's disease, are detectable mammographically. For high-risk young women, the potential benefit of detecting a small, clinically occult breast cancer through screening mammography must be weighed against the possible risks. These risks include the need for biopsy of lesions that prove to be benign, and a false sense of security conveyed by a negative mammogram. Because of the lack of data, it is difficult to make recommendations for mammographic surveillance of these high-risk young women. However, it has been advocated that women who have undergone radiation for Hodgkin's disease should have regular screening mammography beginning 10 years after radiation therapy or at age 30, whichever comes first. It has also been stated that women with a first-degree relative with premenopausal breast cancer should begin screening mammography at an age 5–10 years earlier than the age of the relative at the time of diagnosis. The optimal interval between screening examinations is another question that has not been resolved. It is conjectured that because cancers in younger women tend to be faster growing, a shorter screening interval (i.e., yearly) may be warranted.

In the patient presented in this case, the screening mammogram revealed a tiny cluster of calcifications (Fig. 1). The next step in the management of this patient would be to obtain magnification views of these calcifications to better characterize their morphology. On these magnified images, the calcifications were seen to be heterogeneous in shape and therefore suspicious for malignancy. The patient underwent needle localization and excisional biopsy of the calcifications and was found to have ductal carcinoma in situ without evidence of invasive tumor. Because of the prior radiation,

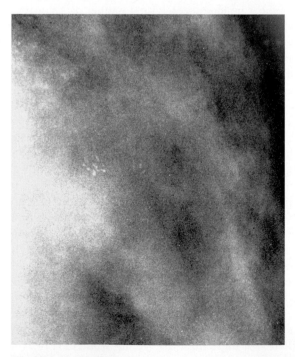

Figure 1 Screening mammogram in a young woman revealing cluster of microcalcifications.

the patient was not considered a candidate for breast-conserving surgery and radiation and underwent simple mastectomy. She has had yearly mammograms of the contralateral breast and is alive and well with no evidence of disease 9 years later.

BIBLIOGRAPHY

Bhatia S, Robison LL, Oberlin O, et al. Breast cancer and other second neoplasms after childhood Hodgkin's disease. N Engl J Med 1996; 334:745–751.
Cook KL, Adler DD, Lichter AS, et al. Breast carcinoma in young women previously treated for Hodgkin disease. AJR 1990; 155:39–42.
Hancock SL, Tucker MA, Hoppe RT. Breast cancer after treatment of Hodgkin's disease. J Natl Cancer Inst 1993; 85:25–31.
Meyer JE, Kopans DB, Oot R. Breast cancer visualized by mammography in patients under 35. Radiology 1983; 147:93–94.

A Second Opinion

KIRBY I. BLAND and DANIEL S. KIM

Exposure to ionizing radiation has been shown clearly to increase the risk of breast cancer in women. This has been documented in women treated with low-dose radiotherapy for postpartum mastitis, in women who received multiple chest fluoroscopies, and in Japanese women exposed to radiation during atomic bomb explosions at Hiroshima and Nagasaki. The development of secondary malignancies following treatment of Hodgkin's disease has also been documented. However, until two recent reports, the increased risk of breast cancer following treatment of Hodgkin's disease was thought to be only minimally elevated.

In 1993, Hancock et al. reported a 4.1 overall relative risk of developing invasive breast cancer among women treated for Hodgkin's disease. However, for those women diagnosed and treated before 30 years of age, the relative risk was 19. And in women treated before age 15, the relative risk was 136. In 1996, Bhatia et al. reported an increased risk of breast cancer, following treatment for Hodgkin's disease, 75 times the risk in the general population. The estimated actuarial cumulative probability of breast cancer was 35% at 40 years of age. Bhatia et al. found increasing radiation dose, usually above 2000 cGy, and age at diagnosis and treatment between 10 and 16 years to be correlated with increased risk of breast cancer. The incidence of bilateral breast cancer has also been reported to be as high as 22%. The majority of these patients are less than 40 years of age, and the prognosis for younger women with breast carcinoma has been shown to be worse.

There are no defined guidelines for mammographic screening in this high-risk population. Most breast cancers following Hodgkin's disease treatment occurred 10–15 years later but ranged from 4 to 34 years. Physical examination and screening mammography are of utmost importance in these patients. We would encourage monthly breast self-examination, begin yearly clinical examination, and start annual mammographic screening 10 years after treatment, or at age 30, whichever comes first. This high-risk population may benefit from prophylactic tamoxifen.

We would not offer this patient any further therapy (radiotherapy/chemotherapy). Although the risk of bilateral disease has been reported, we would *not* perform a "mirror" contralateral biopsy. If she had invasive disease, we would offer her a modified radical mastectomy.

BIBLIOGRAPHY

Baral E, Larsson LE, Mattsson B. Breast cancer following irradiation of the breast. Cancer 1977; 40:2905–2910.

Bhatia S, Robsion LL, Oberlin O, et al. Breast cancer and other second neoplasms after childhood Hodgkin's disease. N Engl J Med 1996; 334:745–751.

Boice JD, Land CE, Shore RE, et al. Risk of breast cancer following low-dose radiation exposure. Radiology 1979; 131:589–597.

Chung M, Chang HR, Bland KI, Wanebo HJ. Younger women with breast carcinoma have a poorer prognosis than older women. Cancer 1996; 77:97–103.

Hancock SL, Tucker MA, Hoppe RT. Breast cancer after treatment of Hodgkin's disease. J Natl Cancer Inst 1993; 85:25–31.

Peters MH, Sonpal IM, Batra MK. Breast cancer in women following mantle irradiation for Hodgkin's disease. Am Surg 1995; 61:763–766.

Shore RE, Hempelmann LH, Kowaluk E, et al. Breast neoplasms in women treated with X-rays for acute postpartum mastitis. J Natl Cancer Inst 1977; 59:813–822.

Tokanuga M, Land CE, Yamamoto T, et al. Incidence of female breast cancer among atomic bomb survivors at Hiroshima and Nagasaki, 1950–1980. Radiat Res 1987; 112:243–272.

Yahalom J, Petrek JA, Biddinger PW, et al. Breast cancer in patients irradiated for Hodgkin's disease: A clinical and pathologic analysis of 45 events in 37 patients. J Clin Oncol 1992; 10:1674–1681.

Case #H.18.7
Goal: To discuss genetic evaluation and counseling for a family history of breast cancer

MONICA MAGEE

A 33-year-old woman seeks advice because of a strong family history of breast cancer (mother had bilateral breast cancer, first diagnosed age 44; maternal grandmother died of breast cancer age 53; sister diagnosed with breast cancer age 38; maternal aunt diagnosed with breast cancer age 47). There is no family history of ovarian cancer.

Ascertaining and interpreting a detailed pedigree remains the cornerstone of assessing family risk factors for breast cancer. Features of a family history that are most suggestive of an inherited risk for breast cancer include the presence of early-onset breast cancer (i.e., premenopausal), bilateral breast cancer, and affected individuals in multiple generations. In addition, ovarian cancer and male breast cancer may be seen in some families and can be associated with a particularly high probability of an inherited risk for breast cancer. Both maternal and paternal histories of breast cancer must be considered.

The proband's history is very suggestive of a strong inherited risk for breast cancer. The early onset of breast cancer in three generations, together with the presence of bilateral disease, suggests a mutation in an autosomal dominant breast cancer susceptibility gene. While risk assessment models, including the Claus and Gail models, are useful in low- to moderate-risk families, the use of such models given this very strong family history is not indicated. Based on the pedigree, we can make the reasonable assumption that there is an autosomal dominant gene mutation in her family and that her risk of inheriting that mutation, and its associated cancer risks, is 50%.

Having identified this family as likely to carry a mutation in a breast cancer susceptibility gene, it is reasonable to offer genetic testing for inherited mutations of *BRCA1* and *BRCA2*. Inherited mutations in *BRCA1* and *BRCA2* account for the majority of autosomal dominant predisposition to breast cancer. To provide accurate interpretation of test results, the approach to genetic testing is to first test one of her living affected relatives (i.e., preferably her mother, sister, or maternal aunt) for *BRCA1* and *BRCA2* mutations. Therefore, genetic testing of the proband requires not only her interest in testing, but also the interest, consent, and cooperation of at least one affected family member.

There are several possible outcomes of genetic testing in the family: (a) If no mutation is found in the proband's affected relatives, the family history remains compelling and one would assume that there is a cancer-predisposing mutation in a different gene or an undetected mutation in either *BRCA1* or *BRCA2*. In this case, testing of our patient would *not* be helpful and she should be counseled that her risk of developing cancer remains significantly increased. (b) If one of her affected relatives tests positive for a *BRCA1* or *BRCA2* mutation, the proband could then be offered targeted testing for that specific mutation. If the proband tests positive for the familial mutation, her lifetime risk for breast cancer could be as high as 85%. In addition, her lifetime risk of ovarian cancer could also be increased by varying amounts depending on the gene mutation. (c) If one of her affected relatives tests positive for a *BRCA1* or *BRCA2* mutation and the proband subsequently tests negative for the familial mutation, her lifetime risk for breast cancer would go down to the general population risk (assuming there is no paternal history). The testing of a living affected relative is very important to the informativeness of a negative test result. Had neither the mother nor the aunt been available for testing, a negative test result in our patient would *not* have significantly lowered her assessed risk.

Having identified the proband as being at high risk for breast cancer, either through pedigree analysis alone or in concert with genetic testing, the question arises as to what interventions can be offered to help her. Heightened breast cancer surveillance, including increased mammograms, clinical examinations, and breast self-examination, are appropriate suggestions, keeping in mind that no prospective trials are available to assess the efficacy of such interventions in women at increased genetic risk. Prophylactic mastectomy may also be considered as an option for the proband and could potentially provide some benefit in terms of her risk for breast cancer. However, there are insufficient data to recommend for or against prophylactic mastectomy to reduce the breast cancer risk in our patient. Prophylactic mastectomy remains a major surgical procedure, with medical, cosmetic, and psychological implications. If the proband is strongly considering prophylactic surgery, genetic testing could be especially helpful. A negative result in the proband following the identification of a mutation in her family could avoid unnecessary surgery. If she tested positive for the family's mutation, prophylactic oophorectomy might also be a consideration. Neither prophylactic mastectomy nor oophorectomy reduces the associated cancer risks to zero.

Given the complexities of cancer risk assessment, genetic counseling is a crucial component in allowing individuals to make informed choices. Genetic counseling is an ongoing process of education and support that allows the proband to understand her risk assessment, her options for surveillance and risk reduction, and the options of genetic testing, while also providing supportive counseling. Apart from the previously described limitations of interventions to decrease her breast cancer morbidity and mortality and the limitations of genetic testing, genetic counseling would also include a discussion of implications of the risk assessment for other family members and the potential psychological consequences and risks for insurance and employment discrimination associated with genetic testing. The many needs of this high-risk patient may best be addressed in a specialized cancer genetics clinic where risk assessment, surveillance and surgical options, supportive counseling, and education can be provided through a collaborative effort of multiple health care providers.

BIBLIOGRAPHY

Burke W, Daly M, Garber G, Botkin J, Kahn MJ, Lynch P, McTiernan A, Offit K, Perlman J, Peterson G, Thomson E, Varricchio C. Recommendations for follow-up care of individuals with an inherited predisposition to cancer. II. *BRCA1* and *BRCA2*. JAMA 1997; 277:997–1003.

Claus EB, Risch N, Thompson WD. Autosomal dominant inheritance of early onset breast cancer. Cancer 1994; 73:643–651.

Ford D, Easton DF, Bishop DT, Narod SA, Goldgar DE, and the Breast Cancer Linkage Consortium. Risk of cancer in *BRCA1* mutation carriers. Lancet 1994; 343:692–695.

Ford D, Easton DF. The genetics of breast and ovarian cancer. Br J Cancer 1995; 72:805–812.

Gail MH, Brinton LA, Bryar DP, et al. Projecting individualized probabilities of developing breast cancer for white females who are being examined annually. J Natl Cancer Inst 1989; 81:1879–1886.

Hoskins KF, Stopfer JE, Calzone KA, Merajver SD, Rebbek TR, Garber JE, Weber BL. Assessment and counseling for women with a family history of breast cancer, A guide for clinicians. JAMA 1995; 273:577–585.

Wooster R, Neuhausen S, Mangion J, et al. Localization of a breast cancer susceptibility gene, *BRCA2*, to chromosome 13q12–13. Science 1994; 265:2088–2090.

Case #H.18.8
Goal: To discuss the indications for genetic testing

BARBARA L. WEBER

A 29-year-old Ashkenazi Jewish woman engaged to be married seeks counseling regarding her risk for developing breast cancer. She is nulliparous. She has had two prior breast biopsies that revealed fibroadenomas with no atypia. There is a family history of breast cancer in her maternal grandmother (age 53 at time of diagnosis) and a maternal aunt (age 62). Her 37-year-old sister recently underwent a breast biopsy that revealed atypical lobular hyperplasia, but no cancer. The patient requests information regarding genetic testing for breast cancer susceptibility.

The process of risk assessment and genetic counseling in this woman should cover several areas including: (a) her lifetime and age-adjusted risk for developing breast cancer using epidemiological modeling, (b) the likelihood that she carriers a germline alteration in the breast cancer susceptibility genes *BRCA1* and/or *BRCA2*, and (c) the pros and cons of undergoing predictive genetic testing.

The patient's breast cancer risk can be estimated based on several models in common use. The Claus model was developed to estimate breast cancer risk based solely on family history of breast cancer. This model was derived using family history data from the Cancer and Steroid Hormone (CASH) study, which included almost 5000 women with breast cancer and an equal number of age-matched controls. The basis of this model is that the women most likely to carry inherited genetic alterations that predispose to breast cancer are those women with multiple close relatives who developed breast cancer at young ages. The model has been adapted into a series of published tables that estimate breast cancer risk in decade increments based on the relationship of family members with breast cancer to the individual being evaluated and the age when breast cancer was diagnosed in those relatives. The Claus model estimate for this patient is 0.6% at her current age, already exceeding the 0.5% average risk of a 40-year-old American woman and the level at which annual screening mammography has now been recommended. Her risk increases to 5.3% by age 50, and reaches an 18.8% lifetime risk. This is compared to the average lifetime breast cancer risk of American women of 11%.

The major advantages of the Claus model include the ability to consider both maternal and paternal relatives and the structuring of the tables to allow risk information to be delivered based on current age. The need to include paternal relatives is obvious when considering the possible inheritance of breast cancer susceptibility genes that are equally likely to be inherited from the father (although there is no history to suggest this scenario in this case). The ability to estimate current risk also is quite valuable to avoid the perception of excess risk in young women. The major disadvantage of this model is that it may significantly underestimate the risk of developing breast cancer in a *BRCA1* or *BRCA2* mutation carrier and overestimate breast cancer risk for a woman in such a family who has not inherited a disease-related mutation. Additionally, this model was developed in 1994, before the knowledge that the Ashkenazi Jewish population has a significantly higher mutation carrier rate for deleterious mutations in *BRCA1* and *BRCA2* than unselected Caucasian populations. This is another source of underestimating breast cancer risk in this patient.

Another commonly used means of estimating breast cancer risk is the Gail model, which calculates risk using a formula that considers age at menarche, age at first live birth, number of first-degree relatives with breast cancer, number of previous breast biopsies, and current age as pertinent risk factors. The effect of each factor on breast cancer risk was estimated using data from the Breast Cancer Detection Demonstration Project (BCDDP). This model also predicts a cumulative risk over the next 30 years and corrects for other causes of mortality. The Gail model breast cancer risk estimates for this patient are 3.3% by age 40, 11.9% by age 50, and 18.1% by age 80. The Gail model was used to calculate risk for women considering entry into the NSABP Breast Cancer Chemoprevention Trial. Like the Claus model, the Gail model may underestimate risk for *BRCA1* and *BRCA2* mutation carriers and overestimate risk for their noncarrier relatives. Additionally, the Gail model allows other risk factors to significantly modify breast cancer risk in the presence of a family history, which is currently unsubstantiated by other studies. In addition, this model does not take age of diagnosis of breast cancer in relatives into consideration, nor does it consider the presence of breast cancer in second-degree relatives, negating any contribution to risk from paternal relatives. Finally, its use requires the software containing the necessary formulas. As is true for the Claus model, the Gail model is most accurate when used to predict risk for women without a striking family history of breast cancer.

Nonfamilial risk factors also may be considered in estimating breast risk, and as noted above, the accuracy with which they may be mixed with familial risk factors is unknown. Such factors for this patient might include early menarche (which she does not report), nulliparity or first pregnancy after age 30 (which she is too young to assess for), previous breast biopsies (generally considered risk predictors in the presence of atypia, which was not present in the fibroademonas), and use of oral contraceptives (which she does not report). Thus this patient appears to have no significant nonfamilial risk factors for breast cancer, and her risk is perhaps best assessed using the Claus model.

Finally, one should consider the likelihood that this woman carries a deleterious mutation in *BRCA1* or *BRCA2*. Based solely on her Ashkenazi Jewish heritage, without consideration of her family history of breast cancer, the population risk predicted by several studies is approximately 2.5%. Taking the family history into consideration, one can use recently published tables that predict the likelihood of finding a *BRCA1* mutation based primarily on the median age of diagnosis of breast cancer in the family, the presence or absence of ovarian cancer in a family member, and Ashkenazi

Jewish ancestry. Using this model, the likelihood that a *BRCA1* alteration explains the breast cancer occurrence in this patient's family is estimated at 8–10%. To estimate the likelihood that this patient herself carries such a mutation, the familial risk is assigned to the closest relative affected with breast cancer (her mother) and that risk multiplied by 0.5 (as she has a 50/50 chance of having inherited the familial mutation, if one exists, from her mother). Thus the likelihood that this patient carriers a *BRCA1* alteration is approximately 4–5%. Tables are not yet available for predicting the likelihood of finding a *BRCA2* mutation in this family, but preliminary data suggest that the likelihood will be approximately half that predicted for *BRCA1*. At this low level of risk, many women will opt not to be tested.

BIBLIOGRAPHY

Claus EB, Risch N, Thompson WD. Autosomal dominant inheritance of early-onset breast cancer. Cancer 1994; 73:643–651.

Couch FJ, Blackwood MA, DeShano ML, et al. *BRCA1* mutations in women attending clinics that evaluate the risk of breast cancer. N Engl J Med 1997; 336(20):1409–1415.

Gail MH, Brinton LA, Byar DP, et al. Projecting individualized probabilities of developing breast cancer for white females who are being examined annually. J Natl Cancer Inst 1989; 81:1879–1886.

H.19. BREAST CANCER IN THE ELDERLY

Case #H.19.1
Goal: To discuss the management of high-risk breast cancer in elderly patients

DANIEL F. HAYES

An 88-year-old woman presents with stage II breast cancer (T2N1M0). The tumor is hormone receptor negative, aneuploid, and has a high S phase. The past medical history is remarkable for hypertension that is well controlled on calcium channel blockers. Physical examination reveals an elderly woman who appears younger than her stated age. There are no signs of metastatic disease.

Treatment of elderly women with breast cancer is a poorly studied issue for which there are few evidence-based guidelines or data on which to draw conclusions. For example, women over the age of 70 have rarely been included in prospective, randomized trials of adjuvant chemotherapy, and few, if any, women in their ninth decade are included in such studies. Therefore, decisions regarding adjuvant systemic therapy in such women must be based on extrapolations from data regarding other age groups and logical assumptions. Although both of these approaches are fraught with bias and potential error, we are unfortunately left with making decisions for this older age group in such a manner.

This patient's prognosis is relatively poor, given that she has positive axillary lymph nodes, and her tumor is greater than 2 cm, ER/PR negative, and has a high S-phase fraction. Therefore, I would estimate her odds of distant recurrence over the subsequent 10 years after surgery to be approximately 50%.

Of course, this patient's potential of suffering recurrence and death from breast cancer must be weighed against her overall life expectancy. Even a healthy 88-year-old woman has a reasonably high chance of suffering death from a non-breast-cancer-related cause, such as stroke or coronary artery disease. This is especially true for a patient who has hypertension (although this patient's hypertension appears well controlled). Let us assume that this patient has a 50% chance of mortality due to non-breast-cancer-related causes over the next 10 years. Thus, if only 50% of women in her age group will live the next 10 years (unrelated to breast cancer), and 50% of them will suffer distant recurrence and death from their stage II breast cancer, overall only 25% of such patients would be expected to die from breast-cancer-related causes. Indeed, this may be an overestimate, since her odds of dying of non-breast-cancer-related causes is probably even higher than 50%.

Subset analysis of several initial studies of adjuvant chemotherapy, which rarely contained doxorubicin, versus observation in postmenopausal women failed to demonstrate a substantial reduction in mortality at 5, 10, and even 15 years of follow-up. Furthermore, when divided into subsets by decade, the relative benefits of adjuvant chemotherapy decreased in an almost stepwise fashion between the sixth, seventh, and even eighth decade. Thus, it is difficult to suggest that a woman in her 80s is likely to substantially benefit from non-doxorubicin-based adjuvant chemotherapy. For example, let us assume that a premenopausal patient gains a 25–30% proportional reduction in mortality from chemotherapy versus observation. For a 50-year-old postmenopausal woman, that reduction is decreased to approximately 15–20% and for a 60–70-year-old woman, the proportional reduction is decreased even further to approximately 10%. If this decrease in proportional reduction is extended into the 70s and 80s, one can only assume that the proportional reduction in mortality for a woman in this patient's age group approaches, at most, 10%. Thus, if she has a 25% chance of dying of breast cancer, treating 100 such women will result in two or three being alive and disease free 10 years later who would not have been had they only been observed.

A few studies have suggested that doxorubicin-containing regimens may result in a reduction in distant disease recurrence and perhaps mortality in postmenopausal patients that was not observed in the early clinical trials. In NSABP B-16, analysis of older women suggested a small, but statistically significant reduction in mortality in women who received AC plus tamoxifen versus those who received tamoxifen alone. More recently, in a U.S. Intergroup study in which postmenopausal ER-positive women all received tamoxifen, and then were randomly assigned to CAF + tamoxifen versus tamoxifen alone, a 5% disease-free survival benefit was observed with 6 years of follow-up for the CAF arm. In this study, no difference in overall survival has emerged.

Of note, retrospective analyses of older women have suggested that if carefully selected, healthy women over the age of 70 have no increased risk of significant therapy-related mortality than do younger women. The M.D. Anderson experience suggests that doxorubicin can be given to these women reasonably safely, although there is a slight increase in the incidence of congestive heart failure.

In summary, the decision as to whether to treat this patient must be considered individually. The potential benefits are extraordinarily small, given this patient's expected non-breast-cancer mortality over the next 10 years, her potential benefit from chemotherapy, and the potential side effects and possible major toxicities. However, it appears that an otherwise healthy female has a reasonable chance of tolerating chemotherapy. I personally would recommend that this patient be observed without adjuvant chemotherapy. On the other hand, other physicians and patients would consider the 1–2% survival benefit sufficient to outweigh the concerns over side effects and toxicities. Ultimately, of course, the patient will have to choose.

BIBLIOGRAPHY

Albain K, Green S, Osborne K, Cobau C, Levine E, Ingle J, et al. Tamoxifen vs. cyclophosphamide, adriamycin, and 5FU plus either concurrent or sequential T in postmenopausal receptor positive, node positive breast cancer: a Southwest Oncology Group Phase III Intergroup Trial. Proc Am Soc Clin Oncol 1997 (in press).

Early Breast Cancer Trialists' Collaborative Group T. Systemic treatment of early breast cancer by hormonal, cytotoxic, or immune therapy: 133 randomised trials involving 31,000 recurrences and 24,000 deaths among 75,000 women. Lancet 1992; 339:1–15, 71–85.

Fisher B, Redmond C, Legault-Poisson S, Dimitrov NV, Brown AM, Wickerham DL, et al. Postoperative chemotherapy and tamoxifen compared with tamoxifen alone in the treatment of positive-node breast cancer patients aged 50 years and older with tumors responsive to tamoxifen: results from the National Surgical Adjuvant Breast and Bowel Project B-16. J Clin Oncol 1990; 8:1005–1018.

Ibrahim N, Frye D, Buzdar A, Walters R, Hortobagyi G. Doxorubicin-based chemotherapy in elderly patients with metastatic breast cancer: tolerance and outcome. Arch Intern Med 1996; 156:882–888.

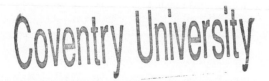

Index

Page numbers in *italics* indicate figures. Page numbers followed by "t" indicate tables.

473

About the Editors

WILLIAM N. HAIT is Professor of Medicine and Pharmacology at the University of Medicine and Dentistry of New Jersey/Robert Wood Johnson Medical School, New Brunswick, New Jersey, and Director of The Cancer Institute of New Jersey, New Brunswick. Dr. Hait is the author or coauthor of nearly 200 articles, abstracts, and books, and holds several patents and inventions. A member of numerous societies, including the American Cancer Society, the American Association of Cancer Research, and the American Society of Clinical Oncology, he has given numerous lectures and received many awards and honors. Dr. Hait received the B.A. degree (1971) from the University of Pennsylvania, and the M.D. (1978) and Ph.D. degrees (1978) from the Medical College of Pennsylvania, Bedford.

DAVID A. AUGUST is Acting Chief of the Division of Surgical Oncology, Department of Surgery, the University of Medicine and Dentistry of New Jersey/Robert Wood Johnson Medical School, New Brunswick, New Jersey. Dr. August is the author or coauthor of over 100 scientific journal articles, book chapters, abstracts, and other publications. A Fellow of the American College of Surgeons and a member of the Society of Surgical Oncology, among several other societies, he has participated in numerous scientific, teaching, and research activities. Dr. August received the B.S. degree (1976) from the Massachusetts Institute of Technology, Cambridge, and the M.D. degree (1980) from the Yale University School of Medicine, New Haven, Connecticut.

BRUCE G. HAFFTY is Associate Professor of Therapeutic Radiology at the Yale University School of Medicine, New Haven, Connecticut. Dr. Haffty is the author or coauthor of over 160 abstracts, articles, reviews, and book chapters and is a member of numerous societies, including the American Medical Association and the American Society of Therapeutic Radiology and Oncology. The recipient of several awards and honors, he has given lectures and participated in many national and international professional activities and funded researches. Dr. Haffty received the B.S. degree (1972) from the University of Massachusetts, Amherst, the M.S. degree (1976) from Worcester Polytechnic Institute, Massachusetts, and the M.D. degree (1984) from the Yale University School of Medicine, New Haven, Connecticut.